T0256415

HEALTH MATTERS

Evidence, Critical Social Science, and Health Care in Canada

In *Health Matters*, contributors from a range of disciplinary and interdisciplinary traditions address multiple dimensions of health care, such as nursing, midwifery, home care, pharmaceuticals, medical education, and palliative care. Through their explorations, the book poses questions about the role that the forms of expertise associated with evidence-based health care play in shaping how we understand and organize health services. Authors critique instrumental, managerial ways of knowing health care and focus on how such ways of knowing limit our understandings of and responses to health care problems and are linked with the growing commodification, individualization, and privatization of Canadian health services. Working with analytic perspectives such as feminism, Marxist political economy, critical ethnography, science and technology studies, governmentality studies, and institutional ethnography, the volume demonstrates how critical social science perspectives contribute alternative perspectives about what counts as health care problems and how to best to address them.

ERIC MYKHALOVSKIY is a professor in the Department of Sociology at York University.

JACQUELINE CHOINIERE is an associate professor in the School of Nursing in the Faculty of Health at York University.

PAT ARMSTRONG is a Distinguished Research Professor of Sociology, Fellow of the Royal Society of Canada, and a professor in the Department of Sociology at York University.

HUGH ARMSTRONG is a Distinguished Research Professor and professor emeritus of Social Work, Political Economy, and Sociology at Carleton University.

Health Matters

Evidence, Critical Social Science, and Health Care in Canada

EDITED BY ERIC MYKHALOVSKIY,
JACQUELINE CHOINIERE, PAT ARMSTRONG,
AND HUGH ARMSTRONG

UNIVERSITY OF TORONTO PRESS
Toronto Buffalo London

Toronto Buffalo London
utorontopress.com
Printed in the U.S.A.

ISBN 978-1-4875-0779-4 (cloth)
ISBN 978-1-4875-2538-5 (paper)
ISBN 978-1-4875-3697-8 (EPUB)
ISBN 978-1-4875-3696-1 (PDF)

Library and Archives Canada Cataloguing in Publication

Title: Health matters : evidence, critical social science, and health care in Canada / edited by Eric Mykhalovskiy, Jacqueline Choiniere, Pat Armstrong, and Hugh Armstrong.
Other titles: Health matters (2020)
Names: Mykhalovskiy, Eric, editor. | Choiniere, Jacqueline, 1952– editor. | Armstrong, Pat, 1945– editor. | Armstrong, Hugh, 1943– editor.
Description: Includes bibliographical references and index.
Identifiers: Canadiana (print) 20200192108 | Canadiana (ebook) 20200192124 | ISBN 9781487507794 (cloth) | ISBN 9781487525385 (paper) | ISBN 9781487536978 (EPUB) | ISBN 9781487536961 (PDF)
Subjects: LCSH: Social medicine – Canada. | LCSH: Medical care – Research – Canada. | LCSH: Medical care – Canada – Evaluation. | LCSH: Evidence-based medicine – Canada. | LCSH: Medical policy – Canada.
Classification: LCC RA418.3.C3 H43 2020 | DDC 362.1/0420971 – dc23

This book has been published with the help of a grant from the Federation for the Humanities and Social Sciences, through the Awards to Scholarly Publications Program, using funds provided by the Social Sciences and Humanities Research Council of Canada.

University of Toronto Press acknowledges the financial assistance to its publishing program of the Canada Council for the Arts and the Ontario Arts Council, an agency of the Government of Ontario.

Canada Council for the Arts
Conseil des Arts du Canada

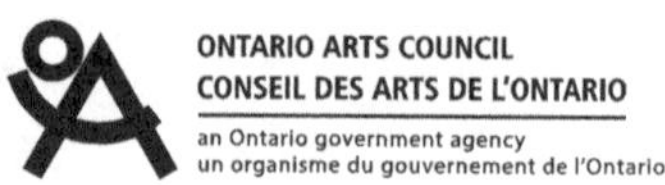

Funded by the Government of Canada
Financé par le gouvernement du Canada
Canada

Contents

HEALTH MATTERS

1 Introduction

ERIC MYKHALOVSKIY, JACQUELINE CHOINIERE, PAT ARMSTRONG, AND HUGH ARMSTRONG

Health Matters: Evidence, Critical Social Science, and Health Care in Canada is an edited collection of original research on the Canadian health care system that intervenes in the applied, instrumental turn in Canadian health research. The contributors to this volume come from disciplinary and institutional sites that traverse sociology, anthropology, health policy, the health professions, universities, community agencies, and trade unions. They address multiple dimensions of health care, including intensive care nursing, midwifery, home care, long-term care, the pharmaceutical industry, medical device research, palliative care, and much more.

What unites their contributions is the authors' engagement with social science theory and methods to call into question the dominant neoliberal rationalities that shape applied health care policy and health scholarship in Canada. Contributors do not explore their empirical research sites with a view to improving the cost-effectiveness of health services or enhancing market-based reform strategies. They do not encourage us to become even more responsible for our individual health, nor do they contribute to health care outcomes research in terms of conventional metrics of accountability. Instead, they critique instrumental, managerial ways of knowing health care. They focus on how such ways of knowing limit our understandings of and responses to health care problems and are linked with the growing commodification, individualization, and privatization of Canadian health services.

The contributors to this volume come to social science theory and methods from different locations. Some occupy university positions in the social sciences and are trained in critical social science traditions that they bring to bear in their writing. Others work in the health sciences or in community-based research environments and provide examples of how scholars working in these settings make use of critical social science approaches in their work. Rather than suggest that there is a single best framework, or an approach that is properly critical against others that are ill informed, this volume displays various ways Canadian scholars make sense of critical social science and use it to produce alternatives to neoliberal, managerial ways of knowing health care.

The term "neoliberalism" is employed here and elsewhere to capture several ideas in social science as well as practices in the social world. It consists of three central and related aspects (Armstrong 2013). It is an *ideology* that champions markets free of state intervention as the principal guarantor of individual freedom. It is a set of *policy* measures centred on freeing markets from state regulation and on promoting the penetration of markets into fields previously considered public goods, such as electricity, water, mass transit, education and training, and health care. Finally, it is a mode of *governance* that understands and reinforces the notion that power is and can be exercised outside the state sector. So-called governing at a distance can involve "lean" governments that shed direct service delivery while extending the reach of both market-based law and individual responsibility. Governing at a distance has also been used to describe the activities of non-state actors and the forms of technology and expertise with which they are associated that seek to govern people's conduct through a form of "regulated autonomy" (Rose and Miller 1992). Since the 1970s, neoliberalism has come to pervade public and social science discourse on both the left and the right across the world, as well as political and economic practice, albeit with uneven application (Harvey 2007). The critique of neoliberalism made by contributors to this collection focuses on marketization and individualization in health care as well as the role played by various forms of authoritative knowledge and evidence in organizing health care services.

In this introduction we explain our rationale for bringing this collection together. We argue that an applied, instrumental turn in health research has created challenges for the pursuit of critical social science research on health care in Canada. We share our understanding of the forms of knowledge that characterize the applied turn in health research as well as the institutional and discursive relations that have encouraged it. Finally, we describe how we orient to the notion of critical social science research on health care and give an overview of the chapters that make up the collection.

Why This Book?

For decades, Canadian social scientists have produced an important body of research that critically explores the network of knowledges, technologies, devices, practices, institutions, funding mechanisms, policies, and people that form our health care system. Some Canadian scholars have critiqued the consequences of the move to privatize medicare and restructure health services (Armstrong and Armstrong 2010; Coburn 2010; Rachlis 2007; Williams et al. 2001), while others have explored inequities in health care organization, training, delivery, and access, and how they are structured by relations of gender, race, class, and other bases of social differentiation (Beagan 2000; Brotman et al. 2002; Hankivsky 2011; Harbin, Beagan, and Goldberg 2012; Hennebry, McLaughlin, and Preibisch 2016; Koehn et al. 2013; Nestel 2006; Penning and Zheng 2016; Tang and Brown 2008; Webster et al. 2016).

Canadian social scientists have examined the implications of new forms of accountability and management on physicians (Coburn, Rappolt, and Bourgeault 1997), nurses (Campbell and Rankin 2017; Choiniere 2011; Rankin and Campbell 2006), midwives (Bourgeault 2000, 2006; Katherine 2015; MacDonald 2007), paramedics (Corman 2017), and other health professions and workers, both paid and unpaid (Armstrong et al. 1997, 2008; Baines 2015; Laxer 2015; Porter and Gustafson 2012). Some Canadian scholars have critiqued the politics of knowledge associated with evidence-based decision making and the standardization of health care (Bell 2017; Knaapen 2014; Laforest and Orsini 2005; Mykhalovskiy 2001, 2003; Rappolt 1997; Thille and Russell 2010), while others have turned their attention to the biopolitics of health-related social movements (Batt 2017; Costa et al. 2012; King 2006; Titchkosky and Michalko 2009; Orsini and Smith 2010; Poland, Dooris, and Haluza-Delay 2011; Titchkosky and Michalko 2009).

Canadian social scientists have contributed to critiques of medicalization (Malacrida 2004; Moss and Dyck 2002; Paterson 2010), explored the displacement of Indigenous health knowledges and practice by biomedicine (Adelson 2000; Kaufert and O'Neil 2009), and offered novel ways of conceptualizing care and caring (Armstrong and Braedley 2013; Grant, Amaratunga, and Armstrong 2004; Neysmith et al. 2012). Others have sought to reorient biomedical and policy discourses through research on lay experiences of health, illness, and care (Etowa et al. 2017; Husbands et al. 2019; Johnson et al. 2004; McCoy 2005, 2009; Mykhalovskiy, McCoy, and Bresalier 2004; Sinding, Barnoff, and Grassau 2004; Whelan 2007) and through critical analyses of pharmaceutical industry practices (Ford and Saibil 2009; Holloway 2014; Lexchin 2016), home care (Aronson 2004; Denton et al. 2002; England et al. 2007; Grigorovich 2015; Thériault, Low and Luke, 2014), long-term care (Armstrong and Daly 2017; Armstrong and Day 2017; Ronald et al. 2016; Tanuseputro et al. 2015), and other areas of health care delivery (Deber 2018; Hindmarch, Orsini, and Gagnon 2018; Martin 2017; Morrow and Weisser 2012).

We were motivated to edit this collection out of a concern for how an instrumental turn in Canadian health research is marginalizing this rich tradition of critical social science scholarship on health care. For over a decade, we have listened to colleagues describe and have ourselves experienced serious challenges to the pursuit of critical health scholarship. We have heard countless stories from health scholars whose theoretically driven approaches to social science research have been misunderstood and rejected in the peer review process of government-funded research agencies. Those who pursue qualitative modes of enquiry have described how their research has been deemed to lie outside the relevancies of health care policymakers and been dismissed as ungeneralizable or anecdotal (Eakin 2016). We have heard stories about serious difficulties finding mainstream publication venues in the health sciences for research that critiques rather than contributes to dominant trends in health care policy. Colleagues who work in health sciences environments have described feeling pressured to "dumb down" their social science research to make it palatable to their peers, and struggling to make their work recognized as legitimate and worthwhile (Kontos and Grigorovich 2018).

These and similar stories share a common narrative about the institutional and discursive challenges faced by health scholars who work from critical social science traditions. They gesture to forms of judgment and authority that position critical enquiry, its modes of research, and its forms of evidence as irrelevant, esoteric, and "outside" the main business of Canadian health research. These stories are about relations of knowledge and power that tell us that critical social science research on health care doesn't matter. *Health Matters* opposes and intervenes in these relations. It brings together examples of scholarship that refuse to pose only those questions predetermined by conventional health care policy agendas and that avoid the rush to identify quick fixes for health care problems. The chapters that form this collection question how health care issues are formulated by applied research; critique current arrangements; and explore, rather than avoid, the complexity of the social, political, technological, and other relations that form the health care system. *Health Matters* speaks back to the applied turn, claiming that critical scholarship does matter; in fact, that it matters very much to our understanding of the health care system, what its problems are, and what can be done about them. We hope that the book will be of interest to social science academics and graduate students who work on Canadian health care, health services researchers and health scientists curious about critical social science perspectives, health policymakers, health practitioners, and other readers concerned about health care in Canada.

The Applied, Instrumental Turn in Canadian Health Research

Science and technology studies and other forms of scholarship have exposed the myth of a pure, free-floating science that exists apart from social, political, or economic contexts and interests (Goldenberg 2006; Haraway 1991; Latour and Woolgar 1986; Mintzberg 2017; Smith 1987; Stone 2001). Other scholarship argues against making sharp binary distinctions in favour of modes of analysis that emphasize the deconstruction of rigid categories and the fluidity of boundaries (Anzaldua 1987; Bowker and Star 1999; Learmonth 2003; Travers 2015). Notwithstanding these intellectual trends, it is common to distinguish between applied and basic or pure research in both scholarly and public discourse about scientific research (Flexner 2017). In general terms, applied research is understood to focus, in a narrow and immediate way, on solving discrete problems that are of concern to an external stakeholder or research sponsor. Pure, basic, or theoretical research, by contrast, is framed as curiosity-driven knowledge that is unfettered by the pursuit of any specific practical aim (Freeman and Rossi 1984).

This book is not a statement against all forms of applied health research. Indeed, many of the contributors, ourselves included, have worked with social movements, trade unions, and other partners on research that addresses the practical problems they face or that otherwise attends to their knowledge needs and interests. Among the contributions to this collection, important examples are provided by Anne Rochon Ford's research on the health risks faced by racialized women working in the nail salon industry, Christianne Stephens's community-informed research on structural violence and Indigenous peoples' experiences of health care, and Vicki Van Wagner and Elizabeth Darling's analysis of the use of evidence in policy debates about midwifery care.

At the same time, this book is not a collection that venerates so-called pure knowledge pursued for "its own sake" without practical or public aims. All of the contributors to this volume link their scholarly pursuits with a concern to improve health care for Canadians. Often, however, their suggestions for improvement challenge conventional policy understandings of what it means to intervene in health care. For example, Ariel Ducey and colleagues respond to the overuse of vaginal mesh surgery not by calling for better regulations, guidelines, or clinical trials, but by recommending interventions that heighten practitioners' reflexivity about how their decisions are situated within specific organizational, professional, and institutional trajectories.

Institutional and Discursive Sources of the Applied Turn in Health Research

The growing popularity of applied health care research is an important feature of the contemporary social organization of knowledge about health care in Canada. The turn to applied, instrumental health care research has three principle sources: changes in the function of knowledge in the context of a capitalist knowledge economy, shifts in the public role of universities and the emergence of new forms of university managerialism and accountability relations, and changes in state funding of health research.

At the broadest level, the applied, instrumental turn reflects large-scale transformations in the role played by knowledge in a neoliberal context. Scholars have used such terms as the "knowledge economy" (Olssen and Peters 2005) and "knowledge capitalism" (Burton-Jones 1999) to refer to the central role played by scientific, technical, and related forms of knowledge in post-industrial economies. They argue that such knowledge is not only a growing source of economic growth, but has itself become the leading form of global capital (Burton-Jones 1999).

The knowledge economy has propelled new ideas about the relationship between knowledge and capital accumulation and the relationship between research, education, and the economy (Olssen and Peters 2005). In the health context, Rossiter and Robertson (2014, 199) argue that the political, economic, and ideological shifts associated with knowledge capitalism have promoted ends-oriented health research that is "driven by the demands of the economized knowledge market." They suggest that the neoliberal knowledge economy has reoriented the entire field of health research in Canada away from emergent, reflexive enquiry towards research that is predictable and that can be immediately applied to solve discrete health care problems.

The applied turn has also been propelled by transformations in how universities operate and are governed. In Canada, universities are increasingly being understood as centres for producing commercial, applied, and other forms of knowledge that will drive the economy (Polster 2015; Polster and Newson 2015; Slaughter and Rhoades 2004; Turk 2017). This changed conception of the public role of universities has coincided with an unprecedented growth of university administration relative to the resources committed to teaching and learning, the installation of professional managers at upper levels of university administration, and the growing representation of the corporate sector on university governance boards (Ginsberg 2011; Metcalfe 2010). Accountability relations have taken hold in universities that are similar to those that have restructured the health care sector. University teaching and research are increasingly the object of a managerial gaze consumed with understanding the "value added" of institutional activities through a host of performance indicators, quality assurance schemes, and outcomes assessments (Olssen and Peters 2005). Most recently, the Ontario Progressive Conservative government announced in its 2019 budget that 60 per cent of funding for colleges and universities will be tied to performance indicators (Jones 2019). Under the weight of such forms of managerialism and accountability, traditional emphases on open scholarship and critique lose ground to an emerging focus on entrepreneurialism and research pursued in partnership with industry and other knowledge users to address their immediate practical problems. In this volume, Kelly Holloway and Matthew Herder consider how these relations are at play in the growing emphasis on commercialization in the training of Canadian biomedical researchers. They suggest that a new ethic of commercialization is being established in Canadian biomedical training that discourages critical discussion of the contradictions of commercialization, including the taken-for-granted assumption that it leads to better health care.

Finally, the turn to applied, instrumental health research has resulted from changes in the organization of funding for Canadian university-based research. One of the most significant of these changes was the establishment of the Canadian Institutes of Health Research (CIHR) in 2000 and the decision in 2009 by the Social Sciences and Humanities Research Council (SSHRC) to stop funding health research (Albert and Laberge 2017). The CIHR is not a monolithic funding agency; indeed, some of the contributors to this volume have received support from the CIHR for their research. Nevertheless, the CIHR is primarily driven by an applied mandate to use federal funds to support research that enhances the health of Canadians and builds a more "effective" health care system (Canadian Institutes of Health Research Act, 2000). At the time the CIHR was established, senior Canadian scholars made a case for the importance of social sciences and humanities health research, even as they expressed anxiety that the new funding body might marginalize the distinct theories, methods, and research strategies of the social sciences and their characteristic commitment to reflexivity and critique (Grant et al. 1999). Some eighteen years into the CIHR mandate, their concerns appear prescient.

Many researchers have argued that the integration of the social sciences within the CIHR has produced serious barriers to the practice of critical social science research on health care in Canada (Albert 2014; Albert and Laberge 2017; Albert et al. 2009; Graham et al. 2011; Rossiter and Robertson 2014). They have noted that while the CIHR is mandated to fund social science research, its intellectual and organizational culture has not adapted to recognize the epistemological specificity of social research on health and health care. Social scientists are barely present on CIHR review committees, meaning that those who apply for institute funding often face standards of judgment and rules of evidence that prevail in the biomedical and applied health sciences (Albert et al. 2009). Social scientists are also marginalized from CIHR's key leadership and decision-making structures. A recent study reports that they have been largely absent from CIHR's Governing Council and the leadership of CIHR's thirteen institutes and its College of Reviewers. As a result, they have little power to shape internal decisions and policies that direct CIHR's approach to research funding (Albert and Laberge 2017). The unique problems social scientists encounter when seeking funding through CIHR were formally acknowledged in the most recent international review of the funder (Gluckman et al. 2017). *The International Peer Review Expert Panel Report* found that CIHR has no transparent mechanism for allocating funds to its four pillars and that social scientists face particular challenges related to "different review cultures at CIHR and SSHRC," the "different lenses that health scientists and social scientists/humanities researchers may bring to research questions," and different approaches to performance assessment used by social scientists/humanities researchers and clinical and biomedical researchers (Gluckman et al. 2017, 29–30).

While some social science scholars have succeeded in securing CIHR funding for their research, their success may come at some cost to the unique character of critical social science enquiry. Recent study findings by Albert (2014) suggest that social science applicants often efface social science theory and methods from their CIHR applications in anticipation of reviews informed by the conventions of natural and medical science. Concerns have also been raised about the erosion of critical social science health research under the weight of CIHR's commitment to narrow conceptions of applied research. In a detailed analysis of a recent CIHR request for proposals, Rossiter and Robertson (2014, 205) argue that what appears as a neutral call for research favours research "amenable to use or application in terms of making specific measurable changes to current policies and systems of care and provision [that are] necessarily bound to the *rationalization* of care." Other conventions of CIHR funding, including the requirement to establish elaborate knowledge translation plans in advance of conducting research and the use of targeted funding priorities that favour applied research pursued in partnership with commercial, policymaking, and other end users, have led some social scientists to question whether there is a viable future for critical social science health research in Canada (Graham et al. 2011).

Towards an Alternative

The turn to applied, instrumental health research in Canada and the relations of knowledge, university governance, and external research funding that support it have not squelched or drowned out critical social science health research. But they have created serious impediments to critical social enquiry of health care, particularly for emerging social scientists. Recent suggestions that SSHRC will return to funding health research hold much promise in this regard, and a recent CIHR call for proposals geared towards social scientists who have not previously held CIHR grants as principal investigators is another step in the right direction.[1] But much more work needs to be done. This book contributes to securing a future for social science health research by creating a discursive home for scholarship that treats health care as an object of critical enquiry. We use the term "critical social science" as a general orienting term. It groups together a range of interdisciplinary and disciplinary work that draws on social science theory and methods to call into question the dominant managerial rationality through which health care is increasingly understood and governed and that commits to principles of social justice, equity, and struggles against marginalization and oppression.

We are wary of using the term in ways that suggest something that is sharply demarcated or entirely novel. Over the years, scholars from various social science disciplines who engage diverse theoretical perspectives in the pursuit of distinct intellectual projects have used "critical" to refer to their work.[2] In the Canadian context, the phrase "critical social science in health" appears to have been first used by Joan Eakin and colleagues in their critique of the displacement of health promotion by population health perspectives in the early 1990s (Eakin et al. 1996; Poland et al. 1998; Robertson 1998). Eakin et al. (1996) critique population health for its reliance on objectivist epidemiology, its hostility towards social theory, and its implicit support of neoliberal policies of retrenchment from the welfare state. They describe critical social science as a reflexive analytic practice that works against the grain of established approaches to health research and that grapples with relations of power at play in all forms of knowledge making. While their work drew principally on political economy perspectives and insights from Foucault, we do not suggest by the term "critical social science" an exclusive relationship to any particular established tradition of critical social enquiry (Carroll 2004). The strength of this volume does not lie in its adherence to a singular conceptual scheme or theoretical framework throughout its chapters, but in the range of critical perspectives addressed. The contributors to this volume use a variety of perspectives in their critical analyses of health care, including Marxism, feminism, political economy, Foucauldian work, institutional ethnography, and science and technology studies.

Neoliberalism and Health Care Research

While the chapters in this volume employ various approaches to critical analysis, they are united in offering a counter-voice to instrumental applied research that serves neoliberal health reform. We view neoliberalism as a political project that transforms how societies are governed and organized and, consequently, how states, markets, and citizens are related one with another. Neoliberalism is not simply about the retrenchment of the welfare state or the rejection of government involvement in the economy (Harvey 2007). It is about a "revamping of the state" (Wacquant 2012, 66) as a mechanism that directs the extension of market and commodity relations throughout society, promotes self-reliance and individual responsibility for one's life and fate, and exacerbates social inequities and marginalization.

In the context of Canadian health care, neoliberal relations take shape as reform efforts that introduce and extend market-based practices and forms of reasoning, albeit unevenly. Canadian political economists have taken the lead on research exploring these market-based health reforms. Some have researched the growing use of flexible contracts and other forms of casualization of labour in health care and how they aggravate workplace inequalities and worsen the working conditions faced by an increasingly racialized workforce that occupies the lower end of the health care occupational hierarchy (Armstrong et al. 1997; Armstrong, Armstrong, and Scott-Dixon 2008; Das Gupta 2009). Political economists have called attention to the transformations that occur in how health and health care are understood and how health services are delivered when models of management developed in the private sector are increasingly incorporated into the governance of health care institutions (Armstrong et al. 1997; Balka, Messing, and Armstrong 2006; Kamp and Hvid 2012; Meagher and Szebehely 2013). Others have focused on processes of privatization in hospital and clinic settings and their implications for how care is delivered and experienced (Barlow 2002; Leduc Browne 2000). Ross Sutherland's chapter extends this tradition of political economy analysis with a critique of privatization in an understudied area of the Canadian health care sector, medical laboratory services. By contrast, Christine Kelly's chapter in this volume offers a view onto neoliberal health reform that focuses on its impact on agencies that work with people with disabilities.

In Canada, neoliberal relations of health care also manifest as the growing treatment of health as an individual responsibility. The decline of resources and staff in the formal health care sector is one way that individual responsibility for health care is produced, as the burden of caring for people with illnesses has been transferred onto private individuals, typically family members, often with profound gender consequences (Benoit and Hallgrímsdóttir 2008; Feldberg and Vipond 1999; Neysmith 2000;). The explosion of web-based sources of health information and the growing popularity of shared decision-making models in the formal health care sector also encourage people to become educated about their potential health problems and to act as informed consumers of health services (Henwood, Harris, and Spoel 2011; Sinding et al. 2012; Wathen, Wyatt, and Harris 2008). In this volume, critical analyses of the individualization of responsibility for health and health care are extended by Kirsten Bell's discussion of the assumptions about individual behaviour embedded in tobacco control and by Mary Ellen Macdonald and David Kenneth Wright's analysis of shifts in discourses about decision making in the palliative care sector.

Finally, neoliberal relations of health care are characterized by the proliferation of new forms of accountability that rest on the capacity of numerically based forms of expertise to represent health care activities in a form that is standardized and governable across time and place (Harvey 2007; Miller and Rose 1990; Mykhalovskiy 2001; Rankin and Campbell 2006). Foucauldian scholars in particular have emphasized how neoliberal governance is increasingly organized through the operation of accounting, audit, and related technologies that make it possible to "know" and, therefore, govern state-funded and other services in terms of their efficiency and effectiveness (Katz and Green 2005; Power 1994; Shore and Wright 2004).

In the context of health care, in recent decades a "medico-administrative" way of knowing has taken hold as the predominant way of understanding health care. This managerial way of knowing reduces our understanding of health care to a matter of its performance along a narrow set of numerically based indicators (Mintzberg 2017; Rankin 2003). Quantification, evaluation, measurement, and benchmarking are its mainstay and narrow discourses of quality, excellence, efficiency, effectiveness, and patient satisfaction are its primary modes of representation.

When it becomes aligned with evidence-based decision making in health care (Mykhalovskiy and Weir 2004; Timmermans and Berg 2010), this managerial way of knowing is lent an air of scientific authority that renders its modes of representation neutral and taken for granted. Rather than working with understandings informed by people's day-to-day experiences of health care, medico-administrative knowledge creates a universe of abstract discourse for the purpose of governing health care neoliberally (Jackson et al. 2006; Mykhalovskiy et al. 2008). A number of contributors to this volume explore the workings and implications of medico-administrative rationality. Craig Dale provides a compelling account of the challenges that evidence-based hospital management poses to hands-on nursing care. Alisa Grigorovich critically assesses the limitations of quality assurance mechanisms in the home care sector. The chapter by Tamara Daly and colleagues focuses on the implications of quality management for working conditions in long-term care facilities.

Taken as a whole, the chapters in *Health Matters* express a counter-discourse to health research in the service of neoliberalism. Over fifty years ago, Robert Straus (1957) introduced to the scholarly lexicon the classic distinction between a sociology *in* and *of* medicine. For Straus, sociology *in* medicine was applied research pursued in collaboration with health practitioners that addressed problems they encountered in teaching and clinical care. Sociology *of* medicine, by contrast, was pure research that treated medicine as an object of enquiry. Extending Straus's trope to the current research context, we view this volume as a critical response to health research *in* neoliberalism. The chapters stand together in refusing instrumental, applied research on health care that takes up a client relationship to the neoliberal state. They counter research *in* neoliberalism by critically exploring managerial ways of knowing and the marketization, commodification, and individualization of Canadian health care.

In Canada, health research *in* neoliberalism has been advanced by many disciplines and interdisciplinary mixes. However, in our experience, one of its most prominent homes, particularly for work concerned with efficiency and effectiveness, is established health services research. Health services research is not a specific discipline, but a project of empirical enquiry that addresses the structure, processes, and organization of health care services (Crombie 1996). While it is a diverse inter- and multi-disciplinary project, critical social science has a minor presence within it (Lohr and Steinwachs 2002). The most entrenched form of health services research has developed as an applied response to state demands for evaluative knowledge about the performance of the health care system (Institute of Medicine 1995). Mainstream health services research emphasizes evidence-based decision making and the use of medico-administrative data sets to produce accountable, outcomes-oriented knowledge about the efficiency and effectiveness of health services. This book pushes at the intellectual boundaries that constrain that project of enquiry.

The Organization of the Book

Health Matters is divided into two main sections. The first section of the book, entitled "What Counts as Evidence? Managerial Knowledge, Visibility, and Experience," groups together chapters that critically explore and offer alternatives to dominant forms of knowledge and research associated with the relations that govern and manage the Canadian health care system. Drawing on examples from a range of sites, authors examine how the applied turn in health research produces ways of understanding health care that undermine alternative perspectives, align with neoliberal rationalities, and objectify patients' actual concerns with and experiences of health care.

In his chapter, Craig Dale argues that neoliberal reform has produced stressful, overworked hospital environments in which nurses find it difficult to practise essential bodily care. Drawing on institutional ethnography (Smith 2006) and eight years of observation of critical care nursing, he describes how managerial discourses of quality and efficiency have made matters worse by creating new documentary burdens for nurses that turn their attention away from patients and towards the information needs of hospital administration. He further argues that the new institutional vocabulary of quality, efficiency, and effectiveness produces sanitized representations of care that obscure the problem of sick patients whose needs are unmet. Dale's ethnographic work pierces through the gloss of medico-administrative rationality and exposes the dirty, messy reality of illness while championing the importance of hands-on nursing care for maintaining the health of hospital patients.

Mary Ellen Macdonald and David Kenneth Wright's chapter offers a critique of evidence-based decision-making discourses in palliative care and how they foreground a managerial approach to dying. The authors focus specifically on the discursive shift from "making a decision" to "decision making." They locate this shift in the apparently conflicting yet parallel contexts of the move to patient autonomy, with its subjective, value-related connotations, and the move to evidence-based medicine, with its objective, statistical orientation to medical practice. They select the hospice setting for their case because, unlike the hospital, it partially disrupts the individualized autonomy model of biomedical ethics and the clinical language of medical efficiency. Choices turn out to be constrained in the pursuit of a "good death," as the moment of decision making eclipses any structural critique.

Tamara Daly, Jacqueline Choiniere, and Hugh Armstrong provide a critical assessment of quality management in Ontario's long-term residential care sector. Using a feminist political economy lens, they explore how the introduction of a clinically focused assessment instrument has significantly altered the working conditions of the nurses, aides, and others who care for the very vulnerable residents in this sector. Introduced in response to quality concerns, the instrument tracks residents' clinical indicators, utilizing these assessments to extrapolate workload and, subsequently, funding levels for each facility. Drawing on interviews and observations with front-line staff and managers in two Ontario long-term care facilities, the authors surface several tensions, such as increased staff workload, intensified divisions of labour, and reduced team work among nurses, care aides, and others. They also identify the implications for residents' quality of life, as social and relational aspects of care are devalued with the enhanced priority on clinical or medical assessments.

The remaining chapters in this section explore knowledge relations associated with the project of evidence-based decision making. Vicki Van Wagner and Elizabeth Darling discuss how evidence is interpreted and debated within the context of interprofessional interests and relationships at the site of midwifery care. Research on childbirth has historically been dominated by medicine, and Van Wagner and Darling explore how the hierarchy of evidence comes into play when the tools of applied health research are used by midwives. They demonstrate that reliance on randomized clinical trials and systematic reviews varies with professional interests. The application of research is, in other words, seldom straightforward and, as their chapter so clearly portrays, has to be understood within the context of power relations and established hierarchies.

Christianne Stephens's chapter examines the limitations of epidemiological ways of knowing and proposes community-devised research as an alternative way to understand Indigenous peoples' experiences of health and health care. Her chapter draws on ethnographic research produced in collaboration with members of an Ontario First Nation over a period of seventeen years. Stephens's broader research develops culturally appropriate ways of measuring baseline health data for Indigenous peoples that are produced in collaboration with community partners and that stand as an alternative to standardized, bureaucratic measures of health outcomes. Drawing from this work, Stephens focuses on a case study of the illness and health care experiences of multiple members of a single family. She weaves a careful and powerful analytic narrative about how structural violence, syndemic suffering, and intergenerational trauma lie at the root of the health inequities experienced by those First Nation community members.

In her chapter, Alisa Grigorovich argues that the quality assurance mechanism in home care treats care as an abstract, disaggregated commodity and presupposes that quality is enhanced when care is standardized and homogenized. As an alternative, she develops a context-specific analysis of quality informed by the experiences of care receivers. Extending Mol's (2008) work on the logic of care, she draws on the results of qualitative research with a group that is under-represented in research on home care: older lesbian and bisexual women. Grigorovich shows how, for her participants, quality is not about standardized outcomes, but is a contingent phenomenon based on their ongoing interactions with specific providers. She highlights how the intersectional structural inequalities of heterosexism, homophobia, sexism, and ageism shape care recipients' understandings of good care. At the same time, she exposes the pretence of technical, standardized medico-administrative judgment and shows how quality is an affective and relational phenomenon.

The book's second section, "Health Markets, Individualization, and Commodification," explores substantive issues that stand outside the established foci of applied health research, namely, the processes and impacts of the growing privatization and commodification of health care in Canada. Chapters in this section traverse a range of topics including the health-related regulation of consumption, the health impacts of precarious work, and the implications of market relations and commercialization in medical education and health care delivery.

Kirsten Bell's chapter exposes tensions in the efforts of health promotion experts to intervene in packaging used to market cigarettes to smokers, contributing to an important body of research on critiques of health promotion interventions that govern behaviour by encouraging people to manage their health risks (Lupton 1995; Petersen and Lupton 1996; Polzer and Power 2016; Robertson 2001). Bell augments research on healthy citizenship and moralizing risk discourses by moving past analyses of the formal articulation of health governance. Extending poststructuralist approaches to discourse, she draws on interviews with sixty smokers from Vancouver to explore how people actually respond to health promotion messages. Bell's chapter is an important example of how a critical approach that departs from the cessationist focus of applied tobacco research can surface important tensions between how smokers respond to warnings on tobacco packages and how smoking and smokers are imagined in public health interventions.

Kelly Holloway and Matthew Herder critically examine the commercialization of biomedical training in Canadian universities. Working from a political economy perspective and drawing on survey research, observation at science policy conferences, and interviews with thirty biomedical researchers, they argue that through everyday practices of teaching, research, and mentorship, commercialization is quickly becoming a normative expectation among emerging Canadian biomedical researchers. They suggest that biomedical scientists are increasingly being encouraged to understand themselves as entrepreneurs and that distinctions between science as a public good and science that can be commercialized are rapidly being erased. Commercialization is supported by government policymakers, they argue, and is rarely the subject of critical discourse in biomedical training.

In their chapter, Ariel Ducey, Barry Hoffmaster, Magali Robert, and Sue Ross analyse the significance of the introduction and widespread use of privately manufactured kits for the treatment of women's pelvic floor disorders and the challenge the kits pose for established approaches to regulating medical practice. The chapter describes how working with an interdisciplinary research team that included a surgeon (Robert), an ethicist (Hoffmaster), and a health services researcher (Ross) led Ducey to rethink the complexities involved in transvaginal mesh surgery and how sociological research might help to address them. Ducey and her colleagues expose the limits of conventional resources of critical medical sociology that position surgeons as deficient and ignore the practical, everyday reasoning through which they navigate clinical practice and make sense of the moral grounds of their decisions. They argue that developing better interventions requires beginning from the specificities of a given setting and facilitating surgical judgment through heightened practitioner reflexivity.

Christine Kelly documents how neoliberal strategies of governing from a distance affect non-profit agencies. Neoliberal governance has meant contracting out social and other services formerly provided directly by governments to non-profit and for-profit organizations that successfully compete for government contracts (Osborne and Gaebler 1993). In the process, non-profit agencies tend to lose core funding. Their project funding is less stable, their staff is consequently less secure, and the advocacy work that was once their raison d'être is curtailed if not eliminated. Kelly analyses the effects of this neoliberal shift on agencies serving people with disabilities. Under the Harper government, managed competition restricted financial support for these agencies, and privileged large service-oriented agencies over rights-based agencies oriented to social justice and embedded in social movements. All the while, governments extended their control over the agencies involved as they governed from a distance through detailed requests for proposals (RFP) and reporting requirements.

Ross Sutherland's chapter explores processes of privatization in the medical laboratory sector. He describes how the sector has changed, from one dominated by non-profit facilities at the time medicare was established to one now controlled by large, privately owned firms. He shows how neoliberal arguments about the benefits of competition used to support privatization are contradicted by the dramatic monopolization of the private laboratory market. Drawing on an analysis of policy developments in Ontario, Alberta, and British Columbia, Sutherland suggests that provincial governments have actively supported monopolization, largely by treating the private sector as a "privileged stakeholder," with detrimental consequences for access, public control, and quality of care.

Finally, Anne Rochon Ford critically examines the workplace hazards posed by the use of toxic chemicals in private nail salons. She describes her work with the Toronto-based Healthy Nail Salon Network to document the health risks faced by racialized women working in the nail salon industry. Her chapter demonstrates how social science research on health care has been enlisted in advocacy efforts to establish toxins in the nail salon industry as a priority for federal and provincial governments. Ford also demonstrates the importance of capturing the voices and experiences of those most at risk in this sector, of surfacing the health costs of these exposures, and of building capacity for primary prevention.

Closing Remarks

Critical social science research on health and health care is often received within policy or applied circles as an unwelcome distraction from the main business of responding to serious health care issues. Social science research that calls into question authoritative ways of knowing, critiques professional expertise and practice, or exposes the operation of sexism, racism, homophobia, and other forms of domination in health care can be viewed by applied readers as a trivial nuisance or an unwanted hostility. Such responses can build a conception of critical research as an enterprise that only tears down, negates, or finds fault. They can reinforce a vision of critical social science as a kind of ceaseless nagging, while locating positive, productive scholarship within the limited and established confines of existing forms of applied health research (Mykhalovskiy and Namaste 2019).

To counter such thinking, the concluding chapter to *Health Matters* incorporates material from interviews we conducted with our contributors in which we encouraged them to express their own understandings of the contributions their research makes. While they varied in content, the interviews explored how authors responded to particular challenges in their research, how they came to understand what is important or valuable about their research, and how their work has been used. We draw on the interviews in our conclusion in a discussion of the importance of health care context and of tensions in the research process for the work collected in this volume. We have also integrated interview material in a discussion of the communication of research results. Here we emphasize that critical social science research on health care is not simply about negation; it is also about envisioning alternatives, developing solutions, and creating knowledge that moves into the world broadly. Our conclusion offers backstories to the volume's chapters that help readers to understand our contributors' research and that give them insight into how social science contributes to improved health care in ways that transcend the managerial discourses of neoliberal health reform.

NOTES

1 See "Progress in Supporting Health Social Sciences," https://www.researchnet-recherchenet.ca/rnr16/vwOpprtntyDtls.do?prog=2620&view=currentOpps&org=CIHR&type=EXACT&resultCount=25&sort=program&all=1&masterList=true#ipph.

2 Among a long list of candidates one might include Luc Boltanski's (2011) sociology of emancipation, Dorothy Smith's (2006) approach to studies in the social organization of knowledge and institutional ethnography, Flyvberg's (2001) phronetic sociology, and the many contributors to critical realism, critical race theory, postcolonial studies, critical theory, critical disability studies, critical legal studies, and decolonizing and Indigenous methodologies.

REFERENCES

Adelson, N. 2000. *"Being Alive and Well": Health and the Politics of Cree Well-Being.* Toronto: University of Toronto Press.

Albert, K. 2014. "Erasing the Social from Social Science: The Intellectual Costs of Boundary-Work and the Canadian Institute of Health Research." *Canadian Journal of Sociology* 39 (3): 393–420.

Albert, M., and S. Laberge. 2017. "Confined to a Tokenistic Status: Social Scientists in Leadership Roles in a National Health Research Funding Agency." *Social Science & Medicine* 185: 137–46. https://doi.org/10.1016/j.socscimed.2017.05.018.

Albert, M., S. Laberge, and B.D. Hodges. 2009. "Boundary Work in the Health Research Field: Biomedical and Clinician Scientists' Perceptions of Social Science Research." *Minerva* 47 (2): 171–94. https://doi.org/10.1007/s11024-009-9120-8.

Anzaldua, G. 1987. *Borderlands/La Frontera: The New Mestiza.* San Francisco: Aunt Lute.

Armstrong, H. 2013. "Neoliberalism and Official Health Statistics: Towards a Research Agenda." In *Troubling Care: Critical Perspectives on Research and Practices,* edited by P. Armstrong and S. Braedley, 187–99. Toronto: Canadian Scholars' Press.

Armstrong, P., and H. Armstrong. 2010. *Wasting Away: The Undermining of Canadian Health Care.* New York: Oxford University Press.

Armstrong, P., H. Armstrong, J. Choiniere, E. Mykhalovskiy, and J.P. White. 1997. *Medical Alert: New Work Organizations in Health Care.* Toronto: Garamond.

Armstrong, P., H. Armstrong, and K. Scott-Dixon. 2008. *Critical to Care: The Invisible Women in Health Services.* Toronto: University of Toronto Press.

Armstrong, P., and S. Braedley. 2013. *Troubling Care: Critical Perspectives on Research and Practices.* Toronto: Canadian Scholars Press.

Armstrong, P., and T. Daly. 2017. *Exercising Choice in Long-Term Care: Ideas Worth Sharing.* Ottawa: Canadian Centre for Policy Alternatives.

Armstrong, P., and S. Day. 2017. *Wash, Wear, and Care: Clothes and Laundry in Long-Term Residential Care.* Montreal: McGill-Queen's University Press.

Aronson, J. 2004. "'Just Fed and Watered': Women's Experiences of the Gutting of Home Care in Ontario." In *Caring Possibilities: Women's Work, Women's Care,* edited by K. Grant, C. Amaratunga, P. Armstrong, M. Boscoe, and A. Pederson, 167–84. Aurora: Garamond.

Baines, D. 2015. "Neoliberalism and the Convergence of Non-Profit Care Work in Canada." *Competition and Change* 19 (3): 194–209. https://doi.org/10.1177/1024529415580258.

Balka, E., K. Messing, and P. Armstrong. 2006. "Indicators for All: Including Occupational Health in Indicators for a Sustainable Healthcare System." *Policy and Practice in Health and Safety* 4 (1): 46–61. https://doi.org/10.1080/14774003.2006.11667675.

Barlow, M. 2002. *Profit Is Not the Cure.* Toronto: McClelland and Stewart.

Batt, S. 2017. *Health Advocacy Inc.* Vancouver: UBC Press.

Beagan, B. 2000. "Neutralizing Differences: Producing Neutral Doctors for (Almost) Neutral Patients." *Social Science & Medicine* 51 (8): 1253–65. https://doi.org/10.1016/s0277-9536(00)00043-5.

Bell, K. 2017. *Health and Other Unassailable Values: Reconfigurations of Health, Evidence and Ethics.* New York: Routledge.

Benoit, C., and Hallgrímsdóttir, H.K. 2008. "Engendering Research on Care and Care Work across Different Social Contexts. *Canadian Journal of Public Health* 99 (S2): S7–S10. https://doi.org/10.1007/bf03403797.

Boltanski, L. 2011. *On Critique: A Sociology of Emancipation.* Cambridge: Polity.

Bourgeault, I. 2000. "Delivering the 'New' Canadian Midwifery: The Impact on Midwifery of Integration into the Ontario Health Care System." *Sociology of Health and Illness* 22 (2): 172–96. https://doi.org/10.1111/1467-9566.00198.

Bourgeault, I. 2006. *Push! The Struggle for Midwifery in Ontario.* Montreal: McGill-Queen's University Press.

Bowker, G., and S.L. Star. 1999. *Sorting Things Out: Classification and Its Consequences.* Cambridge, MA: MIT Press.

Brotman, S., B. Ryan, Y. Jalbert, and B. Rowe. 2002. "The Impact of Coming Out on Health and Health Care Access: The Experiences of Gay, Lesbian, Bisexual, and Two-Spirit People." *Journal of Health & Social Policy* 15 (1): 1–29. https://doi.org/10.1300/j045v15n01_01.

Burton-Jones, A. 1999. *Knowledge Capitalism: Business, Work, and Learning in the New Economy.* Oxford: Oxford University Press.

Campbell, M., and J. Rankin. 2017. "Nurses and Electronic Health Records in a Canadian Hospital: Examining the Social Organisation and Programmed Use of Digitised Nursing Knowledge." *Sociology of Health & Illness* 39 (3): 365–79. https://doi.org/10.1111/1467-9566.12489.

Canadian Institutes of Health Research Act SC. 2000, c. 6.

Carroll, W.K. 2004. *Critical Strategies for Social Research.* Toronto: Canadian Scholars Press.

Choiniere, J. 2011. "Accounting for Care: Exploring Tensions and Contradictions." *Advances in Nursing Science* 34 (4): 330–44. https://doi.org/10.1097/ans.0b013e3182356c31.

Coburn, D. 2010. "Health and Health Care: A Political Economy Perspective." In *Staying Alive: Critical Perspectives on Health, Illness, and Health Care,* edited by T. Bryant, D. Raphael, and M.H. Rioux, 65–91. Toronto: Canadian Scholars Press.

Coburn, D., S. Rappolt, and I. Bourgeault. 1997. "Decline vs. Retention of Medical Power through Restratification: An Examination of the Ontario Case." *Sociology of Health & Illness* 19 (1): 1–22. https://doi.org/10.1111/1467-9566.ep10934208.

Corman, M. 2017. *Paramedics On and Off the Streets: Emergency Medical Services in the Age of Technological Governance.* Toronto: University of Toronto Press.

Costa, L., J. Voronka, D. Landry, J. Reid, B. Mcfarlane, D. Reville, and K. Church. 2012. "'Recovering our Stories': A Small Act of Resistance." *Studies in Social Justice* 6 (1): 85–101. https://doi.org/10.26522/ssj.v6i1.1070.

Crombie, I.K. 1996. *Research in Health Care: A Practical Approach to the Design, Conduct and Interpretation of Health Services Research.* New York: John Wiley & Sons.

Das Gupta, T. 2009. *Real Nurses and Others: Racism in Nursing.* Black Point, NS: Fernwood Publishing.

Deber, R. 2018. *Treating Health Care: How the Canadian System Works and How It Could Be Better.* Toronto: University of Toronto Press.

Denton, M., I.U. Zeytinoglu, S. Davies, and J. Lian. 2002. "Job Stress and Job Dissatisfaction of Home Care Workers in the Context of Health Care Restructuring." *International Journal of Health Services* 32 (2): 327–57. https://doi.org/10.2190/vyn8-6nky-rkum-l0xw.

Eakin, J. 2016. "Educating Critical Qualitative Health Researchers in the Land of the Randomized Controlled Trial." *Qualitative Inquiry* 22 (2): 107–18. https://doi.org/10.1177/1077800415617207.

Eakin, J., A. Robertson, B. Poland, D. Coburn, and R. Edwards. 1996. "Towards a Critical Social Science Perspective on Health Promotion Research." *Health Promotion International* 11 (2): 157–65. https://doi.org/10.1093/heapro/11.2.157.

England, K., J. Eakin, D. Gastaldo, and P. McKeever. 2007. "Neoliberalizing Home Care: Managed Competition and Restructuring Home Care in Ontario." In *Neoliberalization: Networks, States, Peoples,* edited by K. England and K. Ward, 169–94. Oxford: Blackwell.

Etowa, J.B., B.L. Beagan, F. Eghan, and W.T. Bernard. 2017. "'You Feel You Have to Be Made of Steel': The Strong Black Woman, Health, and Well-Being in Nova Scotia." *Health Care for Women International* 38 (4): 379–93. https://doi.org/10.1080/07399332.2017.1290099.

Feldberg, G., and R. Vipond. 1999. "The Virus of Consumerism." In *Health Reform: Public Success, Private Failure,* edited by D. Drache and T. Sullivan, 48–64. London: Routledge.

Flexner, A. 2017. *The Usefulness of Useless Knowledge.* Princeton: Princeton University Press.

Flyvbjerg, B. 2001. *Making Social Science Matter: Why Social Inquiry Fails and How It Can Succeed Again.* Cambridge: Cambridge University Press.

Ford, A.R., and D. Saibil. 2009. *The Push to Prescribe: Women and Canadian Drug Policy.* Toronto: Women's Press.

Freeman, H.E., and P.H. Rossi. 1984. "Furthering the Applied Side of Sociology." *American Sociological Review* 49 (4): 571–80. https://doi.org/10.2307/2095470.

Ginsberg, B. 2011. *The Fall of the Faculty: The Rise of the All-Administrative University and Why It Matters.* New York: Oxford University Press.

Gluckman, P, M. Ferguson, A. Glover, J. Grant, T. Groves, M. Lauer, and M. Ulfendahl. 2017. *International Peer Review Expert Panel Report: A Report to the Governing Council of the Canadian Institutes of Health Research.* http://www.cihr-irsc.gc.ca/e/documents/peer_review_international-report-en.pdf.

Goldenberg, M. 2006. "On Evidence and Evidence-Based Medicine: Lessons from the Philosophy of Science." *Social Science and Medicine* 62 (11): 2621–32. https://doi.org/10.1016/j.socscimed.2005.11.031.

Graham, J., N. Adelson, S. Fortin, G. Bibeau, M. Lock, S. Hyde, M.E. Macdonald, I. Olazabal, P. Stephenson, and J. Waldram. 2011. "The End of Medical Anthropology in Canada? A Manifesto." *University Affairs.* 7 February. http://www.universityaffairs.ca/opinion/in-my-opinion/the-end-of-medical-anthorpology-in-canada/.

Grant, K., N. Adelson, P. Armstrong, L. Biggs, S. de Grosbois, M. Koninck, P. Downe, et al. 1999. *Integrating the Social Sciences and Humanities in the*

Canadian Institutes for Health Research. http://www.cfhi-fcass.ca/migrated/pdf/researchreports/commissionedresearch/grant.pdf.

Grant, K., C. Amaratunga, and P. Armstrong. 2004. *Caring For/Caring About: Women, Home Care and Unpaid Caregiving.* Aurora: Garamond.

Grigorovich, A. 2015. "Restricted Access: Older Lesbian and Bisexual Women's Experiences with Home Care Services." *Research on Aging* 37 (7): 763–83. https://doi.org/10.1177/0164027514562650.

Hankivsky, O. 2011. *Health Inequities in Canada: Intersectional Frameworks and Practice.* Vancouver: UBC Press.

Haraway, D. 1991. *Simians, Cyborgs, and Women: The Reinvention of Nature.* New York: Routledge.

Harbin, A., B. Beagan, and L. Goldberg. 2012. "Discomfort, Judgment, and Health Care for Queers." *Journal of Bioethical Inquiry* 9 (2): 149–60. https://doi.org/10.1007/s11673-012-9367-x.

Harvey, D. 2007. *A Brief History of Neoliberalism.* New York: Oxford University Press.

Hennebry, J., J. McLaughlin, and K. Preibisch. 2016. "Out of the Loop: (In) access to Health Care for Migrant Workers in Canada." *Journal of International Migration and Integration* 17 (2): 521–38. https://doi.org/10.1007/s12134-015-0417-1.

Henwood, F., R. Harris, and P. Spoel. 2011. "Informing Health? Negotiating the Logics of Choice and Care in Everyday Practices of 'Healthy Living.'" *Social Science & Medicine* 72 (12): 2026–32. https://doi.org/10.1016/j.socscimed.2011.04.007.

Hindmarch, S., M. Orsini, and M. Gagnon. 2018. *Seeing Red: HIV/AIDS and Public Policy in Canada.* Toronto: University of Toronto Press.

Holloway, K. 2014. "Uneasy Subjects: Medical Students' Conflicts over the Pharmaceutical Industry." *Social Science & Medicine* 114: 113–20. https://doi.org/10.1016/j.socscimed.2014.05.052.

Husbands, W., D. Miller, L.T. McCready, C. Williams, L. Guy, A. Harriott, C.E. James, et al. 2019. "Sexuality and Sexual Agency among Heterosexual Black Men in Toronto: Tradition, Contradiction, and Emergent Possibilities in the Context of HIV and Health." *Canadian Journal of Sociology,* 44 (4): 399–424. https://journals.library.ualberta.ca/cjs/index.php/CJS/article/view/29506/21493.

Institute of Medicine. 1995. *Health Services Research: Work Force and Educational Issues.* Washington, DC: National Academy Press.

Jackson, B.E., A. Pederson, P. Armstrong, M. Boscoe, B. Clow, K.R. Grant, N. Guberman, and K. Willson. 2006. "'Quality Care Is Like a Carton of Eggs': Using a Gender-Based Diversity Analysis to Assess Quality of Health Care." *Canadian Woman Studies* 24 (1): 15–22. https://cws.journals.yorku.ca/index.php/cws/article/view/6171.

Johnson, J.L., J.L. Bottorf, A.J. Browne, S. Grewal, B.A. Hilton, and H. Clarke. 2004. "Othering and Being Othered in the Context of Health Care

Services." *Health Communication* 16 (2): 255–71. https://doi.org/10.1207/s15327027hc1602_7.

Jones, A. 2019. "Ontario to Tie Post-secondary Funding to Grads' Employment and Earnings." *Toronto Star*, 18 April. https://www.thestar.com/news/canada/2019/04/18/ontario-to-tie-post-secondary-funding-to-grads-employment-and-earnings.html.

Kamp, A., and H. Hvid. 2012. "Introduction: Elderly Care in Transition." In *Elderly Care in Transition: Management, Meaning and Identity at Work: A Scandinavian Perspective*, edited by A. Kamp and H. Hvid, 13–28. Copenhagen: Copenhagen Business School Press.

Katherine, W. 2015. "Midwifery in Ontario: Opportunities for Women's Health Policy Research." In *Women's Health: Intersections of Policy, Research, and Practice*, 2nd ed., edited by P. Armstrong and A. Pederson, 278–86. Toronto: Women's Press.

Katz, S., and B. Green. 2005. "The Government of Detail: The Case of Social Policy on Aging." In *Cultural Aging: Life Course, Lifestyle, and Senior Worlds*, edited by S. Katz, 53–69. Peterborough: Broadview.

Kaufert, P.A., and J.D. O'Neil. 2009. "Cooptation and Control: The Reconstruction of Inuit Birth." *Medical Anthropology Quarterly* 4 (4): 427–42. https://doi.org/10.1525/maq.1990.4.4.02a00040.

King, S. 2006. *Pink Ribbons, Inc.: Breast Cancer and the Politics of Philanthropy.* Minneapolis: University of Minneapolis.

Knaapen, L. 2014. "Evidence Based Medicine or Cookbook Medicine? Addressing Concerns over the Standardization of Care." *Sociology Compass* 8 (6): 823–36. https://doi.org/10.1111/soc4.12184.

Koehn, S., S. Neysmith, K. Kobayashi, and H. Khamisa. 2013. "Revealing the Shape of Knowledge Using an Intersectionality Lens: Results of a Scoping Review on the Health and Health Care of Ethnocultural Minority Older Adults." *Ageing & Society* 33 (3): 437–64. https://doi.org/10.1017/s0144686x12000013.

Kontos, P., and A. Grigorovich. 2018. "'Sleight of Hand' or 'Selling Our Soul'? Surviving and Thriving as Critical Qualitative Health Researchers in a Positivist World." *Forum Qualitative Sozialforschung/Forum Qualitative Social Research* 19 (2): 15. http://dx.doi.org/10.17169/fqs-19.2.2990.

Laforest, R., and M. Orsini. 2005. "Evidence-Based Engagement in the Voluntary Sector: Lessons from Canada." *Social Policy & Administration* 39 (5): 481–97. https://doi.org/10.1111/j.1467-9515.2005.00451.x.

Latour, B., and S. Woolgar. 1986. *Laboratory Life: The Social Construction of Scientific Facts.* Princeton: Princeton University Press.

Laxer, K. 2015. "Who Counts in Care: Gender, Power, and Aging Populations." In *Women's Health: Intersections of Policy, Research, and Practice*, 2d ed., edited by P. Armstrong and A. Pederson, 215–37. Toronto: Women's Press.

Learmonth, M. 2003. "Making Health Services Management Research Critical: A Review and a Suggestion." *Sociology of Health and Illness* 25 (1): 93–119. https://doi.org/10.1111/1467-9566.00326.

Leduc Browne, P. 2000. *Unsafe Practices: Restructuring and Privatization in Ontario Health Care.* Ottawa: Canadian Centre for Policy Alternatives.

Lexchin, J. 2016. *Private Profits vs. Public Policy: The Pharmaceutical Industry and the Canadian State.* Toronto: University of Toronto Press.

Lohr, K., and D. Steinwachs. 2002. "Health Services Research: An Evolving Definition of the Field." *HSR: Health Services Research* 37 (1): 15–17. https://doi.org/10.1111/1475-6773.01020.

Lupton, D. 1995. *The Imperative of Health: Public Health and the Regulated Body.* Thousand Oaks: Sage.

MacDonald, M. 2007. *At Work in the Field of Birth: Midwifery Narratives of Nature, Tradition and Home.* Nashville: Vanderbilt University Press.

Malacrida, C. 2004. "Medicalization, Ambivalence and Social Control: Mothers' Descriptions of Educators and ADD/ADHD." *Health: An Interdisciplinary Journal for the Social Study of Health, Illness and Medicine* 8 (1): 61–80. https://doi.org/10.1177/1363459304038795.

Martin, D. 2017. *Better Now: Six Big Ideas to Improve Health Care for All Canadians.* Toronto: Allen Lane.

McCoy, L. 2005. "HIV-Positive Patients and the Doctor-Patient Relationship: Perspectives from the Margins." *Qualitative Health Research* 15 (6): 791–806. https://doi.org/10.1177/1049732305276752.

McCoy, L. 2009. "Time, Self and the Medication Day: A Closer Look at the Everyday Work of 'Adherence.'" *Sociology of Health & Illness* 31 (1): 128–46. https://doi.org/10.1111/j.1467-9566.2008.01120.x.

Meagher, G., and M. Szebehely. 2013. *Marketization in Nordic Eldercare: A Research Report on Legislation, Oversight, Extent and Consequences.* Stockholm: Stockholm University.

Metcalfe, A.S. 2010. "Revisiting Academic Capitalism in Canada: No Longer the Exception." *Journal of Higher Education* 81 (4): 489–514. https://doi.org/10.1080/00221546.2010.11779062.

Miller, P., and N. Rose. 1990. "Governing Economic Life." *Economy and Society* 19 (1): 1–31. https://doi.org/10.1080/03085149000000001.

Mintzberg, H. 2017. *Managing the Myths of Health Care.* Oakland: Barrett-Koehler.

Mol, A. 2008. *The Logic of Care: Health and the Problem of Patient Choice.* London: Routledge.

Morrow, M., and J. Weisser. 2012. "Towards a Social Justice Framework of Mental Health Recovery." *Studies in Social Justice* 6 (1): 27–43. https://doi.org/10.26522/ssj.v61.1067.

Moss, P., and I. Dyck. 2002. *Women, Body and Illness.* Oxford: Rowman & Littlefield.

Mykhalovskiy, E. 2001. "Troubled Hearts, Care Pathways and Hospital Restructuring: Exploring Health Services Research as Active Knowledge." *Studies in Cultures, Organizations, and Societies* 7 (2): 269–96. https://doi.org/10.1080/10245280108523561.

Mykhalovskiy, E. 2003. "Evidence-Based Medicine: Ambivalent Reading and the Clinical Recontextualization of Science." *Health: An Interdisciplinary Journal for the Social Study of Health, Illness and Medicine* 7 (3): 331–52. https://doi.org/10.1177/1363459303007003005.

Mykhalovskiy, E., P. Armstrong, H. Armstrong, I. Bourgeault, J. Choiniere, E. Lexchin, S. Peters, and J.P. White. 2008. "Qualitative Research and the Politics of Knowledge in an Age of Evidence: The Possibilities and Perils of Immanent Critique." *Social Science and Medicine* 67 (1): 195–203. https://doi.org/10.1016/j.socscimed.2008.03.002.

Mykhalovskiy, E., L. McCoy, and M. Bresalier. 2004. "Compliance/Adherence, HIV, and the Critique of Medical Power." *Social Theory & Health* 2 (4): 315–40. https://doi.org/10.1057/palgrave.sth.8700037.

Mykhalovskiy, E., and V.K. Namaste. 2019. *Thinking Differently about HIV/AIDS: Contributions from Critical Social Science.* Vancouver: UBC Press.

Mykhalovskiy, E., and L. Weir. 2004. "The Problem of Evidence-Based Medicine: Directions for Social Science." *Social Science and Medicine* 59 (5): 1059–69. https://doi.org/10.1016/j.socscimed.2003.12.002.

Nestel, S. 2006. Obstructed Labour: Race and Gender in the Re-Emergence of Midwifery. Vancouver: UBC Press.

Neysmith, S.M. 2000. *Restructuring Caring Labour: Discourse, State Practice, and Everyday Life.* Toronto: Oxford University Press.

Neysmith, S.M., M. Reitsma-Street, S. Baker-Collins, and E. Porter. 2012. *Beyond Caring: Labour to Provisioning Work.* Toronto: University of Toronto Press.

Olssen, M., and M.A. Peters. 2005. "Neoliberalism, Higher Education and the Knowledge Economy: From the Free Market to Knowledge Capitalism." *Journal of Education Policy* 20 (3): 313–45. https://doi.org/10.1080/02680930500108718.

Orsini, M., and M. Smith. 2010. "Social Movements, Knowledge and Public Policy: The Case of Autism Activism in Canada and the U.S." *Critical Policy Studies* 4 (1): 38–57. https://doi.org/10.1080/19460171003714989.

Osborne, D., and T. Gaebler. 1993. *Reinventing Government.* New York: Penguin.

Paterson, S. 2010. "Feminizing Obstetrics or Medicalizing Midwifery? The Discursive Constitution of Midwifery in Ontario, Canada." *Critical Policy Studies* 4 (2): 127–45. https://doi.org/10.1080/19460171.2010.490635.

Penning, M.J., and C. Zheng. 2016. "Income Inequalities in Health Care Utilization among Adults Aged 50 and Older." *Canadian Journal on Aging* 35 (1): 55–69. https://doi.org/10.1017/s0714980815000562.

Petersen, A., and D. Lupton. 1996. *The New Public Health: Health and Self in the Age of Risk*. London: Sage.

Poland, B., D. Coburn, A. Robertson, and J. Eakin. 1998. "Wealth, Equity and Health Care: A Critique of a 'Population Health' Perspective on the Determinants of Health." *Social Science & Medicine* 46 (7): 785–98. https://doi.org/10.1016/s0277-9536(97)00197-4.

Poland, B., M. Dooris, and R. Haluza-Delay. 2011. "Securing 'Supportive Environments' for Health in the Face of Ecosystem Collapse: Meeting the Triple Threat with a Sociology of Creative Transformation." *Health Promotion International 26* (suppl. 2): ii202–15. https://doi.org/10.1093/heapro/dar073.

Polster, C. 2015. "The Privatization of Knowledge in Canada's Universities and What We Should Do about It." In *Free Knowledge: Confronting the Commodification of Human Discovery*, edited by P.W. Elliot and D.H. Hepting, 56–66. Regina: University of Regina Press.

Polzer, J.S., and E. Power. 2016. *Neoliberal Governance and Health: Duties, Risks, and Vulnerabilities*. Montreal: McGill-Queen's Press.

Porter, M., and D. Gustafson. 2012. *Reproducing Women: Family and Health Work across Three Generations*. Halifax, NS: Fernwood.

Power, M. 1994. *The Audit Explosion*. London: Demos.

Rachlis, M. 2007. *Privatized Health Care Won't Deliver*. Toronto: Wellesley Institute

Rankin, J.M. 2003. "'Patient Satisfaction': Knowledge for Ruling Hospital Reform: An Institutional Ethnography." *Nursing Inquiry* 10 (1): 57–65. https://doi.org/10.1046/j.1440-1800.2003.00156.x.

Rankin, J., and M. Campbell. 2006. *Managing to Nurse: Inside Canada's Health Care Reform*. Toronto: University of Toronto Press.

Rappolt, S. 1997. "Clinical Guidelines and the Fate of Medical Autonomy in Ontario." *Social Science & Medicine* 44 (7): 977–87. https://doi.org/10.1016/s0277-9536(96)00223-7.

Robertson, A. 1998. "Shifting Discourses on Health in Canada: From Health Promotion to Population Health." *Health Promotion International* 13 (2): 155–66. https://doi.org/10.1093/heapro/13.2.155.

Robertson, A. 2001. "Biotechnology, Political Rationality and Discourses on Health Risk." *Health*. 5 (3): 293–309. https://doi.org/10.1177/136345930100500302.

Ronald, L.A., M. McGregor, C. Harrington, A. Pollock, and J. Lexchin. 2016. "Observational Evidence of For-Profit Delivery and Inferior Nursing Home Care: When Is There Enough Evidence for Policy Change?" *PLOS Medicine* 13 (4): e1001095. https://doi.org/10.1371/journal.pmed.1001995.

Rose, N., and P. Miller. 1992. "Political Power beyond the State: Problematics of Government." *British Journal of Sociology* 43 (2): 173–205. https://doi.org/10.2307/591464.

Rossiter, K., and A. Robertson. 2014. "Methods of Resistance: A New Typology for Health Research within the Neoliberal Knowledge Economy." *Social Theory & Health* 12 (2): 197–217. https://doi.org/10.1057/sth.2014.2.

Shore, C., and S. Wright. 2004. "Whose Accountability? Governmentality and the Auditing of Universities." *Parallax* 10 (2): 100–16. https://doi.org/10.1080/1353464042000208558.

Sinding, C., L. Barnoff, and P. Grassau. 2004. "Homophobia and Heterosexisms in Cancer Care: The Experiences of Lesbians." *Canadian Journal of Nursing Research* 36 (4): 170–88.

Sinding, C., P. Miller, P. Hudak, S. Keller-Olaman, and J. Sussman. 2012. "Of Times and Troubles: Patient Involvement and the Production of Health Care Disparities." *Health: An Interdisciplinary Journal for the Social Study of Health, Illness and Medicine* 16 (4): 400–17. https://doi.org/10.1177/1363459311416833.

Slaughter, S., and G. Rhoades. 2004. *Academic Capitalism and the New Economy: Markets, State, and Higher Education.* Baltimore: Johns Hopkins University Press.

Smith, D.E. 1987. *The Everyday World as Problematic: A Feminist Sociology.* Toronto: University of Toronto Press.

Smith, D.E. 2006. *Institutional Ethnography as Practice.* Toronto: Rowman & Littlefield.

Stone, D. 2001. *The Policy Paradox: The Art of Political Decision-Making.* New York: W.W. Norton.

Straus, R. 1957. "The Nature and Status of Medical Sociology." *American Sociological Review* 22 (2): 200–4. https://doi.org/10.2307/2088858.

Tang, S.Y., and A.J. Brown. 2008. "'Race' Matters: Racialization and Egalitarian Discourses Involving Aboriginal People in the Canadian Health Care Context." *Ethnicity & Health* 13 (2): 109–27. https://doi.org/10.1080/13557850701830307.

Tanuseputro, P., M. Chalifoux, C. Bennett, A. Gruneir, S.E. Bronskill, P. Walker, and D. Manuel. 2015. "Hospitalization and Mortality Rates in Long-Term Care Facilities: Does For-Profit Status Matter?" *Journal of the American Medical Directors Association* 16 (10): 874–83. https://doi.org/10.1016/j.jamda.2015.06.004.

Thériault, L., J. Low, and A. Luke. 2014. "Negotiating the System: Social Workers in Home Support in New Brunswick." *Canadian Review of Social Policy* 70: 64–77.

Thille, P. and G. Russell. "Giving Patients Responsibility or Fostering Mutual Response-ability: Family Physicians' Constructions of Effective Chronic Illness Management." *Qualitative Health Research* 20 (10): 1343–52. https://doi.org/10.1177%2F1049732310372376.

Timmermans, S., and M. Berg. 2010. *The Gold Standard: The Challenge of Evidence-Based Medicine and Standardization in Health Care.* Philadelphia: Temple University Press.

Titchkosky, T., and R. Michalko. 2009. *Rethinking Normalcy: A Disability Studies Reader.* Toronto: Canadian Scholars Press.

Travers, A. 2015. "The Health of Sexual Minority Women and Trans People: An Ontario Perspective." In *Women's Health: Intersections of Policy, Research, and Practice,* 2nd ed., edited by P. Armstrong and A. Pederson. 173–92. Toronto: Women's Press.

Turk, J.L. 2017. "Foreword: The Landscape of the Contemporary University." *Canadian Journal of Communication* 42 (1): 3–12. https://doi.org/10.22230/cjc.2017v42n1a3202.

Wacquant, L. 2012. "Three Steps to a Historical Anthropology of Actually Existing Neoliberalism." *Social Anthropology* 20 (1): 66–79. https://doi.org/10.1111/j.1469-8676.2011.00189.x.

Wathen, N., S. Wyatt, and R. Harris. 2008. *Mediating Health Information: The Go-Betweens in a Changing Socio-Technical Landscape.* Basingstoke: Palgrave Macmillan.

Webster, F., K. Rice, J. Christian, N. Seemann, N. Baxter, C.A. Moulton, and T. Cil. 2016. "The Erasure of Gender in Academic Surgery: A Qualitative Study." *American Journal of Surgery* 212 (4): 559–65. https://doi.org/10.1016/j.amjsurg.2016.06.006.

Whelan, E. 2007. "'No One Agrees Except for Those of Us Who Have It': Endometriosis Patients as an Epistemological Community." *Sociology of Health and Illness* 29 (7): 957–82. https://doi.org/10.1111/j.1467-9566.2007.01024.x.

Williams, A.P., R. Deber, P. Baranek, and A. Gildiner. 2001. "From Medicare to Home Care: Globalization, State Retrenchment, and the Profitization of Canada's Healthcare System." In *Unhealthy Times: Political Economy Perspectives on Health and Care in Canada,* edited by P. Armstrong, H. Armstrong, and D. Coburn, 7–30. Toronto: Oxford University Press.

PART ONE

What Counts as Evidence? Managerial Knowledge, Visibility, and Experience

2 The Dematerialization of Fundamental Nursing Care in an Era of Managerial Reform

CRAIG DALE

The CBC news headline "Man's Teeth Left to Rot While He Was in Hospital's Care" (Ireton 2016) may sound like a caption lifted from a nineteenth-century tabloid. In fact, the accompanying report addresses a contemporary event and heralds a serious disorder plaguing hospitals in Canada and internationally. It relays the astonishing case of Michael Neve, a twenty-six-year-old man with autism and developmental disability who had been in care at the Ottawa Hospital for twenty-four months. The inability of nurses to attend to Michael's oral health during hospitalization led to painful abscesses throughout his mouth. Delays in the medical team's linking his declining physical state with rampant oral infection resulted in protracted suffering. Neve had twenty-six teeth extracted and was fitted for dentures. However, the hospital refused to reimburse his family for the cost of these procedures. Unsettling assumptions regarding the provision of "basic" care in hospital, Neve's story offers a compelling entry point to the shocking dematerialization of nursing care.

Since Florence Nightingale's time, nurses have struggled to build support and visibility for fundamental patient care. Aligned with basic human needs, fundamental care frequently centres on the concept of nursing hygiene – a set of practices associated with maintaining health, preventing disease, and ameliorating suffering (Kitson 2010). Often taken as synonymous with "hands-on" bodily care, fundamental nursing activities apply to all hospitalized patients. They include, but are not limited to, bathing, oral care, toileting, nutrition, and comfort. Nightingale (1860) emphasized that failing to deliver fundamental care contributed to pain, infection, prolonged hospitalization, and even death. Her training protocols and organization of nursing transformed the possibilities of medical intervention by setting a hygienic foundation for all hospital services. Nightingale's campaign to improve hospital staffing, hygienic standards, and rates of patient mortality encouraged nurses to develop an intimate knowledge of the ill body through observation. Use of all senses supported the expert ministrations of the nurse as she tailored treatments to the body's exudate, temperature, and odours as well as its discomforts.

The repercussions of inattention to the body come into view when we consider the fate of vulnerable patients such as Michael Neve. As readers survey his story, I invite them to consider his experience as a window into a larger problem afflicting the health care system. Patients in the modern high-tech hospital are now at risk of injury and death from a lack of hands-on bodily care (Kalisch 2015). A wave of managerial reforms aiming to improve hospital care has not resolved this issue. In fact, I have discovered that managerialism is a source of the problem. Nightingale (1860, 6) understood that "bad administrative arrangements often make it impossible to nurse." In the inexorable drive for efficiency, hospitals increasingly find it necessary to add new administrative duties to nursing work. The resultant time compression experienced by nurses impedes the delivery of fundamental care and has dangerous consequences for patients.

In this chapter I appropriate the economic concept of dematerialization to both define and explain the disappearance of fundamental nursing care. Dematerialization, in economic terms, is often described as the expectation to increase productivity with fewer material resources. I argue that managerial reform disrupts nursing care of the sick both materially and discursively. By bringing the reader to the point-of-care through ethnographic data, I attempt to rematerialize what managerial discourses elide. Abstract managerial ideals of efficiency function to remove the bodies of patients and nurses in ways that limit how the world of the hospital can enter into public knowledge. Materially requiring nurses to feed the growing administrative machinery of the hospital, through various forms of documentation, has introduced new forms of precarity for patient care (Krichbaum et al. 2007).

The focus of this chapter emerges from my decades of clinical experience as an intensive care unit (ICU) nurse in a large academic hospital in Ontario, Canada. Ever-increasing managerial expectations for greater productivity alongside fewer resources mobilized my pursuit of an academic voice to articulate the inability of nurses to perform fundamental patient care. The data and analysis I present emerged over eight years of ethnographic research activity. In the sections that follow I use media stories, observational field notes, interview excerpts, documents, and photographs as empirical evidence supporting my argument. In materializing events that are not so readily observable, I make explicit the connection between managerialism and instances where nursing agency is routinely deflected from fundamental patient care.

Research Context

The turn to managerialism in the Canadian health system has been critically explored by a number of researchers who ask important questions regarding economic modes of health governance reshaping the patient-clinician encounter (Bourgeault et al. 2001). Particular attention has been paid to the consequential impact of private-sector managerial strategies on hospital services. This includes the conceptualization of nursing as a budget "cost" rendering it a target for efficiencies through bed closures, layoffs, standardized work processes, and mandated collection and reporting of quality indicators (Aiken 2008). An important strand of analysis emerging from this body of enquiry focuses on how nursing work intensifies when specific managerial activities are downloaded to nurses. Researchers have identified a growing misalignment between managerial prioritization of efficiencies and the ability of nurses to meet these expectations (Allen 2015).

Campbell and Rankin (2017) have explored the massive infusion of public money for health information technology (IT) in the Canadian hospital system, which has facilitated the ability of health managers and policymakers to generate and circulate numeric performance data. Neoliberal ideals embedded in these activities include the surveillance of health information as the best solution to providing cost-effective patient care. Investigating these assumptions has led to the discovery of new clinician requirements to produce documentary information that renders the health care encounter quantifiable. For example, hospital nurses' expanding responsibility for generating patient data for administrative use has emerged as a serious conflict with their role in caring for the sick. Choiniere (2011) explains how this evolving role may paradoxically leave nurses little time to implement the high-quality patient care espoused in hospital quality targets.

In my experience, numerical data cannot penetrate the material and social actualities that unfold when efficiency is the gold standard of excellence (Holmes et al. 2008). The narrow conception of valid and reliable evidence, as originating in calculable data, is seriously flawed: it eschews patient and clinician experiences. In contrast to a purported neutrality embedded in such evidence, Timmermans and Berg (1997) point out how the generation of managerial health data requires the assignment of actual work to real people. Work requires time, concentration, reminders, and sometimes the reprioritization of other duties. When assigned to nurses, the collection of health data may place bodily care in a lower order of importance. However, all of this effort is invariably transformed and displaced in the abstract traces of work within large institutions.

One way researchers can challenge managerialism in health care is by conducting research that places the body at the centre of health reform. As a nurse, I have found that critical ethnographic and qualitative analyses best meet this goal. Ethnographic and qualitative analyses have also helped me to identify the contraction of thinking, writing, and speaking about illness that is typical of managerial perspectives. My research is particularly informed by institutional ethnography (IE) (Smith 2005), the benefit of which is its ability to open up an alternative formulation of the everyday. IE investigations begin with work activity and aim to explicate "how things happen." IE reveals less visible features of everyday work and assists in clarifying how those activities are both organized and obscured by institutional discourses and texts (McCoy 2008).

My research contributes to this volume by returning to the body in illness (Casper and Moore 2009). Bodies circulate meaning and place important demands on caregivers. Twigg et al. (2011) contend that the low visibility of body care in the contemporary health context limits our understanding of hygiene and its practitioners. The assumption that this work is uncomplicated or always the same is primary in this regard. Diamond (1992) suggests that wider social and economic forces are implicated in these misconceptions as they continually reorient attention away from the body to managerial issues. In the next section, I pull back the proverbial bedside curtain to demonstrate how managerial reform has obscured the visibility of nursing care, added new administrative duties for nurses, and contributed to a troubling phenomenon of missed patient care.

Pulling Back the Curtain

If one were to review the public website of a Canadian hospital, one would likely find the vision or aims of health services expressed in a language of efficiency, safety, and transparency. While these objectives sound perfectly reasonable, one might pause to consider the absence of ill, diseased, and dependent people in such public communications. I view the rhetorical abandonment of the sick as a serious problem, given that it actively diminishes public awareness of the bodily problems presented by illness and the central role of hospitals in skilfully addressing these difficulties. As hospitals shorten lengths of stay and discharge patients "sicker and quicker," the remaining patients have more need for nursing care. However, hospitals have not increased nursing staff in response. In fact, nursing layoffs are often the first strategy hospitals turn to in pursuit of cost efficiencies (Armstrong 2001).

The evidence I have accumulated suggests the discursive turn from ill bodies to the bottom line has had devastating consequences for patient care and outcomes. Withdrawing nursing care means dependent and vulnerable patients struggle to meet the most basic of human needs. I had only vague notions about the scope of this problem when I began conducting field study in a Canadian hospital about eight years ago. My concern with hygienic work emerged from my own clinical practice as an ICU nurse. Limited solutions to the problems I confronted in practice propelled me down a path to investigate oral care – one of the many hygienic accountabilities of nursing. I wanted to know why it was so difficult to perform an act that fell under the rubric of "basic care" in a high-tech hospital setting. The frequent impossibility of oral care, in particular, made me wonder what others knew about this issue and how it could be resolved.

Oral care is now considered a "canary in the coal mine": international research has confirmed that it is the first act of bodily care to perish in time-pressured health settings (Ausserhofer et al. 2014). However, our collective awareness of this disappearance has been delayed. In contrast to the advanced scientific therapies that reach the health care headlines, oral care is routinely relegated to the ordinary, and therefore the background. Liaschenko and Peter (2004, 490) argue that bodily care is conceptually and discursively labelled a "housekeeping" issue, which means it is easily ignored. For example, I was recently speaking with a renowned physician-researcher who conceded in passing that "motherhood" issues such as oral care have received insufficient attention. The intellectual and gendered myopia embodied in such language relegates bodily care to the private or domestic sphere, well outside of public visibility.

Canadians depend upon nurses' work with ill bodies. Yet they may not be compelled to think about that work until they need it. Although oral care may appear to be a particularly mundane set of hospital-based activities, I contend that it is anything but ordinary. Consider the following excerpt from my field notes from an investigation into ICU oral care work:

> The nurse, a physiotherapist, and I (acting as a participant observer) were struggling to turn the critically ill adult patient onto his side. Physically turning a dependent patient in bed is something nurses are expected to do every two hours in this ICU. The patient's body weight, flailing arms, and a heaving mass of tubes, drains, and monitoring cables made this seemingly banal task a herculean effort. As if that were not enough trouble, the patient began to gag, cough, and spasm mid-turn, which triggered the mechanical ventilator to alarm at full pitch. I looked down at the patient's flushed face and his mouth full of tubes. Saliva and sputum flowed freely from his gaping mouth, forming grey pools of liquid on his gown and bed linen. To quell the alarm, the nurse identified the need to "suction the patient." Trading places, I took over her position, holding the patient around

> his middle as she raced to advance a hard plastic suction device into the dark recesses of his mouth to vacuum out the loose secretions. The nurses on this unit explained that poor oral health advances in a bizarre and precipitous manner in critical illness and often results in the accrual of dental plaque and oral bacteria in large quantities. As aspiration of bacteria-laden oral secretions into the lungs can precipitate pneumonia, oral care is a critical intervention. Before the nurse could advance the tool more than an inch inside his mouth, the patient bit down hard with his teeth, impeding her efforts. Oblivious to the unfolding chaos, a harried physician appeared in the doorway to enquire about the patient's laboratory results, which had not yet been inscribed by the nurse into the bedside medical record called the "flowsheet." He was soon replaced by another physician shouting similar questions above the din of an alarm. Both were concerned about a possible infection. The nurse eyeballed her wristwatch and announced the need to forsake our physical care efforts. She had to address the mountain of documentary forms and checklists outside the room before medical team rounds.

This field note is not about nurses not doing their jobs or delivering haphazard care. Instead, it brings a particular set of institutional relations into focus. It is an example of what Diamond (1992, 209) calls the "enterprise of industrial production" and suggests how all nursing work is subject to an overwhelming sense of time compression, or what Krichbaum et al. (2007, 86) refer to as "complexity compression." It also exemplifies conflicting nursing duties that translate into some care activities being omitted while others are prioritized. In the drive to elevate managerial concerns over illness, institutions are implicit in requiring nurses to refocus their activities away from the physical body, thus dematerializing care.

When I sat down with the ICU nurse to discuss what was happening, we spoke at length about her patient's poor oral health and how providing oral care is fraught with challenges, including insufficient time to address her patients' physical needs. The ever-growing pressure to complete standardized documentation competed for her time and attention. She explained that the number of paper and computerized forms, safety checklists, communication tools, and workload measures has grown exponentially alongside the requirement to continuously monitor hospital capacity. In this case, nursing turns away from the patient towards the information needs of administrative decision makers:

> I do recall, you know, when initially coming to this unit, being overwhelmed by looking, even looking at the flowsheet [the patient care record] for the

> first time, having that urgency of writing things down and putting it on paper early because of the other nurses, because of the round times, because of the doctors, because of the teams ... Especially since time doesn't wait for anybody, it flies on its own. And so like you can maybe be eight o'clock one minute and you look at the clock, it's, you know, time for lunch. So you definitely want to try and get those things on paper especially when they're fresh in your mind. But also, there are a lot of teams that are looking for that information specifically on that nurse's flowsheet. And so if you don't get it on there, it's probably more work for you because everybody comes and asks you those things specifically.

Her reference to doctors, teams, and medical rounds is important for understanding the link between nursing documentation and managerial concern for the smooth processing of patients. It is helpful to think about the world of hospital work as a dynamic social system. The connections or links between people are set in a wider field of action. Central to this experience is global awareness of the need to reduce hospital length of stay while increasing the volume of patients treated. For those who work in the ICU, this includes limiting the time patients spend on mechanical ventilators, which requires decision making on medical rounds about weaning from technologic devices. From a nursing perspective, incomplete documentary information could impede such decisions and frustrate managerial expectations to quickly move patients in and through the ICU.

Historically, the inscription work of nurses has safeguarded patients, as it facilitates medical interpretation, diagnosis, and treatment. For example, the documentation of vital signs and laboratory results on special forms can function to identify the onset of threatening problems and prompt early treatment (Jefferies, Johnson, and Griffiths 2010). This is especially important in the ICU where patients are often considered "unstable," meaning their breathing, heart function, and consciousness change unexpectedly. In their understanding of how physicians are trained to read and respond to textual displays, nurses have demonstrated that they cannot significantly deviate from their ongoing documentary work, as it would render the patient vulnerable. ICU nurses have clarified how the dominant managerial perspective pervading health care has contributed to a different reading of their work. Superseding attention to the patient body, all nursing activities are now fused on a concern about the continuous generation of data to support the timely processing of patients.

Diamond (2006) argues that much of what occurs at the point-of-care remains unspoken and therefore invisible. The following observational field note brings to the fore an important contradiction when considering how data collection can dematerialize oral care:

> As I was observing a nursing student struggle to access an ICU patient's mouth with cleaning instruments, the curtains surrounding the bedside parted and the clinical care leader (CCL) entered. As one of the most experienced nurses on the unit, the CCL conveyed a sense of authority. Like dozens of other CCLs across the hospital's units, she is responsible for "patient flow" data collection over a twelve-hour period. This means she has only a short time to collect and organize a diverse range of patient information on this unit for distribution through scheduled in-person meetings, phone calls, and computerized surveillance systems. Knowing the disposition of each patient is part of her assignment. In lay terms, this requires knowledge of who is waiting to be admitted and who is ready to be discharged. The large white form on her clipboard suggests that this work is structured. The student suspended her oral care efforts to give her full attention to the CCL. They exchanged information regarding the invasive technologies in use. This resulted in a number of items being inscribed on the white form. Then as quickly as she had arrived, the CCL and her clipboard departed without enquiring about the student's need for oral care support.

This field note provides a clear instance of the broadly systematic organization of nursing agency away from fundamental patient care to administrative ends. In following the CCL, I was able to examine the form she was completing in detail. A close reading disclosed the requirement that the form be executed by a nurse. Interestingly, its contents audit medical treatments and problems (e.g., infection) rather than nursing care. Over time, I discovered hundreds of nurses enrolled in similar textual work across hospital units. In mapping the trajectory of information on this and other forms, I was led to a complex nexus of institutional activity involving multimillion-dollar computer networks, bed-flow specialists, data analysts, and managers. I learned how nurses are now enrolled in a burgeoning network accountable to the generation of numeric performance indicators reviewed by hospital and government stakeholders.

ICU nurses who provide patient care are now said to spend between 20 and 35 per cent of their time in documentation (Douglas et al. 2013). Presumably, nurses who are recruited into managerial roles, such as the CCL, spend even more time in the collection and distribution of numeric information. The average hospital now collects and reviews between one hundred and several hundred quality indicators and benchmarks; one study reports that an urban trauma hospital tracks more than eighteen hundred indicators (Disch and Sinioris 2012). The flourishing work of hospital performance management is conditioned by a growing desire to detect system problems as they unfold (French and Mykhalovskiy 2013). The prevailing logic holds that ongoing surveillance is necessary to ensure a circuit of continuous feedback and targeted performance improvement.

Some analysts suggest that this evolution of nursing away from bodily care to managerial roles is to be expected. In this case, the growing nursing assignment to organizational tasks is simply an inevitable change in an evolving clinical world (Allen 2015). In this line of thinking, bodily care would be reassigned to a lower grade of worker. However, nurses have not been replaced in the hospital setting. In direct contradiction of the notion of a smooth evolution, nurses are actually expected to do more with the same or fewer resources. The emergence of managerial surveillance is a potent example of social expectations to reduce the incidence of problems (e.g., infection) that may contribute to inefficiencies in the flow of patients. A burgeoning array of guidelines for the prevention of infection requires nurses to perform interventions such as oral care at intensifying intervals. Increasing pressure to simultaneously collect data for surveillance purposes is in tension with the demands of nursing time spent in preventive care.

The downloading of managerial data collection to the unit level invariably draws senior nurses, such as CCLs, away from a leadership role in bedside hygiene and further into the intricacies of statistical reports. As a type of reverse reading of the care encounter, managerial surveillance reports do not bring forward the people, work, and problems behind oral care. In the sections that follow, I further explore the challenge of oral care and the problematic invisibility cloaking this work.

Invisible Work

Critics of managerialism contend that it obscures on-the-ground realities (Mykhalovskiy et al. 2008). Smith (2005) explains that the flat, factual rendering of managerial metrics functions to suppress our awareness of people, activity, and context. Importantly, numeric data can contribute to an inversion of visibility in patient care. For example, nurses are routinely in contact with sputum, saliva, emesis, blood, and many foul odours in the conduct of oral care. Some of this material is dangerous. However, the nature of this work and the conditions under which it plays out are not brought to public attention. By removing excess detail, managerial data is capable of erasing our awareness of this activity and what we might know about it.

As a counterpoint to a discourse of "basic" nursing care, I have discovered that ICU nurses confront serious complexity in the delivery of oral care. First, mouths crowded with tubes are difficult to access with sponge swabs, tooth brushes, and suction devices. Second, orally placed devices such as breathing and feeding tubes are very uncomfortable for patients. Oral tubes in particular require patients to maintain an open mouth, which rapidly dries the mucosa and may lead to painful inflammation, oral lesions, and infection (Dale et al. 2013). In recent observations, I discovered that some ICU patients have up to four orally placed devices (Figure 2.1). Importantly, critically ill patients are not passive recipients of oral care. Common patient reactions include gagging, mouth closing, biting, and attempting to pull out oral devices. These highly reactive behaviours indicate pain and the need for increased nursing time spent in the prevention of oral health deterioration.

As an underestimated dimension of nursing, the labour involved in oral care is given at best passing mention in hospital communication. Wiltshire and Parker, in contrast, illuminate both the necessity and challenge of understanding the physical and social complexity of this work:

> Nurses work with people who have fragile boundaries – people whose skin breaks down; people for whom eating, drinking, breathing, voiding or defecating are rendered problematic; people who are in pain or cannot sleep. When such basic bodily functions become questionable, nursing is required. "To nurse" and "nurse" are relational not definitive or exclusionary concepts ... The broken-down boundaries of the sick body are stanched, augmented and supplemented, by the enabling body of the nurse. Such dealings with the dysfunctional, broken down or transgressed body in turn afflict the nurse, and draw from her/his bodily capacities. (1996, 23)

Implicit in this description is a particular knowledge of the ill body as skilled boundary work. Nursing undoubtedly transgresses the norms of bodily concealment, particularly in terms of touch, smell, or sight. The ill body requires proximity to strangers, intrusive examinations, and assistance with the control of bodily effluvia. Managing the patient's embarrassment at losing control over his or her body is one challenge. The other is managing an innate sense of disgust as well as the fear of contagion attendant on bodily fluids. Not surprisingly, nursing is often synonymous with dirty work, as nurses must negotiate "matter out of place" (Douglas 1966, 50).

The abject nature of bodily hygiene in illness has been the subject of ongoing debates, which invariably touch upon its low visibility; people are reluctant to observe it. I would add that the turn to managerialism simply compounds an invisibility problem. Vested in nursing curriculum, hospital policy, and professional regulations, the concealment of ill bodies is an expectation of nursing. Motivated by an ethos of privacy

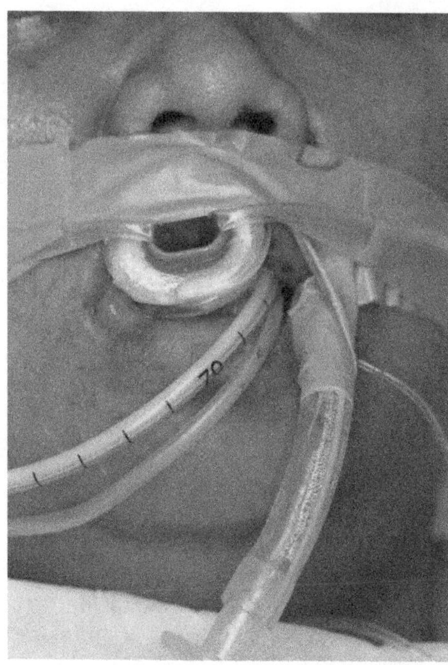

Figure 2.1. This photograph of an ICU patient provides evidence of multiple indwelling oral devices of life support. Oral crowding complicates visual and instrumental nursing access for delivery of preventative oral care and demands greater nursing time.

and ethics, both the patient and onlookers must have their sensibilities considered. Propriety problematically contributes to the obscuring of a complex nursing enterprise in the form of washing, moisturizing, suctioning, catheterizing, disimpacting, delousing, decontaminating, and dressing patients. The rules governing the collection and reporting of managerial performance data further remove this key activity from view in the abstract rendering of care.

Virginia Henderson (1964), an influential nurse theorist and researcher, notes that "there are few more complex arts than keeping a patient well-nourished and his mouth healthy during a long comatose period" (66). The social and material complexity of oral care was well exemplified during my fieldwork visit with an ICU patient with unfortunate changes to her oral health. I spoke at length with one of her assigned nurses, who relayed a sequence of events that were personally "traumatizing." The patient in question had a serious brain injury resulting in coma and an abnormal bite reflex. As is sometimes seen in neurological injury, the patient had bitten her own tongue. However, in this case she had amputated its tip and bisected it lengthwise. The nurse struggled to open her mouth, contain the bleeding, and protect her from further oral trauma (Figure 2.2). The nurse's efforts were further hampered by the perceived indifference of her physician colleagues, who viewed the

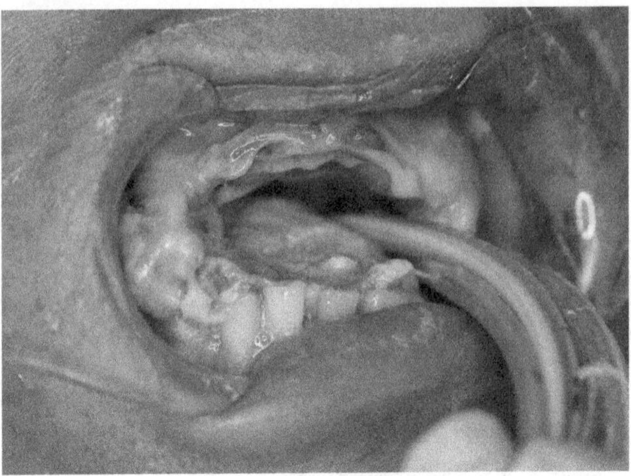

Figure 2.2. This photograph demonstrates oral injury that may arise from indwelling oral devices, insertion of hygienic instruments, and self-inflicted lip or tongue biting. Oral injury may contribute to inflammatory pain, infection, tooth loss, and dental disease. Such issues can require extensive nursing consultation with medical and dental professionals.

issue as of low priority in their list of duties, which formally prioritized the admission and discharge of patients.

While this case may seem extraordinary, similar events have been witnessed by all of the experienced ICU nurses with whom I spoke over several years. They report difficulty getting help to address the overall deterioration in patient oral health during hospitalization. ICU patients, like most hospitalized adults, are typically over the age of sixty-five and experience the highest burden of oral disease in the population (Canadian Academy of Health Sciences 2014). The oral health of older adults is often compromised at entry to the hospital because they lack employment-related dental insurance, which places costly preventative and restorative dental services out of reach. The failure to integrate dental professionals into hospitals and other public health institutions further reduces patients' access to oral care. This long-standing inequity is a growing nursing concern, as considerable scientific knowledge now demonstrates that poor oral hygiene can advance to life-threating conditions during hospitalization (Azarpazhooh and Leake 2006).

Nettleton (1991) notes how women have historically been made accountable for maintaining oral health and preventing costly disease in the domestic sphere. The nursing profession, which remains primarily composed of women, is similarly accountable in the hospital context. Oral care guidelines, doctors' orders, and nursing documentation routinely identify oral care as a nursing accountability. A recent report by the Canadian Academy of Health Sciences (2014) suggests that nurses are well positioned to address inequitable access to dental health services in Canadian hospitals. Despite its good intentions, this recommendation invites nurses to intervene without due consideration of the ongoing dematerialization of nursing work and the problem of missed nursing care explored in the following section.

Missed Nursing Care

Missed or insufficient body care has recently emerged as a new and a pressing international crisis and a key indicator that fundamental nursing care is in serious trouble. The reality of hospital nurses being too busy to carry out oral and bodily hygiene pervades the discussion and has generated considerable hand-wringing among people who advocate for better use of evidence to improve health services. Recent analyses demonstrate how nurses working in time-pressured care settings are frequently forced to make very difficult choices about what care they can realistically accomplish, delay, or not deliver at all. Care omission takes on added importance because increasing patient acuity warrants more time-intensive and skilled nursing.

The problem of omissions in nursing care identifies a growing dissonance between the promise of managerial reform and the harms emerging during hospitalization. For example, individuals now frequently emerge from hospital with a new diagnostic entity called "post-hospital syndrome" – a set of new health problems that may interfere with their recovery and lead to long-term disability (Krumholz 2013, 100). Recently discharged patients have a heightened risk of new ailments, which appear to have little in common with the original admitting diagnosis. Readmission conditions include, but are not limited to, pneumonia, infection, gastrointestinal conditions, cognitive impairment, and metabolic derangements. Kalisch (2015, 84) has linked this phenomenon to missed nursing care, otherwise defined as the "required and standard nursing care that is not being completed."

In speaking with patients who have experienced hospitalization, I am often confronted by the spectre of missed oral care. I recently interviewed a man who sustained a spinal cord injury that resulted in quadriplegia. The inability to move his arms and legs left him in a state of terrified dependency. Throughout his hospital encounter, he experienced how nurses were frequently unable to attend to his mouth, which was persistently dry, unclean, and painful. He developed xerostomia (a severely dry mouth), throat pain, and weeping lesions at the corners of his lips. Subsequent to his discharge home, he spent thousands of dollars on dental restoration, including extraction of several teeth, a root canal, filling of multiple cavities, and the fitting of partial dentures. Because he is no longer employed, he lacks dental insurance to cover these private services. In his case, emotional, physical, and financial costs are the less evident burdens devolving from missed nursing care. As oral health problems are relegated to the world of private dental practice, the true scope of post-hospital syndrome evades public awareness.

In my investigations, I have also discovered family members performing oral hygiene and incurring costs to hire private caregivers to complete this essential work. For example, I recently spoke with a woman who discovered her husband had lost eight teeth during a prolonged admission to Kingston General Hospital. In response to the inability of hospital nurses to deliver oral care, she hired a private dental hygienist to intervene (Pearce 2018). Some family members, however, are not able to afford paid caregivers. For example, the wife of the man experiencing quadriplegia instead chose to remain in hospital at night when she observed hurried nurses being unable to care for her husband's oral health needs. "That's why I've learned how to do [mouth care]," she said. The social reassignment of oral care to family members reinforces arguments that managerial reform is quietly redefining fundamental nursing in hospital as a private responsibility (Armstrong 2001).

Discussion

From the story of Michael Neve to my encounters with ICU patients and family caregivers, it is clear that nursing work is in trouble. Hospitals are now stressful and overloaded environments where nurses have insufficient time and support for fundamental patient care. The oral health of seriously ill patients definitively worsens during hospitalization. However, the manner in which managerial interests are implicated in this problem has received insufficient attention. In surveying historical concerns in oral care, Exley (2009, 1097) writes that "inequalities in oral health and health care [highlight] how, as with medicine, those with the greatest need for preventative dental services were – and continue to be – less likely to access services." Providing the oral and bodily care vulnerable patients need now appears to be subverted by the informational needs of management. My research confirms we are leaving the sick behind.

Concerns over poor oral care have definitively opened the nursing profession to public and political scrutiny. Some argue the professionalization of nursing through baccalaureate entry to practice has led to an overqualified and undertrained cohort of nurses who are "too posh to wash." This line of argument contends that when care falls short of expectations, nurses shoulder much of the responsibility (Scott 2004). While some individuals can be criticized for providing poor care, the main antecedents are to be found beyond individual nurses and their patients. Nurses in Canada are primarily employed in hospitals as front-line caregivers and are therefore subject to managerial dictates (Canadian Institute for Health Information 2017). In the absence of positions consolidating hygienic expertise (e.g., oral hygiene nurse specialist), hospital nurses must turn to managerial roles for professional and financial advancement. Such limitations may perpetuate stigmatizing divisions of labour, sometimes conceptualized as the difference between gross physical needs of the patient ("dirty work") and cleaner tasks that involve less touching of other people's bodies ("informational work"). These circumstances may further dematerialize fundamental nursing care by encouraging experienced nurses to leave patient care.

Central to my argument in this chapter is a limitation in managerial "ways-of-seeing" that leave bodies, the context of care, and unmet oral health needs of patients out of focus (Murray, Holmes, and Rail 2008, 275). With this point in mind, managerial reform is not living up to its claim of offering greater transparency, safety, and efficiency. In her book *Notes on Nursing*, Nightingale (1860, 8) wrote that "the very elements of nursing are all but unknown." My analysis demonstrates this still to be true. Health reform dependent on work that is poorly understood will definitively run into difficulty. Clinical nursing work, as with any kind of work, has a tendency to disappear at a distance. DeVault and McCoy (2004) note that to examine work in a proximal fashion offers the possibility of seeing and thinking differently.

Characterized by increasing complexities, conflicts, and contradictions, hospital-based nursing is in a vulnerable state. In practice, the managerial drive to improve access and reduce costs has resulted in increased bureaucratic surveillance and centralized managerial powers. Mykhalovskiy et al. (2008) describe how this power is interwoven with the collection and reporting of numeric data. However, such data do not uniformly divulge the care omissions emerging at the patient-provider interface. I concur with Kitson's (2010) assertion that nurses are at risk of losing control of their practice. The rise of statistical data, as a higher form of expertise, can be credited with diminished attention to the sick patient. Persistent misconceptions regarding the nature of body work have undermined nurses' abilities to convey their concerns and generate value for fundamental care.

Having accompanied nurses and patients in my investigations, I have discovered the many benefits of observation as evidence. Benner (1994) suggests that the act of care places the nurse in proximity to the patient such that certain needs show up as relevant. In this case, bodily care should not be appraised at a distance; its constitutive parts include the dynamic interplay of the material, social, and political context. The use of the senses in observing the sick is necessary to appreciate the bodily changes occurring in illness. Unfortunately, an ethos of patient privacy conceals the nature of ill bodies and the demands they place on caregivers. The requirement to collect and report managerial data adds an additional layer of nursing work and abstraction that is important to interrogate. Finally, a discourse of "basic" hygiene underestimates the complexity of this assignment. Highlighting the role of observation as evidence seems particularly relevant for those interested in placing the body back into the centre of health reform.

In this chapter I have argued that fundamental patient care is neither more efficient nor safer in today's reformed environment. The problem of patient care is a consequence of a managerial perspective that obscures it. In many ways, hospital nurses have been recast as purveyors of managerial outcomes. Usurping the patient body is a new focus on the body of the health system. The resultant invisibility of illness work, and the troubling conditions in which it is executed, have resulted in missed nursing care and the requirement for families to take up the slack. The dematerialization of this essential care signals an imprudent dismantling of hospital services that is hidden in the numbers. In this case inequities, rather than improvements, have devolved from health reform. With this point in mind, there are compelling reasons to find alternative ways of knowing and intervening in the problems unfolding in health care delivery.

REFERENCES

Aiken, L.H. 2008. "Economics of Nursing." *Policy, Politics, & Nursing Practice* 9 (2): 73–9. https://doi.org/10.1177/1527154408318253

Allen, D. 2015. *The Invisible Work of Nurses: Hospitals, Organisation and Healthcare.* Abingdon: Routledge.

Armstrong, P. 2001. *Exposing Privatization: Women and Health Care Reform in Canada.* Aurora: Garamond.

Ausserhofer, D., B. Zander, R. Busse, M. Schubert, S. De Geest, A.M. Rafferty, J. Ball, et al. 2014. "Prevalence, Patterns and Predictors of Nursing Care Left

Undone in European Hospitals: Results from the Multicountry Cross-Sectional RN4CAST Study." *BMJ Quality & Safety* 23 (2): 126–35. https://doi.org/10.1136/bmjqs-2013-002318.

Azarpazhooh, A., and J.L. Leake. 2006. "Systematic Review of the Association between Respiratory Diseases and Oral Health." *Journal of Periodontology* 77 (9): 1465–82. https://doi.org/10.1902/jop.2006.060010.

Benner, P. 1994. "The Role of Articulation in Understanding Practice and Experience as Sources of Knowledge." In *Philosophy in a Time of Pluralism: Perspectives on the Philosophy of Charles Taylor*, edited by J. Tully and D.M. Weinstock, 136–56. Cambridge: Cambridge University Press.

Bourgeault, I.L., P. Armstrong, H. Armstrong, J. Choiniere, J. Lexchin, E. Mykhalovskiy, S. Peters, and J. White. 2001. "Everyday Experiences of Implicit Rationing: Comparing the Voices of Nurses in California and British Columbia." *Sociology of Health and Illness* 23 (5): 633–53.

Campbell, M.L., and J.M. Rankin. 2017. "Nurses and Electronic Health Records in a Canadian Hospital: Examining the Social Organisation and Programmed Use of Digitised Nursing Knowledge." *Sociology of Health & Illness* 39 (3): 365–79. https://doi.org/10.1111/1467-9566.12489.

Canadian Academy of Health Sciences. 2014. *Improving Access to Oral Health Care for Vulnerable People Living in Canada.* Ottawa: Canadian Academy of Health Sciences.

Canadian Institute for Health Information. 2018. "Regulated Nurses, 2017: Canada and Jurisdictional Highlights." Ottawa: CIHI. https://www.cihi.ca/sites/default/files/document/regulated-nurses-2017-pt-highlights-en-web.pdf.

Casper, M.J., and L.J. Moore. 2009. *Missing Bodies: The Politics of Visibility.* New York: New York University Press.

Choiniere, J.A. 2011. "Accounting for Care: Exploring Tensions and Contradictions." *Advances in Nursing Science* 34 (4): 330–44. https://doi.org/10.1097/ANS.0b013e3182356c31.

Dale, C., J.E. Angus, T. Sinuff, and E. Mykhalovskiy. 2013. "Mouth Care for Orally Intubated Patients: A Critical Ethnographic Review of the Nursing Literature." *Intensive & Critical Care Nursing* 29 (5): 266–74. https://doi.org/10.1016/j.iccn.2012.09.003.

DeVault, M.L., and L. McCoy. 2004. "Institutional Ethnography: Using Interviews to Investigate Ruling Relations." In *Handbook of Interview Research: Context & Method*, edited by J.F. Gubrium and J.A. Holstein, 751–76. Thousand Oaks: Sage.

Diamond, T. 2006. "'Where Did You Get the Fur Coat, Fern?' Participant Observation in Institutional Ethnography." In *Institutional Ethnography as Practice*, edited by D. Smith, 45–63. Oxford: Rowman & Littlefield.

Diamond, T. 1992. *Making Gray Gold: Narratives of Nursing Home Care.* Chicago: University of Chicago Press.

Disch, J., and M. Sinioris. 2012. "The Quality Burden." *Nursing Clinics of North America* 47 (3): 395–405. https://doi.org/10.1016/j.cnur.2012.05.010.

Douglas, M. 1966. *Purity and Danger*, vol. 2: *An Analysis of Concepts of Pollution and Taboo.* London: Routledge & Kegan Paul.

Douglas, S., R. Cartmill, R. Brown, P. Hoonakker, J. Slagle, K. Schultz Van Roy, J.M. Walker, M. Weinger, T. Wetterneck, and P. Carayon. 2013. "The Work of Adult and Pediatric Intensive Care Unit Nurses." *Nursing Research* 62 (1): 50–8. https://doi.org/10.1097/NNR.0b013e318270714b.

Exley, C. 2009. "Bridging a Gap: The (Lack of a) Sociology of Oral Health and Healthcare." *Sociology of Health & Illness* 31 (7): 1093–108. https://doi.org/10.1111/j.1467-9566.2009.01173.x.

French, M., and E. Mykhalovskiy. 2013. "Public Health Intelligence and the Detection of Potential Pandemics." *Sociology of Health & Illness* 35 (2): 174–87. https://doi.org/10.1111/j.1467-9566.2012.01536.x

Henderson, V. 1964. "The Nature of Nursing." *American Journal of Nursing* 64 (8): 62–8. https://doi.org/10.1097/00000446-196408000-00029.

Holmes, D., S.J. Murray, A. Perron, and J. McCabe. 2008. "Nursing Best Practice Guidelines: Reflecting on the Obscene Rise of the Void." *Journal of Nursing Management* 16 (4): 394–403. https://doi.org/10.1111/j.1365-2834.2008.00858.x.

Ireton, J. February 16 2016. "Man's Teeth Left to Rot While He Was in Hospital's Care." CBC. http://www.cbc.ca/news/canada/ottawa/ottawa-man-with-autism-loses-teeth-after-left-to-rot-1.3442864.

Jefferies, D., M. Johnson, and R. Griffiths. 2010. "A Meta-study of the Essentials of Quality Nursing Documentation." *International Journal of Nursing Practice* 16 (2): 112–24. https://doi.org/10.1111/j.1440-172X.2009.01815.x.

Kalisch, B. 2015. "The Post-Hospitalization Syndrome: Can Nursing Make the Difference?" *Nurse Leader* 13 (1): 84–91. https://doi.org/10.1016/j.mnl.2014.10.006.

Kitson, A. 2010. "Reclaiming Nursing Care." *Collegian* 17 (1): 1–2. https://doi.org/10.1016/j.colegn.2010.02.001.

Krichbaum, K., C. Diemert, L. Jacox, A. Jones, P. Koenig, C. Mueller, and J. Disch. 2007. "Complexity Compression: Nurses under Fire." *Nursing Forum* 42 (2): 86–94. https://doi.org/10.1111/j.1744-6198.2007.00071.x.

Krumholz, H.M. 2013. "Post-Hospital Syndrome – An Acquired, Transient Condition of Generalized Risk." *New England Journal of Medicine* 368 (2): 100–2. https://doi.org/10.1056/NEJMp1212324.

Liaschenko, J., and E. Peter. 2004. "Nursing Ethics and Conceptualizations of Nursing: Profession, Practice and Work." *Journal of Advanced Nursing* 46 (5): 488–95. https://doi.org/10.1111/j.1365-2648.2004.03011.x.

McCoy, L. 2008. "Institutional Ethnography and Constructionism." In *Handbook of Constructionist Research.*, edited by J.A. Holstein and J.F. Gubrium, 701–14. New York: Guilford.

Murray, S., D. Holmes, and G. Rail. 2008. "On the Constitution and Status of 'Evidence' in the Health Sciences." *Journal of Research in Nursing* 13 (4): 272–80. https://doi.org/10.1177/1744987108093529.

Mykhalovskiy, E., P. Armstrong, H. Armstrong, I. Bourgeault, J. Choiniere, J. Lexchin, S. Peters, and J. White. 2008. "Qualitative Research and the Politics of Knowledge in an Age of Evidence: Developing a Research-Based Practice of Immanent Critique." *Social Science & Medicine* 67 (1): 195–203. https://doi.org/10.1016/j.socscimed.2008.03.002.

Nettleton, S. 1991. "Wisdom, Diligence and Teeth: Discursive Practice and the Creation of Mothers." *Sociology of Health & Illness* 13 (1): 98–111. https://doi.org/10.1111/1467-9566.ep11340329.

Nightingale, F. 1860. *Notes on Nursing: What It Is, and What It Is Not.* Edited by J.M. Bridges. London: Harrison.

Pearce, N. 2018. "Nothing to Smile About." 4 August. https://www.thewhig.com/news/local-news/nothing-to-smile-about.

Scott, H. 2004. "Are Nurses 'Too Clever to Care' and 'Too Posh to Wash'?" *British Journal of Nursing* 13 (10): 581. https://doi.org/10.12968/bjon.2004.13.10.13040.

Smith, D. 2005. *Institutional Ethnography: A Sociology for People.* Toronto: AltaMira.

Timmermans, S., and M. Berg. 1997. "Standardization in Action: Achieving Local Universality through Medical Protocols." *Social Studies of Science* 27 (2): 273–305. https://doi.org/10.1177/030631297027002003.

Twigg, J., C. Wolkowitz, R.L. Cohen, and S. Nettleton. 2011. "Conceptualising Body Work in Health and Social Care." *Sociology of Health & Illness* 33 (2): 171–88. https://doi.org/10.1111/j.1467-9566.2010.01323.x.

Wiltshire, J., and J. Parker. 1996. "Containing Abjection in Nursing: The End of Shift Handover as a Site of Containment." *Nursing Inquiry* 3 (1): 23–9. https://doi.org/10.1111/j.1440-1800.1996.tb00005.x.

3 From "Making a Decision" to "Decision Making": A Critical Reflection on a Discursive Shift

MARY ELLEN MACDONALD AND DAVID KENNETH WRIGHT

Over the last few decades, decision making has become a prominent construct across health care research and practice. Clinicians, researchers, and administrators in fields ranging from bioethics to clinical communication to palliative care are concerned with decision-support tools, patient decision aids, and shared decision making. Beginning in the 1980s, entire journals have been dedicated to the theory and practice of decision making in health care (e.g., the Sage journal *Medical Decision Making* started in 1981, *BMC Medical Informatics and Decision Making* in 2001). Professional decision-making associations also began around that time (e.g., the Society for Medical Decision Making held its inaugural meeting in Cincinnati in 1979 and has since grown into an international organization). A perusal of North American funding databases (e.g., the Canadian Institutes of Health Research, National Institutes of Health in the United States) shows how clinical researchers have mobilized the decision-making construct in many areas of health research.

Certain domains of clinical practice are especially enamoured of decision making. Decision support tools, such as decision aids (Stacey et al. 2014) and shared decision-making protocols (Charles, Gafni, and Whelan 1997; Kon 2010) for patients, and computer-based clinical decision support systems for clinicians (Blum et al. 2015) are being used to help clinicians, patients, and families assess the risks and benefits of screening and treatment choices in a variety of domains. Examples of implicated clinical areas include general practice (Peiris et al. 2009), intensive care (Kryworuchko et al. 2013), oncology (Lin et al. 2009; Stacey, Samant, and Bennett 2008), orthopaedics (Arterburn et al. 2012), and palliative care (Werth and Blevins 2009).

Prior to the 1950s, however, this focus on the decision – and particularly the term "decision making" – was uncommon in health care contexts. While clinicians, patients, and families have always "made decisions," the compound noun "decision making" is a relatively recent addition to the health care lexicon. The term seems to have entered the clinical arena via hospital administration starting in the 1950s. Since then, the plethora of decision-making technologies has been compelled by two epistemologically distinct – and at times clashing – social phenomena (May et al. 2006). On one hand, the consumerist "patient autonomy" movement has shifted care models away from a paternalistic physician-driven model to a patient-centred paradigm in which illness narratives and patient choice are celebrated as important drivers of the clinical encounter (May and Mead 1999; Wolpe 1998). On the other hand, the scientistic evidence-based medicine movement has created an imperative explicitly to ground clinical practices in research evidence derived from large populations of experimental subjects (e.g., randomized controlled trials) (Greenhalgh, Howick, and Maskrey 2014). These movements have evolved within an increasingly neoliberal arena focused on economic rationalization in medical practice and hospital administration. Within this context, decision making has come to have importance as a medico-administrative technology with utility in many health care domains.

Following the tradition of social studies scholars – such as the authors in this collection – concerned with how health care norms are produced, routinized, and institutionalized, important empirical work and critical reflection are challenging the normative development and role of decision-making protocols and agendas in clinical and research practice (Berg 1997; Boivin, Légaré, and Lehoux 2008; Drought and Koenig 2002; Glasdam, Oeye, and Thrysoee 2015; Jennings 2006; Molewijk et al. 2003; Mykhalovskiy 2008; Peiris et al. 2011). Our chapter adds to this literature by looking specifically at the discursive shift that enabled "making a decision" to become "decision making." To do so, we look first at the linguistic and discursive transformations: we follow the transformation in biomedical ethics where decision making has become a clinical technology in support of an individualistic, rationalized practice, and then we look at the level of hospital administration where it acts as a managerial technology in the service of an efficient neoliberalism that works to manage subjectivity and heterogeneity. In both locations, decision making is implicated in a movement away from the experiential process of illness as embedded in a frame of relational care and towards a rationalizing medico-administrative imperative compelled by neoliberal governance and efficiency. We specifically query how these social movements compelled this shift to decision making and examine the practices and values that are effaced and replaced as a result of the ubiquity of this technology.

We then test these theoretical arguments with an empirical ethnographic study of end-of-life care in a free-standing hospice. In the hospice, we drill down into local practices where we find decision making being used as a rationalizing practice in the service of a health care ideology; however, the discursive tenor we found is unique to the hospice setting. The prevailing ideological ethos in the hospice partially disrupts the individualized autonomy model of biomedical ethics given how families are also implicated in care; further, this ethos also disrupts neoliberalism with an attentive, humanistic focus on dying. Yet in the hospice, decision-making technologies still serve to channel the management of patient and family behaviour and experiences of dying into a normative model that reproduces the "good death" ideology at the core of palliative care. We then conclude the chapter with a reflection on the fundamental challenges "decision making" brings to models of care.

A Linguistic Shift: Making a Decision Becomes "Decision Making"

While our interest in this transformation is motivated by more than curiosity about how language changes over time, we will begin with a grammar lesson. In the form "making a decision," a verb ("making") precedes a noun ("decision"). In the form "decision making," a gerund phrase has been created. A gerund is a form of a verb ("to make"), and therefore expresses action or a state of being. Yet the gerund functions as a noun and occupies the position in a sentence that a noun would (e.g., "it is important to involve all family members in the decision making before purchasing a new house"). When used to modify a noun, as in "decision-making process," the gerund phrase ("decision making") becomes an adjective, here modifying "process" (when it precedes a noun, the gerund should be hyphenated). In contrast, in the form "decision maker," the entire grammatical form shifts to become a noun.

According to the *Oxford English Dictionary*, both "decision maker" and "decision making" appeared at the turn of the twentieth century, showing up in sporting references. As the dictionary entries indicate, the utility of this term then shifted to include political and managerial administration.

decision maker, *n.*
1902 Lowell (Mass.) Sun 11 June 7/1 Umpire Rudderham was the officiating decision maker.
1938 S. CHASE Tyranny of Words xviii. 233 Mr. Baldwin was long the chief decision-maker for the British Empire.

decision-making, *n.* and *adj.*
1918 Newark (Ohio) Daily Advocate 21 May 3/3 Right now is the proper time for decision-making on the question of attending the auto race meet.

1919 S. PETERSON Democracy & Govt. II. iii. 179 This legislative – that is, this policy-adopting or decision-making – power of the President.

Perusing the WorldCat database (the world's largest network of library-based content), we found this trend continuing. In 1940, a publication appeared titled *Christian Conscience and Military Service: A Guide to Decision-Making from a Lutheran Perspective* (Walther League 1940). A few years later, in 1944, Herbert Simon completed his dissertation on decision making and administrative organization (Simon 1944). Simon's subsequent publications on the topic entrenched this construct in the realm of managerial organization (e.g., *Administrative Behavior: A Study of Decision-Making Processes in Administrative Organization*, first published in 1947 and still being published today; see, for example, Simon 2013). Up to the 1950s, publications with "decision making" in the title were rooted in disciplines such as public administration (McCamy 1947), management (Tannenbaum 1950), legislation (Black 1948), and political economy (Goodman 1950).

Specifically in the domain of health, the term "decision making" appears in the mid-fifties. Starting in 1944, papers began appearing in the psychology literature; however, they were mostly focused on group processes (Horwitz 1953) and decision theory (Edwards 1954) and did not yet focus on health issues. "Decision making" appears in the health and hospital literature in 1953, and through the decade maintained a consistent focus on domains such as community organization (Miller 1953), public administration (Bates 1959), bureaucracy (Lefton, Dinitz, and Pasamanick 1959), and authority (Coser 1958). In perhaps a culmination of this emergent trend, in 1960 James Hamilton published *Decision Making in Hospital Administration and Medical Care: A Casebook.*

Tracking references in Medline from that time, we see a steady increase in the presence of the term "decision making" in article titles (see Table 3.1).

Table 3.1. Medline articles with "decision making" in title

Publication date	Number of articles	Total number of articles in Medline	Relative number of articles	Number of DM articles per 100,000 articles
1950–9	10	781,641	0.000013	1.3
1960–9	107	1,511,815	0.000071	7.1
1970–9	470	2,399,113	0.000196	19.6
1980–9	1,223	3,182,707	0.000384	38.4
1990–9	2,479	4,148,032	0.000598	59.8
2000–9	4,504	5,271,040	0.000854	85.4

Modernity, Scientism, and the Rise of Patient Autonomy

This linguistic overview suggests that "making a decision" was codified into "decision making" in the realm of administration and organization, and crossed over into health care via hospital administration. While this descriptive rendering is interesting, understanding what it means requires an in-depth discursive analysis.

To begin, we can contextualize this transformation historically within modernity, an era that saw a celebration of extreme individualism and instrumental reason. In the modern context, the self-determining individual became an entity unto themselves, seeking and achieving the "good life" through a series of rational calculations (Taylor 1989). Specifically in health care, the development of this modern rational subject compelled two important movements: the patient autonomy movement, unseating medical paternalism as the overriding model of patient care, and evidence-based medicine, challenging and replacing experience-based clinical knowledge (May and Mead 1999; May et al. 2006).

Patient autonomy: The principle of patient autonomy first entered medicine via the Nuremberg Code in 1947 in response to the atrocities carried out in the name of science during the Second World War. Entrenched within the Nuremberg Code are the rights of research subjects to consent or refuse involvement in scientific experimentation (Agledahl, Førde, and Wifstad 2011). Following concerns about medical paternalism and the consumer movement contributed to the transformation of patients into health care "consumers"; in the United States, this was especially motivated by the civil rights movements of the 1960s. In parallel, a growing technological imperative in medicine and an expansion of subspecializations in clinical fields furthered the modern relationship between clinician and patient as grounded in patient autonomy (Agledahl, Førde, and Wifstad 2011; Drought and Koenig 2002). Woven through these sociopolitical processes was "the rise of bioethics as a disciplinary force in medicine" (Kaufman, Shim, and Russ 2006, S175). Patient autonomy became the pillar of modern biomedical ethics (Wolpe 1998).

Within this modern biomedical ethical framework, as codified by Beauchamp and Childress (2001), is a master narrative that constructs the individual as a moral agent who is a self-determining, rational problem solver (Carnevale 2007). Ethical dilemmas are seen as resolvable through rational models that weigh harms and benefits. Patient autonomy is primarily manifest via the principle of respect for autonomous patient choice with a focus on informed consent and decision making (Agledahl, Førde, and Wifstad 2011; Drought and Koeni 2002). With this commitment to the patient as a "moralized" entity developed the patient-centred care movement; however, as moral agents, patients have also become "bearers of responsibility for their actions and blame, fault and culpability for 'bad' consequences related to their decisions" (Carnevale 2007, 574).

Evidence-based medicine: Parallel was the rise of the scientistic "evidence-based medicine" movement starting in the 1960s. Following the growing popularity of statistics, there was a push for medical practice to become more scientifically grounded in the results of controlled, randomized, medical research (May et al. 2006). From this focus developed technologies such as point-of-care "decision support tools" (Berg 1997) and clinical practice guidelines (Boivin, Légaré, and Lehoux 2008); both were embraced by health system planners because of their potential to narrow "evidence-to-practice" gaps by bringing epidemiological and clinical trial evidence more explicitly into everyday practice. Medical practice sought to become less "art" and more science; that is, rational, standardized, and reliable (Berg 1997). Both statistics and artificial computer intelligence contributed to this idealized new medicine in which the clinician became logician and statistician (Berg 1997).

The Rhetoric of Choice

Thus, the impetus for decision making was simultaneously evolving in two parallel yet epistemologically distinct social movements. Evidence-based medicine supported the production of quantitative, generalizable scientific knowledge produced through aggregated data of large populations. Through this frame, the clinician's scientific knowledge held epistemological authority. In contrast, the patient-centred movement privileged the epistemological authority of the patient, located in subjective illness narratives and patient values expressed during the clinical encounter. In an attempt to bring these disparate forms of knowledge together, the "evidence-based patient choice" paradigm was born (Ford, Schofield, and Hope 2002). Within this new paradigm, patients' values were ostensibly to be respected from within a scientific evidence-based framework (Mykhalovskiy 2008). It thus became both the right and the responsibility of patients to direct their own care (Drought and Koenig 2002). Decision-making technologies became essential: within the "choice" paradigm, patients needed access to options from which they could make autonomous, informed decisions.

Choice, however, is never unbridled "free choice" (Drought and Koenig 2002). As Agledahl and colleagues (2011, 212) contend, "patients cannot generally choose any treatment they desire, and only have a formal right to refuse treatment. These are the conditions of the health care system in our society, and they are often underplayed in the autonomy debate. The right to choose presupposes a kind of open choice that is, in fact, rare in health care, and this makes 'patient choice' a misleading way of characterising clinical practice." Choice is necessarily constrained by numerous complexly related "sociomedical" elements (Kaufman, Shim, and Russ 2006). The options from which one can choose are greatly predetermined and circumscribed by elements such as market forces (e.g., insurance companies); the routinization that occurs when treatments become normalized as "standard of care" and embedded in clinical practice guidelines (e.g., heart valve stents); the cultures of care (e.g., the multiple specialists assigned to patients with comorbid conditions creating discrete choices and decisional moments); clinicians' opinions, experiences, and professional power; the legal system (e.g., in many jurisdictions one can choose how to die but not when); the technologies, resources, and social supports available in different care contexts; and the limits of biological processes (Agledahl, Førde, and Wifstad 2011; Allen et al. 2015; Borgstrom and Walter 2015; Kaufman, Shim, and Russ 2006; Wolpe 1998).

The concept of choice is then rendered more complex by a moral responsibility on the part of both clinician and patient to not just choose, but choose correctly. Kaufman and colleagues (2006, S175) write that in this era of "procedure-driven medical care," "the availability of more options at ever older ages and the normalization of life-extending, life-enhancing treatments at older ages promote the notion that aging and death are not inevitable and foster the assumption that one can, and should, choose to intervene." Thus, for example, it has become morally unjustified to not offer dialysis to all patients with end-stage renal disease. As a result, the dialysis population is growing older; yet this therapy has not changed considerably in its delivery or outcomes since its inception. The option to choose death over dialysis is rarely articulated, and institutional commitments to integrating palliative care into nephrology programs remain largely underdeveloped (Kaufman, Shim, and Russ 2006).

Yet careful ethnographic work peering into the "black box" of choice (Kaufman, Shim, and Russ 2006) suggests that while "choice" may be lauded, it rarely materializes as a robust social practice. Kaufman and colleagues demonstrate that while patients and providers support patient-directed decision making in theory, for practitioners and their elderly patients in the study, choice regarding life-extending therapies was organized, constrained, and mobilized such that standard-of-care treatment options continued to trump patient involvement in treatment decisions. More often than not, clinicians made the choices for patients;

they did not actually offer patients choices and instead proceeded with standard treatment (Kaufman, Shim, and Russ 2006).

During treatment discussions, the use of rhetoric and other persuasive tactics by treating clinicians in the negotiation further affects the choices patients actually make. Turns of phrase, emotion, and patient vulnerability combine to guide the patient towards the medical action preferred by the clinician (Dubov 2015; Kaufman, Shim, and Russ 2006). Given the already heavily biased context, some argue that persuasion can be more ethical than patient autonomy models that treat patients like rational decision-making experts (Dubov 2015). Patients and family are often unable to reason through complex risk calculations or realistically envision long-term goals in the face of medical uncertainty (Dubov 2015); further, medical knowledge is often incommensurate with lay understandings (Drought and Koenig 2002). When a physician is aware that decisions are being made in such compromised states with such complex data, Dubov argues that they have a moral duty to intervene and to use persuasion to sway the patient and family towards the best medical outcome (Dubov 2015).

When a decision is actually made by a patient, exactly what that decision means is up for debate. While theoretically, decision making is premised on a commitment to "rational, individualized conceptions of human action" (Mykhalovskiy 2008, 137–8), when patient preferences are stated they are rarely reliably and validly stable and indeed may seem quite "irrational" to the treating clinician (Dubov 2015). Choice and decision making are both highly dependent on timing and context (Lynn et al. 2000); this may be especially true at end of life (Gauthier and Swigart 2003; Lynn et al. 2000). Semantically framing potential outcomes in probability of survival versus probability of mortality – inversely related – has been shown to alter patient decisions to undergo surgery (Lynn et al. 2000; McNeil et al. 1982). Also, the background education and experience of patients and family affect how they interpret medical information (e.g., when risk is presented in numerical formats) (Keller and Siegrist 2009). Further, as Borgstrom and Walter discuss, patients "are not isolated individuals making rational choices in their own interest, but are social beings embedded in networks of relationships and often concerned for other family members as much as for themselves" (Borgstrom and Walter 2015, 100).

Finally, many of the possibilities that actually make it onto the "choice menu" for patients are then codified through decisional technologies, transformed into "decisional options," and result in expressions of what are labelled "patient preferences." May and colleagues locate these decisional technologies at the intersection of patient and clinician authority, where they interact with a third epistemological authority, what these authors call *technogovernance.* "Technogovernance" is a term meant to capture the transformative framing that occurs as these technologies intersect with systems of practice, a framing infused with power, knowledge, and subjectivity. Technogovernance serves to mediate authoritative tensions within the patient-clinician dyad; for example, shared decision making transforms patient subjective experience into "preferences," in the process both constraining and managing clinical heterogeneity and patient choice (May et al. 2006).

Decision Making: An Administrative Technology in the Service of Managerial Efficiency

Examining the sociomedical movements of patient autonomy and evidence-based medicine helps reveal the discursive shift from "making a decision" to "decision making." In this shift, we see the creation and reproduction of a new discursive object: the clinician-patient unit. By "clinician-patient unit" we refer to both the actual and symbolic relations in which the patient and health care provider(s) converge, mobilized by concern about the patient's health. This unit has become the key phenomenon for bioethics; thus, it also sits at the centre of decision making, taking on importance for a range of expert authorities. Through this discursive movement, decision making has become a clinical technology serving the biomedical ethical focus on the individualistic, rationalized clinical practice in which the clinician-patient dyad sits.

Now we add another key piece of this story, a piece hinted at above and to which we now return. The etymology of the gerund "decision making," as we have seen, harkens back first to military administration and then to health administration. In addition to being a technology of biomedical ethics to support an individualistic, rationalized clinical practice, decision making also acts as an administrative technology. That is, in the struggle of clashing values and epistemologies within a health care setting, decision making can also act as a medico-administrative function in the service of managerial efficiency and control. This argument was glimpsed above in the work of May and colleagues.

In our current neoliberal context, health care, like many social institutions, is being reorganized via market principles that value minimizing public cost, decentralizing government, and privatizing health and social services (Glasdam, Oeye, and Thrysoee 2015; Hamann 2009; McGregor 2001). Within this social ethos is a system that valorizes the neoliberal subject, that is, "an individual who is morally responsible for navigating the social realm using rational choices and cost-benefit calculations grounded on market-based principles to the exclusion of all other ethical values and social interests" (Hamann 2009, 37). Paramount to this subject is rationality and self-determination (Glasdam, Oeye, and Thrysoee 2015; McGregor 2001). In the context of health care, we see the heightened promotion of an individual's own responsibility for their health (Mykhalovskiy 2008): the ideal patient is a consumer (McGregor 2001) who is "responsible, strong, self-determined, controlled, and acknowledges and accepts the responsibility of playing an important part in handling his/her health care-related problems" (Glasdam, Oeye, and Thrysoee 2015, 227). This version assumes patients have "the choice, the capacity, and the obligation to exercise such choices and responsibilities" (Glasdam, Oeye, and Thrysoee 2015, 231). The sick person thus has become a customer who is in charge of choosing their desired *care acts*; they are no longer seen to be a vulnerable patient needing to be *cared for* (Borgstrom and Walter 2015; Mol 2008). As suggested above, with this shift the locus – and thus also the burden – of responsibility for choosing treatment and care and living with the outcomes now sits squarely with the patient (Glasdam, Oeye, and Thrysoee 2015).

Through a Foucauldian lens, decision making can be read as a technology of biopower (Foucault 2008): within neoliberal governmentality, individuals discipline and govern their own bodies and behaviours via the decision-making imperative. Patients seek clinicians to provide expert information, and the patient – as in a consumer marketplace – analyses the information, seeks more information from other sources if required, rationally makes a decision that fits their own best interests, and ultimately accepts responsibility for the outcomes (Glasdam, Oeye, and Thrysoee 2015; Hamann 2009). The clinician also becomes disciplined in this scenario: they are disciplined into professionalized bodies negotiating with rational consumers under an imperative of managerial efficiency.

Moving towards neoliberalism thus takes health care away from a social justice concern for a "public good" or a humanistic commitment to caring about patients (Glasdam, Oeye, and Thrysoee 2015; McGregor 2001). Critics of neoliberalism argue that this new version of the patient as consumer is the antithesis of the frail hospitalized elderly patient who wants to be *cared about*, in addition to being *cared for* (Borgstrom and Walter 2015). Similarly, ethnographic work shows health care providers decrying this version of care, frustrated with how it devalues the "human side" of their interactions with patients (Chan et al. 2017).

Such neoliberal values can be discerned within the decision-making tools being used in clinical management. Contrary to the way that many interact with them, decision technologies such as patient decision aids and clinical practice guidelines are not neutral "carriers of facts" from research evidence to clinical practice (Boivin, Légaré, and Lehoux 2008). Through an empirical normative analysis of interviews with tool developers and tool users, Boivin and colleagues (2008) show how values, such as compliance with professional recommendations, clinical efficiency, and fiscal responsibility, become embedded in these tools. Such values can run counter to clinical and patient values for comprehensive and compassionate care. As Kirmayer (1988, 57) reminds us, "When values are explicit they may be openly debated but rhetoric uses metaphor to smuggle values into discourse that proclaims itself rational, even-handed and value-free." Embedded in the administrative technologies of decision making are meaning and values; exposing these values can require examination of their grammar and rhetoric, as well as their moral, social, and political practices and agendas.

Case Study: Decision Making at the End of Life

Thus far, we have demonstrated how decision making acts as a technology of biomedical ethics to support an individualistic, rationalized clinical practice, while at the same time acting as a managerial technology in the service of an efficient neoliberal administration. Following this theorizing, we now turn to an empirical context to challenge and build this argument.

Palliative care is a model of care that runs counter to many tenets of biomedicine. Yet it is not immune to "rationalizing" medical practices; decision-making technologies and tools influence the work that palliative care clinicians value and perform. In palliative care, the emphasis on decision making has become pronounced through "best practices"; for example, forgoing life-prolonging technologies, discontinuing medical interventions, and encouraging advanced directives and resuscitation protocols have become normative decisional moments at end of life (Belanger, Rodriguez, and Groleau 2011; Drought and Koenig 2002). Even the practice of "doing nothing" has been translated into the decision-making frame: van der Heide and colleagues (2003) refer to "the practice of non-treatment decision-making" as one such decisional moment.

Palliative care is also a specialty that prides itself on being explicitly patient- and family-centred, attentively humanizing death, dying, and bereavement. As such, its modus operandi can clash with both the biomedical ethics focus on patient autonomy and the neoliberal agenda found in institutional health care settings. As Borgstrom and Walter suggest, the discourse of compassion has grown in end-of-life care rhetoric, displacing choice as a way to "rescue socialised health and social care" from the market-oriented reforms brought in via neoliberalism (Borgstrom and Walter 2015, 101). Notwithstanding – or perhaps because of – this "counterculture" stance and practice, our own ethnographic work in a free-standing hospice suggests that palliative care is an interesting location in which to examine decision making.

Palliative care is an approach to care that focuses on alleviating suffering and promoting quality of life for people living with life-threatening illness and for their families. Common caregiving practices in palliative care include aggressive clinical management of pain and other symptoms combined with support for psychological, social, and spiritual needs; such practices are offered by a multidisciplinary team of professionals and volunteers. Residential hospice care is one type of palliative care that, in Canada, is delivered in a free-standing care facility. Patients admitted to hospice are usually at the very end of life (typical length of stay until death is two weeks) and are aware that they are dying. An important element of hospice management and vision is enabled through their status as not-for-profit institutions, funded at least partially through charitable contributions. As such, while hospices must sustain health care practices that align ethically and legally with provincial practice standards, they also have a certain liberty to shape the culture of care within their walls.

Drawing on ethnographic data collected over a period of fifteen months in a residential hospice (Wright 2012), we suggest that decision making indeed acts as a medico-administrative technology in this location. However, it does not always operate in support of biomedicine and, in fact, eschews the use of many biomedical technologies to prolong life. Neither is it linked to the neoliberal pursuit of cost-efficiencies. Rather, decision making in the hospice is a medico-administrative technology that serves a unique ideological commitment to the hospice's vision of "good dying," by which we mean a commitment to accepting finitude and seeking a gentler, less technological ending. In hospice, patient choice and decision making are negotiated in relation to an institutional discourse that values the "good death."

Upon entry to the hospice, the patient has already made at least one major decision: to forgo life-sustaining interventions, which must be agreed to in order to qualify for hospice admission. Metaphors of "changing lanes" and "switching gears" are used to characterize this shift from acute care to end-of-life care (Thompson, McClement, and Daeninck 2006). At the hospice of our study, the referring clinician had to attest to the patient's "understanding" that they were at the end of life, and that goals of further care would not focus on life prolongation. Patients, or family members on their behalf, had to confirm in writing, upon arrival, their agreement that hospice care means end-of-life care, and that should the focus of care shift, the patient could be transferred out of the hospice.

While the choice to transition away from acute treatments and towards palliative care may be thought of as a discrete decisional action, once in the hospice the processes of "changing lanes" and "switching gears" continue to be negotiated throughout the patient's stay. For example, although it was made clear to patients and families that there was no possibility of receiving "life-saving" interventions (e.g., CPR) in the hospice, it was less obvious to some family members why interventions that were perceived to be "life-sustaining" were equally avoided (e.g., IV hydration, encouraging patients to eat). As a nurse said:

> That's one of the things you start working on right away with the family, the minute they walk in the door. Explaining how things work here and what we do here. And the family might say, "Well, I think he's dehydrated. Did you, should [you] start an IV or something?" And then maybe we go into the whole explanation of the palliative care, that we don't do that here.

In the hospice, decision making was guided by health care providers who gently navigated families towards coming "on board" and onto "the same page" with the choices the health care providers believed essential to quality end-of-life care. While choice was rhetorically presented in the spirit of patient volition (Pollock 2015), in reality there were limited choices actually on the hospice "menu"; those choices available were deliberately shaped by an ideological commitment to the "good death:"

> DAVID: If the family accepts, does that go better? Is it a better death?
> HOSPICE NURSE: Definitely. I've seen good deaths where family members start wailing and crying and jumping on their loved ones at time of death because they just weren't, they weren't ready for that one to, their loved one to die.
> DAVID: Sorry, you said those were good deaths?
> HOSPICE NURSE: The good death for the patient, but not for the family member.
> DAVID: Ok, so everything went well and then at that moment, then not so well ...
> HOSPICE NURSE: It collapsed. Everything collapsed. So I think supporting the family, supporting the family members, preparing them, educating them, bringing them to reality, sometimes it's just they're in denial, even though they're in palliative care and this facility is for end-of-life care, they may not really be psychologically ready for their loved ones to pass away, so it's basically making sure that they're on that page that they should be on.

The ideological commitment to the "good death" was infused throughout the hospice, from the architecture through to the hiring practices. A central motif buttressing this commitment was how the hospice was "not a hospital." The architecture underscored this point: the hospice imitated a homelike environment and hospice caregivers referred to it as a "house." The "house" had multiple living spaces with chairs and sofas, fireplace, and bookshelves. On sunny days, light streamed into these living spaces through floor-to-ceiling windows and illuminated the hanging artwork and tapestries. In the evening, soft lighting and beige-painted walls created an orange glow that was warm and inviting. Despite being a place of death, the hospice was lived and described by the hospice caregivers as a "dynamic, living, [and] joyous place."

The hospice caregivers' values continued this motif of "not a hospital." They believed the hospice saved patients and families from experiencing bad deaths in hospital. Contrary to hospital care, patients and families were "cared about" in the hospice, not just "cared for." Hospice caregivers expended considerable energy in helping people to spend their time in whatever ways were most meaningful to them. This creation of a caregiving culture defined by values of comfort and dignity speaks directly back to the "malaise" of modern health care elaborated above. In the hospice, beneficence and family-centred care were valued just as strongly as individual autonomy: conversations took precedence over the "tasks" of caregiving, and hospice caregivers sought to alleviate patients and families of the burden of responsibility that was associated with having to make difficult decisions about end-of-life care.

> DAVID: What is this place all about?
>
> SOCIAL WORKER: ... it's heaven [*smiles*] ... it couldn't be a better place for patients and family to be when they face terminal illness, and also to die in dignity ... to get privacy, to get looked after, not only the patient but also family, to get space.

This social worker's words point to a narrative of moral experience that oriented and directed hospice caregivers in their practice. These caregivers shared a singular and unwavering commitment to specific values that underpinned ideas about what a "good death" should be, values such as comfort and dignity. These values constituted a normative framework that defined the ethical meaning of care in this setting. It was through these values – which pervaded all levels of the organization, including professional and volunteer caregivers, support staff, and senior management – that hospice caregivers held themselves and each other accountable. As a nursing leader said, "And if people don't have those values they find out sooner or later that probably they don't belong working here."

Mobilizing the values of comfort and dignity, in conjunction with acts of explicit "caring about," hospice caregivers could justify constraining patient and family choice. Decision making in the hospice was less about fostering true choice among options than about maintaining an established moral order in the face of impending death. Facilitating such management required hospice caregivers to structure moral experience by conveying to patients and family what was at stake in "bad dying." When families had differing ideas about what was most important or about how care should be organized, the stage was set for a tense caregiving relationship. For example, some families felt that hospice caregivers adopted an overzealous approach to pain management that unduly prioritized comfort over mental alertness. These families wanted to be able to communicate with their loved one, whereas the hospice caregivers wanted to administer levels of medication that could reduce the patient's ability to engage. Some families felt that the tranquillity of the hospice space was unsettling and that it minimized the critical nature of the patient's health status. Families sometimes resisted being positioned by hospice caregivers as recipients of care themselves, preferring to take a more active role in the care of their loved one. As a social worker reflected:

> Because those girls [daughters] were, you know were not respecting boundaries ... So we had ... a meeting ... mentioning that maybe it was time for them to just drop the role as "nurses" but [be] the daughters. So it was difficult for them to let go of that role. But I think towards the end in the last, past week actually, they sort of mellowed, and were more cooperative.

Discussion and Concluding Thoughts

The hospice has provided a clinical location to deepen our understanding of the discursive objects created by the sociomedical movements outlined above. Palliative care – and especially hospice care – originally emerged as an alternative to many of the tenets of biomedicine, continuing to evolve in resistance to many of the values that undergird modern health care reform. Our examination demonstrates, however, a strong ideology at work in this location, one that was bolstered by decision-making technologies with important repercussions for patient and family experience at end of life. The rhetoric of choice was present in the hospice, yet fostering true choice among options was less the focus than maintaining moral order and establishing a good death. Decision making acted in this location as a force of technogovernance (May et al. 2006), mediating tensions in the family-clinician dyad in the service of the "good death" ideology.

Patient autonomy, decision making, and choice have become normative goods within modern biomedical ethics and by extension modern clinical practice. Yet these constructs remain fraught and contested. Patients are not hyper-rational beings, nor do they live discrete illnesses in simple contexts; this is increasingly true as patients age and approach end of life (Borgstrom and Walter 2015). Social research shows that decision making requires "significant cognitive, emotional and moral work" (Drought and Koenig 2002, 119). For such work to improve patient outcomes, it needs to be within a health care context that is structured and invested in this new paradigm of patient autonomy, decision making, and choice. Much empirical research shows that it is not, nor is it moving that way.

Every frame necessarily casts shadows on other views. The current focus on decision making and the micro location of "decisional moments" narrows our gaze to eclipse a structural critique of normative health care models. Decision making is but one moment within an institutional context that surrounds and long precedes it, a context embedded in a sociopolitical reality that predetermines how each patient narrative will actually unfold. While the discourse of patient choice celebrates autonomy and self-determination, the entrenched structural politics and the sociomedical economy and value system greatly restrict and control what is on the choice menu, who gets the power to make the choice, if and how that choice authentically reflects preferences, and how informed it ultimately is. In other words, "the usual course of care will remain the usual course of care" (Lynn et al. 2000, S219).

The individualistic interpretation required of the principle of autonomy elides the moral dimensions of extended familial and interprofessional relationships, as well as a broader gaze on the social institutions within which health care plays out, be it a hospital or a hospice. Has this emphasis on patient autonomy led to the *underdevelopment* of other important moral values, namely beneficence and justice? ask Agledahl and colleagues (2011). These authors sum up this concern: "The prevailing focus on patient choice has created a distinct discourse in bioethics that does not reflect what is at stake in medical care. This may distract our attention away from conditions of greater moral significance in clinical practice" (215).

We wrap up this chapter by pausing on Agledahl and colleagues' reflection: What is at stake and what is eclipsed when we focus on the clinician-patient decisional interaction?

In the hospice, as well as in many other clinical locations, patients and families often resist explicit decision making. When vulnerable and sick, patients want to be "cared about" as well as "cared for," and not necessarily made responsible for outcomes of decisions they did not want to have to make (Drought and Koenig 2002; Glasdam, Oeye, and Thrysoee 2015; Lynn et al. 2000; Mykhalovskiy 2008). While "doing nothing" can still be framed as a choice, it can feel safer; dying patients (and their families) do not necessarily want "aggressive promotion of autonomy" (Lynn et al. 2000, S217). Borgstrom and Walter look at how current health care approaches commodify care into a noun, moving it away from compassion and into a marketization that begets a focus on administrative metrics with accompanying tick-box forms representing performance targets. As we saw in the hospice, end-of-life care discourses can be committed to both choice and compassion with care embedded within a relational ethic of bedside compassion and "presence," that is, "sitting with the person, performing small personal acts of kindness" with unmeasurable "emotional labour" (Borgstrom and Walter 2015, 103). Yet in the hospice, while "caring about" was clearly valued by the hospice caregivers, it was enacted from within an ideological agenda via decisional technologies.

Nussbaum's (2000) analysis of the moral limits of rationalist, administrative frameworks shows how the inherent messiness of the existential and the tragic is eclipsed by technologies such as decision making. Illness can produce "tragic questions" for which there are no good decisions; each option is unthinkable (e.g., should I suffer through more chemotherapy or leave my children without a parent?). In contrast, rationalist models assume a cost-benefit, good-harm balance that can lead to a "right" answer. When the focus is placed on the rational act at one moment in time, then the contemplative life is discursively eclipsed. The focus on the decision ultimately leads us away from the tragedy of the dilemma, leaving moral residue in its wake. As an administrative technology, decision making overlays a managerial imperative onto patient experience and illness trajectories, turning patient "experience" into patient "preferences." As shown in the hospice, the use of this technology controls and constrains the messiness of illness. In so doing, this managerial frame transforms what counts as sought-after outcomes, for instance, the "good death." The locus of patient and family involvement is shifted from a state of being (e.g., experiencing illness) to the state of doing, choosing, preferring (e.g., as decision makers). As decision makers, they are given a degree of control over what is now the important outcome: the decision. Yet, as discussed above, with this control comes the doubled-edged sword of choice and the burden of responsibility. Illness and dying are then set up to be experienced as a series of managed, agreed-upon decisions.

In this chapter, our examination of the discursive shift from making a decision to decision making has revealed a medico-administrative technology in the service of powerful – yet often hidden – ideologies that undergird our health system. In broad strokes, decision making acts to advance the neoliberal rationalization of clinical practice by reproducing individualist, rationalist models of patient autonomy and choice in the service of managerial efficiency. In the clinical context of the hospice, decision making "smuggles in" the values of the palliative care agenda. This agenda, while resistant to many biomedical interventions and less constrained by a neoliberal commitment to patient autonomy and cost-efficiency, is still committed to producing normative decisional moments throughout the end-of-life process. In so doing, this agenda produces and reproduces a version of the patient and family that aligns with the palliative care ideology of "good dying." With this chapter, ultimately, we call for social scientists to continue to cast their critical gaze onto the taken-for-granted to uncover additional hidden products of powerful discourses.

ACKNOWLEDGMENTS

We are grateful for the research assistance offered by Janet E. Childerhose and Laura A. Macdonald in the writing of this paper. Mary Ellen Macdonald was supported by a Fonds de recherche du Québec–Santé (FRQS) Chercheur-Boursier salary award. During his hospice ethnography, David Kenneth Wright received a training fellowship from the Canadian Institutes of Health Research and Canadian Cancer Society Research Institute Strategic Training Program in Palliative Care Research (grant number STI-63286) as well as a fellowship from the FRSQ (award number 17395).

REFERENCES

Agledahl, K.M., R. Førde, and A. Wifstad. 2011. "Choice Is Not the Issue: The Misrepresentation of Healthcare in Bioethical Discourse." *Journal of Medical Ethics* 37 (4): 212–15. https://doi.org/10.1136/jme.2010.039172.

Allen, D., V. Badro, L. Denyer-Willis, M.E. Macdonald, A. Paré, T. Hutchinson, P. Barré, et al. 2015. "Fragmented Care and Whole-Person Illness: Decision-Making for People with Chronic End-Stage Kidney Disease." *Chronic Illness* 11 (1): 44–55. https://doi.org/10.1177/1742395314562974.

Arterburn, D., R. Wellman, E. Westbrook, C. Rutter, T. Ross, D. McCulloch, M. Handley, and C. Jung. 2012. "Introducing Decision Aids at Group Health Was Linked to Sharply Lower Hip and Knee Surgery Rates and Costs." *Health Affairs* 31 (9): 2094–104. https://doi.org/10.1377/hlthaff.2011.0686.

Bates, F.L. 1959. *Authority and Decision-Making in Voluntary Hospitals.* Ithaca: Sloan Institute of Hospital Administration, Cornell University.

Beauchamp, T.L., and J.F. Childress. 2001. *Principles of Biomedical Ethics.* New York: Oxford University Press.

Belanger, E., C. Rodriguez, and D. Groleau. 2011. "Shared Decision-Making in Palliative Care: A Systematic Mixed Studies Review Using Narrative Synthesis." *Palliative Medicine* 25 (3): 242–61. https://doi.org/10.1177/0269216310389348.

Berg, M. 1997. *Rationalizing Medical Work: Decision-Support Techniques and Medical Practices.* Cambridge, MA: MIT Press.

Black, D. 1948. "On the Rationale of Group Decision-Making." *Journal of Political Economy* 56 (1): 23–34. https://doi.org/10.1086/256633.

Blum, D., S.X. Raj, R. Oberholzer, I.L. Riphagen, F. Strasser, and S. Kaasa. 2015. "Computer-Based Clinical Decision Support Systems and Patient-Reported Outcomes: A Systematic Review." *The Patient – Patient-Centered Outcomes Research* 8 (5): 397–409. https://doi.org/10.1007/s40271-014-0100-1.

Boivin, A., F. Légaré, and P. Lehoux. 2008. "Decision Technologies as Normative Instruments: Exposing the Values Within." *Patient Education and Counseling* 73 (3): 426–30. https://doi.org/10.1016/j.pec.2008.07.017.

Borgstrom, E., and T. Walter. 2015. "Choice and Compassion at the End of Life: A Critical Analysis of Recent English Policy Discourse." *Social Science & Medicine* 136–7: 99–105. https://doi.org/10.1016/j.socscimed.2015.05.013.

Carnevale, F.A. 2007. "The Birth of Tragedy in Pediatrics: A Phronetic Conception of Bioethics." *Nursing Ethics* 14 (5): 571–82. https://doi.org/10.1177/0969733007080203.

Chan, L., M.E. Macdonald, F.A. Carnevale, and R. Cohen. 2017. "'I'm Only Dealing with the Acute Issues': How Medical Ward 'Busyness' Constrains Care of the Dying." *Health* 22 (5): 451–68. https://doi.org/10.1177/1363459317708822.

Charles, C., A. Gafni, and T. Whelan. 1997. "Shared Decision-Making in the Medical Encounter: What Does It Mean? (Or It Takes at Least Two to Tango)." *Social Science & Medicine* 44 (5): 681–92. https://doi.org/10.1016/S0277-9536(96)00221-3.

Coser, R.L. 1958. "Authority and Decision-Making in a Hospital: A Comparative Analysis." *American Sociological Review* 23 (1): 56–63. https://doi.org/10.2307/2088624.

Drought, T.S., and B.A. Koenig. 2002. "'Choice' in End-of-Life Decision Making: Researching Fact or Fiction?" *Gerontologist* 42 (Spec. no 3): 114–28. https://doi.org/10.1093/geront/42.suppl_3.114.

Dubov, A. 2015. "Ethical Persuasion: The Rhetoric of Communication in Critical Care." *Journal of Evaluation in Clinical Practice* 21 (3): 496–502. https://doi.org/10.1111/jep.12356.

Edwards, W. 1954. "The Theory of Decision Making." *Psychological Bulletin* 51 (4): 380–417. https://doi.org/10.1037/h0053870.

Ford, S., T. Schofield, and T. Hope. 2002. "Barriers to the Evidence-Based Patient Choice (EBPC) Consultation." *Patient Education and Counseling* 47 (2): 179–85. https://doi.org/10.1016/S0738-3991(01)00198-7.

Foucault, M. 2008. *The Birth of Biopolitics: Lectures at the Collège de France, 1978–1979.* Translated by G. Burchell. New York: Palgrave Macmillan.

Gauthier, D.M., and V.A. Swigart. 2003. "The Contextual Nature of Decision Making Near the End of Life: Hospice Patients' Perspectives." *American Journal of Hospice and Palliative Medicine* 20 (2): 121–8. https://doi.org/10.1177/104990910302000210.

Glasdam, S., C. Oeye, and L. Thrysoee. 2015. "Patients' Participation in Decision-Making in the Medical Field – 'Projectification' of Patients in a Neoliberal Framed Healthcare System." *Nursing Philosophy* 16 (4): 226–38. https://doi.org/10.1111/nup.12092.

Goodman, H.A. 1950. *The Lilienthal Confirmation Controversy: A Study in Legislative Decision-Making.* http://worldcat.org/z-wcorg/database.

Greenhalgh, T., J. Howick, and N. Maskrey. 2014. "Evidence Based Medicine: A Movement in Crisis?" *BMJ* 348. https://doi.org/10.1136/bmj.g3725.

Hamann, T.H. 2009. "Neoliberalism, Governmentality, and Ethics." *Foucault Studies* 6: 37–59. https://doi.org/10.22439/fs.v0i0.2471.

Hamilton, J.A. 1960. "Decision Making in Hospital Administration and Medical Care: A Casebook." *JAMA Network* 174 (18): 2246. https://doi.org/10.1001/jama.1960.03030180066034.

Horwitz, M.B. 1953. *Motivational Effects of Alternative Decision-Making Processes in Groups.* Urbana: Bureau of Educational Research.

Jennings, B. 2006. "The Politics of End-of-Life Decision-Making: Computerised Decision-Support Tools, Physicians' Jurisdiction and Morality." *Sociology of Health and Illness* 28 (3): 350–75. https://doi.org/10.1111/j.1467-9566.2006.00496.x.

Kaufman, S.R., J.K. Shim, and A.J. Russ. 2006. "Old Age, Life Extension, and the Character of Medical Choice." *Journals of Gerontology, Series B, Psychological Sciences and Social Sciences* 61 (4): S175–84. https://doi.org/10.1093/geronb/61.4.S175.

Keller, C., and M. Siegrist. 2009. "Effect of Risk Communication Formats on Risk Perception Depending on Numeracy." *Medical Decision Making* 29 (4): 483–90. https://doi.org/10.1177/0272989X09333122.

Kirmayer, L.J. 1988. "Mind and Body as Metaphors: Hidden Values in Biomedicine." In *Biomedicine Examined,* vol. 13, edited by M. Lock and D. Gordon, 57–93. Dordrecht: Kluwer.

Kon, A. 2010. "The Shared Decision-Making Continuum." *JAMA* 304 (8): 903–4. https://doi.org/10.1001/jama.2010.1208.

Kryworuchko, J., E. Hill, M.A. Murray, D. Stacey, and D.A. Fergusson. 2013. "Interventions for Shared Decision-Making about Life Support in the

Intensive Care Unit: A Systematic Review." *Worldviews on Evidence-Based Nursing* 10 (1): 3–16. https://doi.org/10.1111/j.1741-6787.2012.00247.x.

Lefton, M., S. Dinitz, and B. Pasamanick. 1959. "Decision-Making in a Mental Hospital: Real, Perceived, and Ideal." *American Sociological Review* 24 (6): 822–9. https://doi.org/10.2307/2088570.

Lin, G.A., D.S. Aaronson, S.J. Knight, P.R. Carroll, and R.A. Dudley. 2009. "Patient Decision Aids for Prostate Cancer Treatment: A Systematic Review of the Literature." *CA: A Cancer Journal for Clinicians* 59 (6): 379–90. https://doi.org/10.3322/caac.20039.

Lynn, J., H.R. Arkes, M. Stevens, F. Cohn, B. Koenig, E. Fox, N.V. Dawson, R.S. Phillips, M.B. Hamel, and J. Tsevat. 2000. "Rethinking Fundamental Assumptions: SUPPORT's Implications for Future Reform." *Journal of the American Geriatrics Society* 48 (S1): S214–21. https://doi.org/10.1111/j.1532-5415.2000.tb03135.x.

May, C., and N. Mead. 1999. "Patient-Centredness: A History." In *General Practice and Ethics: Uncertainty and Responsibility*, edited by C. Dowrick and L. Frith, 76–91. London: Routledge.

May, C., T. Rapley, T. Moreira, T. Finch, and B. Heaven. 2006. "Technogovernance: Evidence, Subjectivity, and the Clinical Encounter in Primary Care Medicine." *Social Science & Medicine* 62 (4): 1022–30. https://doi.org/10.1016/j.socscimed.2005.07.003.

McCamy, J.L. 1947. "Analysis of the Process of Decision-Making." *Public Administration Review* 7 (1): 41–8. https://doi.org/10.2307/972353.

McGregor, S. 2001. "Neoliberalism and Health Care." *International Journal of Consumer Studies* 25 (2): 82–9. https://doi.org/10.1111/j.1470-6431.2001.00183.x.

McNeil, B.J., S.G. Pauker, H.C. Sox Jr., and A. Tversky. 1982. "On the Elicitation of Preferences for Alternative Therapies." *New England Journal of Medicine* 306 (21): 1259–62. https://doi.org/10.1056/NEJM198205273062103.

Miller, P.A. 1953. "A Comparative Analysis of the Decision-Making Process in Community Organization toward Major Health Goals." PhD diss., Michigan State College of Agriculture and Applied Science.

Mol, A. 2008. *The Logic of Care: Health and the Problem of Patient Choice.* London: Routledge.

Molewijk, A.C., A. Stiggelbout, W. Otten, H. Dupuis, and J. Kievit. 2003. "Implicit Normativity in Evidence-Based Medicine: A Plea for Integrated Empirical Ethics Research." *Health Care Analysis* 11 (1): 69–92. https://doi.org/10.1023/A:1025390030467.

Mykhalovskiy, E. 2008. "Beyond Decision Making: Class, Community Organizations, and the Healthwork of People Living with HIV/AIDS: Contributions from Institutional Ethnographic Research." *Medical Anthropology* 27 (2): 136–63. https://doi.org/10.1080/01459740802017363.

Nussbaum, M.C. 2000. "The Costs of Tragedy: Some Moral Limits of Cost-Benefit Analysis." *The Journal of Legal Studies* 29 (S2): 1005–36. https://doi.org/10.1086/468103.

Peiris, D.P, R. Joshi, R.J. Webster, P. Groenestein, T.P. Usherwood, E. Heeley, F.M. Turnbull, A. Lipman, and A.A. Patel. 2009. "An Electronic Clinical Decision Support Tool to Assist Primary Care Providers in Cardiovascular Disease Risk Management: Development and Mixed Methods Evaluation." *Journal of Medical Internet Research* 11 (4): e51. https://doi.org/10.2196/jmir.1258.

Peiris, D.P., T. Usherwood, T. Weeramanthri, A. Cass, and A. Patel. 2011. "New Tools for an Old Trade: A Socio-Technical Appraisal of How Electronic Decision Support Is Used by Primary Care Practitioners." *Sociology of Health & Illness* 33 (7): 1002–18. https://doi.org/10.1111/j.1467-9566.2011.01361.x.

Pollock, K. 2015. "Is Home Always the Best and Preferred Place of Death?" *The BMJ* 351: h4855. https://doi.org/10.1136/bmj.h4855.

Simon, H.A. 1944. "Decision Making and Administrative Organization." *Public Administration Review* 4 (1): 16–30. https://doi.org/10.2307/972435.

Simon, H.A. 2013. *Administrative Behavior: A Study of Decision-Making Processes in Administrative Organization.* New York: Simon and Schuster.

Stacey, D., F. Légaré, N.F. Col, C.L. Bennett, M.J. Barry, K.B. Eden, M. Holmes-Rovner et al. 2014. "Decision Aids for People Facing Health Treatment or Screening Decisions." *Cochrane Database of Systematic Reviews* (1): CD001431. https://doi.org/10.1002/14651858.CD001431.pub4.

Stacey, D., R. Samant, and C. Bennett. 2008. "Decision Making in Oncology: A Review of Patient Decision Aids to Support Patient Participation." *CA: A Cancer Journal for Clinicians* 58 (5): 293–304. https://doi.org/10.3322/CA.2008.0006.

Tannenbaum, R. 1950. "Managerial Decision-Making." *Journal of Business of the University of Chicago* 23 (1): 22–39. https://doi.org/10.1086/232927.

Taylor, C. 1989. *Sources of the Self: The Making of the Modern Identity.* Cambridge, MA: Harvard University Press.

Thompson, G.N., S.E. McClement, and P.J. Daeninck. 2006. "'Changing Lanes': Facilitating the Transition from Curative to Palliative Care." *Journal of Palliative Care* 22 (2): 91–8. https://doi.org/10.1177/082585970602200205.

van der Heide, A., L. Deliens, K. Faisst, T. Nilstun, M. Norup, E. Paci, G. van der Wal, P.J. van der Maas, and EURELD Consortium. 2003. "End-of-Life Decision-Making in Six European Countries: Descriptive Study." *The Lancet* 362 (9381): 345–50. https://doi.org/10.1016/S0140-6736(03)14019-6.

Walther League. 1940. *Christian Conscience and Military Service: A Guide to Decision-Making from a Lutheran Perspective.* Chicago: Walther League.

Werth, J., and D. Blevins. 2009. *Decision-Making Near the End of Life: Issues, Developments, and Future Directions.* New York: Routledge.

Wolpe, P. 1998. "The Triumph of Autonomy in American Bioethics: A Sociological View." In *Bioethics and Society: Sociological Investigations of the Enterprise of Bioethics,* edited by R. DeVries and J. Subedi, 38–59. New York: Prentice Hall.

Wright, D.K. 2012. "Delirium and the Good Death: An Ethnography of Hospice Care." PhD diss., University of Ottawa.

4 Code Work: RAI-MDS, Measurement, Quality, and Work Organization in Long-Term Care Facilities in Ontario

TAMARA DALY, JACQUELINE CHOINIERE, AND HUGH ARMSTRONG

Albert Einstein's notion of the role of subjectivity in measurement is highlighted by the Neils Bohr character in Michael Frayn's play *Copenhagen*:

> Measurement is not an impersonal event that occurs with impartial universality. It's a *human act*, carried out from a specific point of view in time and space, from a *particular viewpoint of a possible observer*. (Frayn 1998, 71)

Reflecting on the notion of measurement as a human act, informed by the observer's viewpoint – in terms of what is measured, by whom, and to what ends – raises important questions for health, health services, health outcomes, and care work organization. What conditions and care are measured, what health care data are collected, by whom, in what way and for what ends affects who gets care with public funds, the quantity and quality of that care, the way care work is organized, and the quality of working conditions for those providing care.

In response to growing quality concerns, the Ontario government requires long-term care facilities (LTCFs) to collect clinical assessment data about residents' health conditions and behaviours, using the Resident Assessment Instrument-Minimum Data Set (RAI-MDS) Version 2.0 (Canadian Institute for Health Information 2002). This standardized assessment tool, originally created in the United States and now developed by the non-profit corporation interRAI, tabulates residents' clinical needs and calculates resource allocations. The Ontario government relies mainly on this tool to track quality indicators, to impose care accountability requirements, and to assess funding levels based on acuity measures, which are then pegged to resource utilization groups for resource allocation. The data are collected and collated by nurses and dietary, recreation, and RAI coordinator staff (who are mostly nurses and social workers by training).

Our primary focus in this chapter is to explore the implications of this assessment instrument for the work lives of health care providers in LTCFs. The data for this chapter are drawn from government documents, organizations' newsletters and websites, and fieldwork involving participant observations and key informant interviews conducted during case studies of promising practices and healthy active ageing in two Ontario LTCFs. These case studies were part of a broader exemplary comparative case study conducted in twenty-five LTCFs between 2013 and 2015 in Canada (Ontario, BC, Nova Scotia, and Manitoba), the United States (Texas), Germany (North Rhine-Westphalia), Norway, Sweden, and the United Kingdom.[1] The two Ontario LTCFs that are the focus of this chapter are non-profit, have operated for more than fifty years, and have offered a wide variety of services catering to seniors.

In the field, we conducted rapid team-based ethnographies over four days in each of the LTCFs. Twelve to fourteen researchers working in teams of two conducted observations and interviews on both a secure and an open unit between the hours of 7 a.m. and roughly midnight. In addition to the field notes from individual observations, we conducted ninety-four key informant interviews with management, staff (front-line nurses, personal support workers, and dietary, therapy, and RAI coordinators), residents, family, and volunteers in these two Ontario facilities. Interviews were verbatim transcribed and analysed. For this chapter we draw on observations and interviews with front-line staff and managers only.

Our analysis is framed by feminist political economy (Andrew et al. 2003; Armstrong and Connelly 1989, 5–12; Vosko 2002), reflected first in assumptions that social and political forces offer important contexts for our analysis, including the priority accorded to neoliberal forces that have encouraged new public management–based reforms like RAI-MDS (see Armstrong, Daly, and Choiniere 2016), but also in our assumptions about the research process itself. In our approach, team members surfaced key themes for each jurisdiction by reflecting on the content of interviews and observations, making presentations to the larger group of researchers to discuss emerging themes, collectively identifying where more research was needed, and having smaller subteams take up specific areas of study (such as RAI-MDS).

The chapter is organized as follows. The next section provides an overview of Ontario's LTCF "quality" policy context and the RAI-MDS "data trail." Themes emerging from the observations and interviews are presented in the following section. Our findings show that the tool reorganizes the everyday work of front-line care workers, alters their interactions with residents, and shifts the division of labour between nurses, care aides, and RAI coordinators. The final section discusses the importance of our findings for researchers, policymakers, and professionals.

Ontario Policy Context

In Ontario, there were on any day in 2015–16 about 78,000 residents in 625 long-term care facilities (Health Quality Ontario 2017). Those providing front-line care, housekeeping, dietary, and recreation services to these residents face increasingly precarious, fast-paced, and highly gendered work environments, and work organizations that are task oriented, hierarchical, and medicalized (Daly and Szebehely 2012).

The LTCF sector is publicly funded, with people paying privately for accommodation costs (McDonald 2015). In Ontario, a minimum acuity level, assessed using RAI-MDS, is required for admission into an LTCF, and estimates suggest there are nineteen thousand people awaiting admission (Bronskill et al. 2010). The high demand for care along with stringent medical RAI-MDS assessment criteria have resulted in substantial waiting lists for those assessed as eligible for admittance, and have also contributed to increased resident complexity and acuity over the past decade.

Ontario also differs from the other provinces and territories in that two-thirds of the sector is owned or managed by for-profit chains, with the remainder split nearly evenly by non-profit, or charitable, and municipal facilities. The difference between for-profit and non-profit facilities is complicated by the fact that some non-profit and municipal facilities contract out management, kitchen, laundry, or housekeeping services to for-profit organizations. Evidence suggests that the contracting out of management services is increasing, and is associated in part with the complexity of managing LTCFs within the RAI-MDS data collection regime (Daly 2015), forcing smaller organizations to purchase this capacity.

Assessments for clinical care, management, and accountability for the sector have changed over time. Starting in 1993, Ontario used a made-in-Canada assessment and funding system called the Alberta Classification. In 1998, Ontario's Hospital Services Restructuring Commission (HSRC) – whose controversial mandate was to cut and redesign hospital and long-term-care services – recommended implementation of the RAI-MDS tool. Indeed, as Hoffmann and Leichsenring (2011, 2) point out, applying new public management tools and approaches (such as RAI-MDS) to areas of social and health services is about "increasing efficiency and effectiveness," "reducing costs," and measuring quality in "increasingly market-driven systems" that are composed of users who contribute higher levels of out-of-pocket payments and who want to be able to purchase quality services. In keeping with their neoliberal assumptions, assessment systems such as RAI-MDS enable policy makers to steer and not row (Osborne and Gaebler 1992), or, stated another way, allow the system to be managed from a distance (Armstrong, Daly, and Choiniere 2016).

Again, our interest in this chapter is to explore the implications of RAI-MDS as a new public management approach for attaining quality, for those who work at the point of care and for those who manage that care.

Findings

The selected themes related to RAI-MDS and front-line work that emerged in our fieldwork are presented below.

Workload: Coding and Caring

Workloads in Ontario LTCFs are widely acknowledged to be heavy (about one PSW [personal support worker] for eight to twelve residents on the day shift; closer to one to twenty-five residents on the night shift). These staffing levels are far below those elsewhere, such as in Nordic and European countries. For example, Sweden has a much higher 0.8 care staff per resident ratio (Hansebo et al. 1998).

Echoing the concerns of many, one Ontario PSW reported how difficult it was to complete tasks in the time allotted:

> It's just the fact that you don't have enough time. That's what bothers me. And sometimes you have to cut the corners and, you know, we don't want to do this. You go home and you think and you say, "Oh, you know, I should have done this, I should have done that" but, you know, you have to arrange your day to make it. You don't have a choice, you know. To me I would like to do more.

In the context of lacking time to provide care, a key theme from the observations and interviews concerned the added burden of the RAI-MDS assessments as well as the enhanced division of labour to complete the required assessments. The implications of these assessments included when and how resident needs are coded, who provides hands-on care, and who does the computer work for the coding. Front-line workers described the coding demands as an additional and significant pressure in their already busy day. Many did not see the clinical relevance of the tool. In fact, they often indicated that RAI-MDS assessments were unrelated to the provision of care. Despite this, there is little doubt that they experienced considerable stress and pressure to complete the assessments.

Staff members are typically assigned specific residents who are due for an assessment on a particular day. One registered practical nurse (RPN) spoke for many about the implications of this added workload, describing how the pressures to complete the coding work, in the context of heavy caring loads, meant it sometimes had to be completed outside of paid work hours if there was inadequate time during regular, paid hours.

> The person is assigned to you so you're going to arrange your schedule to be finished on time so if you are late so you know that you are late, you have to catch up sometime. Otherwise you have the [RAI-]MDS coordinator coming telling you, "I need it to be done this day and it has to be done." It's happened to me many times ... sometime we get upset because they say, "You cannot leave if it's not finished." ... I was so upset.

Other nurses spoke of carving out work time to complete the assessments by invoking the authority of the director of care (DOC), especially when the regular demands of the care work might take precedence. One RPN said:

> So ... I do use the [director] too. I tell her [the MDS coordinator], "Well, [director] says that you have to do my noon meds so I can do my MDS. If you don't want to do it, you talk to the DOC." And so she does it so that gives me the time, that extra hour, to do my MDS ... It's hard because you need to find that little time. It's like wow!

Speaking to the tension between doing the care and completing the coding, a PSW noted:

> I do understand it's important, the data, you know, and you have to prove whatever you do so yes, we'll have some money from the government and I do understand that, but down the road there's an impact.

Managers were more likely to report on the importance of the assessment work to capture resident acuity and identify when shifts occur in the case mix index (CMI; a measure of the home's aggregate acuity level). A CMI drop in absolute terms from a 1.0, but also in relative terms compared with the home's previous acuity levels, can result in less funding and fewer people resources. As this manager explains:

> A "1" is considered average, so if you are an average long-term care resident in Ontario you're 1, so when we say, "Oh, this unit is more complex," then you should see a CMI above 1. When you have units that maybe the

> residents are more stable but maybe require physical care but not a lot of treatments you would see an MDS potentially below 1. If you are coding badly, you could score as low as .6. So that means basically for every dollar one home would get, you would get 60 cents, so I hope your resources match the 60 cents you are getting. Because if you are coding badly you'll be in debt.

The link between funding and acuity increases the pressure on coding activities. Coding "poorly" holds significant repercussions, and careful attention is devoted to tracking data and closely monitoring workers to ensure that coding is completed in a timely manner. As one manager noted:

> Because now that it is all tied to finances the data quality is really important, so it means that the MDS coordinators now have to be extremely vigilant about when was a patient admitted, when were they sent out to acute care, all of those dates matter, because when we send it to C[anadian] I[nstitute for] H[ealth] I[nformation] you'll get it rejected, so you know, this has happened in the last couple of quarters that we have to be much, much more vigilant.

As another manager stated:

> We also make sure that there's no assessments missing because all of this now is all linked to our funding. So we don't want to miss any assessments. We don't want to miss any patient dates because that's all linked now to our funding.

Managers and administrators spoke to the implications of the time lag between assessment and funding. When funding drops but residents' needs increase, it becomes more difficult for staff to code well. They reported on the challenges associated with balancing resource inability and incapacity to code properly, and those associated with balancing the coding of residents' changing needs and the immediate and pressing demands of the care work. The negative implications for funding were grave. Managers informed us that once homes "got behind" or "coded badly," they had difficulty making up the delta between their funding levels and the resources required to properly manage both the code work and the care work.

In Ontario, daily care work (bathing, eating, etc.) has traditionally been performed by PSWs and nurses (primarily RPNs). It is clear from our interviews that the introduction of RAI-MDS significantly altered this care. As one manager noted, "Coding in LTC is fairly new ... it's a challenge." Even accounting for its novelty, many workers agreed that the tool had intensified and changed the nature and organization of the work of all staff, exacerbating existing professional divisions of labour. Following its introduction, registered staff became more likely to spend their time in record keeping and medication dispensing, with far less time spent performing hands-on care. The bulk of care work fell to PSWs, who reported having far too many residents per shift, and complained that they could no longer count on nurses for an extra pair of hands, since nurses no longer "did care." PSWs described how RAI-MDS often moved RPNs off the floor and in front of computers to perform the code work, resulting in less time to care for, or get to know, the residents.

For their part, many nurses also lamented this shift, commenting that they did not get into nursing in order to perform computer work. Registered practical nurses (generally with college-level training) reported spending much more time on the computer and far less time working directly with residents. Registered nurses (generally with university-level training) noted that the heightened assessment requirements had increased their workloads, as they covered multiple floors, managing as many as seventy-two residents per shift and working to ensure that the correct information was logged into the computer system. One RPN complained that computer work took nurses' time away from residents.

> Because they take a lot of ... time from the residents to come on the computer ... but I don't think they realize the amount of time it takes from the residents ... Sometimes it's very stressful because there's so many MDS to do.

Most of the personal support workers reported that this division of labour between care work and code work kept them from feeling like a team. Nurses reported feeling torn as they tried to balance the immediacy of the residents' care needs against the managerial expectations driven by ministerial requirements that staff continually document care and changes in care needs, to ensure the financial stability of the home. Lacking any direct experience with the coding work performed by nurses, personal care staff reported being abandoned to care for residents. Teamwork was also complicated by part-time and contract nurses who floated between jobs at various facilities, and who often did not engage in coding activities because the residents and procedures were generally unknown to them.

The centrality of coding work cleaved divisions between full- and part-time RPNs, as the latter were less likely to use the tool. Further divisions occurred as PSWs were "helped" by some part-time nurses who didn't have RAI-MDS coding obligations, while others (full-time or regular part-time nurses) were viewed as "not helpful" because they engaged in the computer work. One RPN commented:

> We do have part-time RPN that are "not coded," which means they don't know anything about the computer ... So they won't do care plans because they can't get into the computer to do the care plans. They can't do MDS because they're not coded for MDS. And they don't do a lot of the things that we do. So what makes the conflict is sometimes the [PSW], which is the one that does care, they will see RPNs like that.

The nurses recognized the challenges for PSWs with this sharper division of labour. As one RPN reported:

> Before in the morning when we didn't have MDS we helped the PSW to do two persons or one ... We get them up, wash and give them their break ... But then when they brought in that MDS and ... we can no longer take residents because with the residents you cannot do MDS. So when they took away the residents so the RPN don't do any more residents ... the [PSW] didn't like that because they didn't get the help from us.

RAI coordinators are tasked with ensuring that care work is coded to best advantage the home in terms of its CMI. We heard that there were many skills required of RAI coordinators. When asked if many small homes were struggling given the complexities of the reporting requirements, one manager nodded vigorously in agreement and then responded:

> The knowledge of the [RAI] coordinators from a computer perspective needs to be much, much higher. It's not just now sending out little memos, and little emails. Like, if you don't have a moderate to high level of computer knowledge you can't move around in these databases, you can't run the reports. A lot of the reports, like you're picking pieces of information and amalgamating it, you might put it in Excel. The people just don't have the skills. What we're hearing from some of the small homes is those positions are turning over.

The interviews point out the ways that RAI-MDS has limited teamwork and reciprocity, exacerbating whatever professional divisions of labour may have already existed. This was, as mentioned, largely because the reporting requirements make it more likely for registered staff to spend their time coding, record keeping, and medication dispensing, with far less time performing hands-on care. PSWs, who were accustomed to having a more team-like relationship with RPNs in particular, and counted on nurses for an extra pair of hands when needed, indicated that they were now alone in hands-on care. Most of the PSWs reported that this division kept them from feeling like a team. Nurses reported being conflicted by the immediacy of the residents' care needs and the managerial requirements that staff continually document care and any care changes so as to ensure the financial stability of the facility. The fact that the part-time and contract nurses, not involved in coding, were considered "more helpful" to PSWs actually served to individualize the structural nature of the increased division of labour. Furthermore, the RAI-MDS coordinators, primarily focused on monitoring for timely assessment and coding, helped shift the focus from care to coding.

A Less Holistic Approach

Both the RAI-MDS and the RUGS-III reward medical complexity, rather than social care needs, with higher scores. The managers who were interviewed did not question the clinical emphasis or express concern that important aspects of care were left out of this assessment. According to one:

> And so we can start looking at not only case mix or resource utilization reports, but there's also a lot of quality indicators that we look at because we want to improve care. So my role as well is to take out some of the information that I can to provide to the staff, to the managers.

Alternatively, more front-line staff expressed concern over the lessened importance accorded the more social aspects of care. Social care such as spending time talking and comforting was often left undone, or performed in a rush while en route to or during the course of some other duty. Residents seem almost frozen in place compared with the swift pace of the staff, who were rushing here and there. It was clear in our interviews with both PSWs and RPNs that this aspect of care is both very important and largely absent. An RPN reports:

> Before MDS ... We used to deal with [residents] more. We used to go there, put them to bed ... talk with them and there's a lot of things that we do ... After a shower I used to blow-dry their hair ... So it's like "[name]" and they put the bell on. "Yes, what can I do for you?" "Do you think you could just sit with me for two minutes?" They just want to talk but I can't talk ... "Can you just sit here? Why do you have to go away?" ... I have to tell you it has happened many times where my residents have asked me to stay for just two minutes. So I will just actually sit and I say, "Okay. Okay, I've got to go now." ... sometimes they try to tell you something ... but you do not

> have time. But sometimes when you [are] with them you realize they mix the words, one or two words, give you the story and so you catch it ... You socialize like when you give pills ... it's not very long.

The lack of time to provide meaningful social care was linked to the time-consuming nature of doing the coding work. One PSW echoed a widely held belief:

> Before, it was more time with the clients. And [now] ... too much information to get data, to get some funding for money. We kind of forget the real picture of nursing ... So we're at the bedside, yeah, but ... non-stop every day, every day. Non-stop ... you know, patients are human beings. I would not appreciate to be pushed like we push the clients.

Another nurse echoed the same sentiment: "they [residents] are more lonely." Another PSW noted how nurses' roles have changed and how this change has pulled nurses away from care in general and social care in particular:

> Eventually it seems like the more you got a [nursing] title the less you have to deal with clients, so who is going to take care of the clients eventually? ... before, everybody was assigned to clients because when you decide to be a nurse it's because you want to touch that client, you want to be close, eh?

Skills, Training, and Careers

Our findings demonstrate how the job of being a nurse in LTCFs was no longer the same type of work that it once was. They also illustrate how the work and focus of administrators and managers have changed. The RAI-MDS requires LTCFs to recruit care workers with different sets of skills, and many interviewees spoke about this. Also, managers noted that, with the implementation of this coding system, it was necessary to hire coordinators but was difficult to attract and retain them given the required computer skills and the intensity of the demands. One manager said:

> You are seeing people go to meetings, and they are in this role, they were talked into it, "You were a really [a] great RN on the unit," and the director of care says, "Would you like to be an MDS coordinator?" and you think "Oh, OK, great, maybe." Then you get into the job and it is all electronic and everything is databases, you have to run reports, the quality of the data that we have to submit almost overnight with this new funding formula we're having data quality issues we didn't even know we had.

A nearly universal concern of managers was the increased regulatory complexity required of LTCF. One of the ways that managers dealt with the regulatory complexity was by forming networks with other homes. This was commonly done through the home's membership in one or both of the representative organizations, one exclusively for the non-profit providers (AdvantAGE) and the other for profit and non-profit providers (The Ontario Long Term Care Association, OLTCA).

Finding staff with training to use the RAI-MDS without disadvantaging the home presented recruitment and reporting challenges, which were exacerbated for small or rural homes. One manager noted:

> I talked to this MDS coordinator about a year and a half ago from a small rural place with sixty beds ... they were affiliated with a community hospital and she said the CEO had called her and he wanted her to run reports on CMI, she said to him, "I don't know what that is." I don't think that there [was] anyone who could instruct her when she start[ed] th[e] job about how important CMI is, how do you make sure that your coding is done properly to maintain your CMI.

Discussion and Conclusions: Assessing the Assessment Tool

According to Hawes and colleagues (2003, 26), the RAI-MDS implementation has resulted in numbers triumphing over anecdote: "The policy experts ... noted that the research findings would lend both scientific legitimacy and the weight of numbers to anecdotal stories from family members and providers." Supporters argue that RAI-MDS has improved staff ability to plan care and monitor interventions (Hawes et al. 2003, 29). American academics see the quality indicators from RAI-MDS and other sources as a bulwark against a sector largely controlled by commercial interests (Ronald et al. 2016), because it provides quality indicators on health data that are publicly reported. Yet many do not see the RAI-MDS indicators as the only quality metrics that need to be considered. For instance, there are important structural indicators, such as staffing hours, staffing mix, and ownership (Harrington et al. 2016) when it comes to residents' quality of life and workers' quality of work. Quality-of-life issues are also critically important and are often cited as most important by residents.

There remains strong support for the resident benefits of RAI-MDS. Hirdes et al. (2013b) indicate that Ontario data collected between 1996 and 2011 are valid and reliable. Despite its benefits (Bowen and Zimmerman 2008; Hirdes et al. 2013a; Estabrooks, Knopp-Sihota, and Norton 2013), its continued use has not been without criticism: for not being sensitive enough to depression (Koehler et al. 2005; McCurren 2002; Shin and Scherer 2009); for not being well-integrated into care planning and quality improvement (Parmelee et al. 2009); for not taking account of residents' social and historical contexts (Kontos, Miller, and Mitchell 2009); and for missing co-morbidities compared with administrative data (Lix et al. 2014). Shin and Scherer (2009) summarize studies that critique the MDS 2.0 for data inaccuracy compared with charts. They note experts' arguments that over 10 per cent of the items have high error rates, with those assessing cognitive functioning, psychosocial well-being, physical functioning, skin condition, and activity engagement as the most error prone.

Shin and Scherer (2009) argue that one of the ways to ensure higher data reliability is to have registered nurses or those specially trained in its use complete it. As our findings suggest, this assessment tool is increasing divisions between the registered staff who do the coding work and the care aides who perform the majority of daily, hands-on care. Generally ignored by RAI-MDS proponents is how this sharpened division of labour affects the quality of teamwork and the overall provision of care. Missing from much of the analysis are the implications for relationship-oriented care or the provision of social care.

Our findings regarding increased workload, deteriorating team relations, and reduced social focus are joined by other criticisms of RAI-MDS. Parmelee and colleagues (2009) found that medical directors and senior clinical staff in veterans' affairs facilities consider the tool less useful than directors of care or RAI coordinators. Despite its being advertised as a clinical tool, Morley (2013) notes its problematic clinical utility because of the questionable validity of individual-level data and the impact on work organization given its time-consuming nature (taking twenty minutes longer than other assessments). As Morley also notes, the original MDS released in 1999 "proved to be a real oxymoron, as it was by no means minimum, but rather excessively extensive" (1). With the release of version 2.0 little was improved, as it remained "overlong, creating a collection burden with little interface with day to day care." There are few Canadian reviews of MDS 2.0 concerning its impact on workload. One study indicates that it is not only onerous for PSWs, but that it also devalues important knowledge of residents' histories and social needs (Kontos, Miller, and Mitchell 2009). An Ontario case study has shown how, as part of a linked set of onerous regulatory changes producing a significant administrative burden, the tool has helped to consolidate commercial hegemony in Ontario (Daly 2015, 28). Currently, the United States utilizes MDS-RAI 3.0, which, though more positively perceived, comes with additional documentation requirements, including resident interviews and additional standardized assessment procedures (Rahman and Applebaum 2009).

According to Banerjee and Armstrong (2015), the new regulatory system in LTC de-centres residents and centres "paperwork." In our research, the focus of the RAI-MDS coordinators (and other managers) on the data, rather than what is happening between residents and workers, is evidence for this claim. While increasing amounts of paperwork have certainly been an aspect of Ontario's health sector reform over the past twenty-odd years, the difference with RAI-MDS concerns its focus on data rigour and statistical oversight. The link to funding means that "data inaccuracies" related to care needs are pursued. For instance, the ministry can track coded events, such as 85 per cent of residents requiring help to lift their legs into bed, and then downgrade the task from a more expensive mobility issue to a less expensive transfer issue (Armstrong, Daly, and Choiniere 2016). The tool's premise is that funding resources are matched to needs or, put another way, that resources, though inadequate, are consistent between facilities given the needs. The challenge here is that staffing resources were reportedly inadequate for care needs before the tool's introduction. Its significant role in bifurcating the care work of front-line staff, and contributing to a heavier workload, further undermines rather than improves the capacity of front-line workers to provide care. The one area where there is little dispute is that the tool enables managers to govern from afar, to redefine how funding is aligned to care, and to shift the focus of care onto immediate activities of daily living and the most medically complex needs (Armstrong, Daly, and Choiniere 2016). Indeed, work organization has changed. Front-line staff have reorganized their work around the collection of the data, making the centrality of the data enterprise in LTCFs highly evident. Managers referred to the data in terms that indicated it was a main organizing principle for their work.

In addition, the purity of the data has been treated as nearly a sacrosanct part of care. As John Hirdes and colleagues (2013b, 2) articulate:

> Examples of factors that can undermine the quality of data in "real-world" situations include: poor training and lack of ongoing education; lack of staff expertise; inadequate "buy-in" by staff; systematic biases in reporting due to financial incentives or avoidance of negative consequences of unfavorable findings; temporary coding problems with the introduction of new systems; declining attention and underfunding; lack of feedback to users; and poor data collection or coding strategies.

For RAI-MDS supporters, the problem has to be with the LTCF and its staff, not with the tool itself. It is a position that centres data collection and code work over care work, placing the blame for poor data quality on individual incompetence. This perspective does not take account of how code work may stand in contrast to care work, or how this kind of activity is the opposite of what attracted many to work with seniors in the first place. In addition, little attention is paid to the structures and systems, such as overwork and underfunding, that may further impede proper coding.

While the CMI aims to predict resource use, it is exceedingly poor at predicting "time use." Medically complex conditions, which trigger nursing or therapy care, are reimbursed at a higher rate, while the care for residents with behaviours related to dementia, in the absence of medical complexity or special therapy needs, has much lower reimbursement rates. This means that very time-consuming work for PSWs, and sometimes also for nursing and managerial staff, is not adequately captured. Yet, residents and families want and need this care, and front-line staff face the tension between these care needs and those valued by the broader system.

In summary, how the RAI-MDS affects workload, the division of labour, and the quality of care and care relationships has been understudied. Care staff in general, but care aides (PSWs) in particular, are facing increased work pressures and growing difficulty in providing care that residents both need and want. Not only are the social and relational aspects of care devalued, but the work required to implement the tool, check the data, understand the coding definitions, and shift practices when definitions change has also been underestimated, which has significant implications for management staff. We argue that it is highly problematic for residents, their families, and staff when decisions that affect funding, in addition to the public reporting of quality, ignore such critical aspects of care and care work within LTCFs.

ACKNOWLEDGMENTS

We would like to acknowledge the members of the "Reimagining Long-Term Residential Care" research project led by Pat Armstrong, and funding from SSHRC, CIHR, Tamara Daly's CIHR Research Chair in Gender, Work and Health, and York University.

NOTE

1 Armstrong, Pat (PI). "Reimagining Long-term Residential Care: An International Study of Promising Practices." SSHRC MCRI grant# 412-2010-1004.

REFERENCES

Andrew, C., P. Armstrong, H. Armstrong, W. Clement, and L.F. Vosko. 2003. *Studies in Political Economy: Developments in Feminism.* Toronto: Women's Press.

Armstrong, H., T. Daly, and J. Choiniere. 2016. "Policies and Practices: The Case of RAI-MDS in Canadian Long-Term Care Homes." *Journal of Canadian Studies* 50 (2): 348–67. https://doi.org/10.3138/jcs.50.2.348.

Armstrong, P., and M.P. Connelly. 1989. "Feminist Political Economy: An Introduction." *Studies in Political Economy* 30 (1): 5–12. https://doi.org/10.1080/19187033.1989.11675504.

Banerjee, A., and P. Armstrong. 2015. "Centring Care: Explaining Regulatory Tensions in Residential Care for Older Persons." *Studies in Political Economy* 95 (1): 7–28. https://doi.org/10.1080/19187033.2015.11674944.

Bowen, S.E., and S. Zimmerman. 2008. "Understanding and Improving Psychosocial Services in Long-Term Care." *Health Care Financing Review* 30 (2): 1–4.

Bronskill, S., M. Carter, A. Costa, A. Esensoy, S. Gill, A. Gruneir, D.A. Henry et al. 2010. *Aging in Ontario.* http://www.ices.on.ca/flip-publication/aging-in-ontario-an-ICES-chartbook-of-health-service/index.html#3/z.

Canadian Institute for Health Information. 2002. "Minimum Data Set 2.0 Canadian Version." https://www.cihi.ca/en/residential-care.

Daly, T. 2015. "Dancing the Two-Step in Ontario's Long-Term Care Sector: Deterrence Regulation = Consolidation." *Studies in Political Economy* (95): 29–58. https://doi.org/10.1080/19187033.2015.11674945.

Daly, T., and M. Szebehely. 2012. "Unheard Voices, Unmapped Terrain: Comparing Care Work in Long-Term Residential Care for Older People in Canada and Sweden." *International Journal of Social Welfare* 21 (2): 139–48. https://doi.org/10.1111/j.1468-2397.2011.00806.x.

Estabrooks, C., J. Knopp-Sihota, and P.G. Norton. 2013. "Practice Sensitive Quality Indicators in RAI-MDS 2.0 Nursing Home Data." *BMC Research Notes* 6: art. no. 460. https://doi.org/10.1186/1756-0500-6-460.

Frayn, M. 1998. *Copenhagen.* New York: Anchor.

Hansebo, G., M. Kihlgren, G. Ljunggren, and B. Winblad. 1998. "Staff Views on the Resident Assessment Instrument, RAI/MDS, in Nursing Homes, and the Use of the Cognitive Performance Scale, CPS, in Different Levels of Care in Stockholm, Sweden." *Journal of Advanced Nursing* 28 (3): 642–53. https://doi.org/10.1046/j.1365-2648.1998.00707.x.

Harrington, C., J.F. Schnelle, M. McGregor, and S.F. Simmons. 2016. "The Need for Higher Minimum Staffing Standards in U.S. Nursing Homes." *Health Services Insights* 9: 13–19. https://doi.org/10.4137/HSI.S38994.

Hawes, C., B.C. Vladeck, J.N. Morris, C.D. Phillips, and H. Fredeking. 2003. "The RAI and the Politics of Long-Term Care: The Convergence of Science and Politics in U.S. Nursing Home Policy." In *Implementing the Resident Assessment Instrument: Case Studies of Policymaking for Long-Term Care in Eight Countries.* Milbank Memorial Fund. https://www.milbank.org/publications/implementing-the-resident-assessment-instrument-case-studies-of-policymaking-for-long-term-care-in-eight-countries/.

Health Quality Ontario. 2017. Measuring Long-Term Care Home Performance in Ontario. http://www.hqontario.ca/System-Performance/MeasuringSystemPerformance/Measuring-Long-Term-Care-Homes.

Hirdes, J.P., D.G. Sinclair, J. King, P. Tuttle, and J. McKinley. 2013a. "From Anecdotes to Evidence: Complex Continuing Care at the Dawn of the Information Age in Ontario." In *Implementing the Resident Assessment Instrument: Case Studies of Policymaking for Long-Term Care in Eight Countries.* Milbank Memorial Fund. https://www.milbank.org/wp-content/uploads/2016/04/ResidentAssessment_Mech2.pdf.

Hirdes, J.P., J.W. Poss, H. Caldarelli, B.E. Fries, J.N. Morris, G.F. Teare, K. Reidel, and N. Jutan. 2013b. "An Evaluation of Data Quality in Canada's Continuing Care Reporting System (CCRS): Secondary Analyses of Ontario Data Submitted between 1996 and 2011." *BMC Medical Informatics and Decision Making* 13, art. no. 27. https://doi.org/10.1186/1472-6947-13-27.

Hoffmann, F., and K. Leichsenring. 2011. "Quality Management by Result-Oriented Indicators: Towards Benchmarking in Residential Care for Older People." Policy brief. European Centre for Social Welfare Policy and Research, Vienna. https://www.researchgate.net/publication/236647474_Quality_management_by_result-oriented_indicators_Towards_benchmarking_in_residential_care_for_older_people_Vienna_European_Centre_Policy_Brief_June.

Koehler, M., T. Rabinowitz, J. Hirdes, M. Stones, G.I. Carpenter, B.E. Fries, J.N. Morris, and R.N. Jones. 2005. "Measuring Depression in Nursing Home Residents with the MDS and GDS: An Observational Psychometric Study." *BMC Geriatrics* 5 (1): 1–8. https://doi.org/10.1186/1471-2318-5-1.

Kontos, P.C., K.L. Miller, and G.J. Mitchell. 2009. "Neglecting the Importance of the Decision Making and Care Regimes of Personal Support Workers: A Critique of Standardization of Care Planning through the RAI/MDS." *The Gerontologist* 50 (3): 352–62. https://doi.org/10.1093/geront/gnp165.

Lix, L.M., L. Yan, D. Blackburn, N. Hu, V. Schneider-Lindner, and G.F. Teare. 2014. "Validity of the RAI-MDS for Ascertaining Diabetes and Comorbid Conditions in Long-Term Care Facility Residents." *BMC Health Services Research* (1): 17–27. https://doi.org/10.1186/1472-6963-14-17.

McCurren, C. 2002. "Assessment for Depression among Nursing Home Elders: Evaluation of the MDS Mood Assessment." *Geriatric Nursing* 23 (2): 103–8. https://doi.org/10.1067/mgn.2002.123796.

McDonald, M. 2015. "Regulating Individual Charges for Long-Term Residential Care in Canada." *Studies in Political Economy* (95): 83–114. https://doi.org/10.1080/19187033.2015.11674947.

Morley, J.E. 2013. "Editorial, Minimum Data Set 3.0: A Giant Step Forward." *JAMDA* 14: 1–3. https://doi.org/10.1016/j.jamda.2012.10.014.

Osborne, D., and T. Gaebler. 1992. *Reinventing Government: How the Entrepreneurial Spirit Is Transforming the Public Sector.* Reading, MA: Addison-Wesley.

Parmelee, P.A., S.E. Bowen, A. Ross, H. Brown, and J. Huff. 2009. "'Sometimes People Don't Fit in Boxes:' Attitudes toward the Minimum Data Set among Clinical Leadership in VA Nursing Homes." *Journal of the American Medical Directors Association* 10 (2): 98–106. https://doi.org/10.1016/j.jamda.2008.08.004.

Rahman, A.N., and R.A. Applebaum. 2009. "The Nursing Home Minimum Data Set Assessment Instrument: Manifest Functions and Unintended Consequences – Past, Present, and Future." *The Gerontologist* 49 (6): 727–35. https://doi.org/10.1093/geront/gnp066.

Ronald, L.A., M.J. McGregor, C. Harrington, A. Pollock, and J. Lexchin. 2016. "Observational Evidence of For-Profit Delivery and Inferior Nursing Home Care: When Is There Enough Evidence for Policy Change?" *PLoS Medicine* 13 (4): e1001995. https://doi.org/10.1371/journal.pmed.1001995.

Shin, J.H., and Y. Scherer. 2009. "Advantages and Disadvantages of Using MDS Data in Nursing Research." *Journal of Gerontological Nursing* 35 (1): 7–17. https://doi.org/10.3928/00989134-20090101-09.

Vosko, L.F. 2002. "The Pasts (and Futures) of Feminist Political Economy in Canada: Reviving the Debate." *Studies in Political Economy* 68 (1): 55–83. https://doi.org/10.1080/19187033.2002.11675191.

5 Disputing Evidence: Canadian Health Professionals' Responses to Evidence about Midwifery

VICKI VAN WAGNER AND ELIZABETH DARLING

Care during pregnancy and childbirth is an ongoing topic of public, professional, and political debate and controversy. In both high- and low-income countries, access to care, variations in rates of intervention, concerns about rising rates of caesarean section, and questions about the roles of midwives and physicians in birth are debated in the professional literature and popular culture. The medicalization and "industrialization" (Gawande 2006, 1) of birth in high- and middle-income countries have given rise to scholarly critique and public activism to lower rates of intervention and to humanize childbirth (Reiger 2001). In low-income countries, concerns about access to care include concerns about quality and appropriateness of care and have inspired movements for kindness and respect in childbirth care that have been taken up across the world (White Ribbon Alliance 2011).

Obstetrics was once awarded the dubious distinction of being the least-evidence-based medical specialty. This changed with the publication of a two-volume compendium of evidence titled *Effective Care in Pregnancy and Childbirth* (Chalmers, Enkin, and Keirse 1989), which is recognized as one of the foundational texts of evidence-based medicine (Godlee 2012, e7017). A substantial body of applied research now informs, but has not lessened, the debate and controversy. This chapter looks at how evidence informs debates in Canada about the organization of care during pregnancy and childbirth, the roles of midwives and physicians, and strategies to improve birth outcomes.

In 2008, the Cochrane Database of Systematic Reviews, widely considered a gold-standard source of health care evidence, published a review of eleven randomized controlled trials (RCTs) on midwife-led care (Hatem et al. 2008, 1). The review identified all of the RCTs on care during pregnancy and childbirth in the world literature and found studies that met the inclusion criteria from the United Kingdom, Ireland, and

Australia. Originally entitled "Midwife-Led versus Other Models of Care for Childbearing Women," the review was updated in 2013 (Sandall et al. 2013) to include two new studies and was renamed "Midwife-Led Continuity Models versus Other Models of Care" to clarify the model being evaluated. It was last updated in 2016 (Sandall et al. 2016) and included fifteen RCTs from the United Kingdom, Ireland, Australia, and Canada.

The Cochrane authors describe standard care in the countries where the research took place as varying within units that may be characterized as more physician-led or more midwife-led. The research examines the impact of supporting midwives to be primary care providers and to work within a relational model that provides continuity of care by a known midwife. They call this model midwifery-led continuity of care. The trials compare midwife-led continuity models (MLCM) to care by unknown care providers, who may be midwives, nurses, or physicians. An understanding of the benefits of this midwife-led model is important in Canada because it is the model of care in which all Canadian midwives currently provide care.

Significantly, these reviews showed high rates of satisfaction with MLCM, which had better outcomes in several important maternal and newborn indicators as well as reduced rates of common interventions, and was less expensive than comparator models. For other outcomes there was no difference between MLCM and the comparator models of care. As the 2016 update says, MLCM "provides benefits for women and babies and we have identified no adverse effects" (Sandall et al. 2016, 3). The Cochrane Review findings, along with those from a large cohort study of place of birth (Brocklehurst et al. 2011, 17), led organizations such as the National Health System and National Institute for Health and Care Excellence (NICE) in the United Kingdom to recommend that midwifery-led care and choice of birthplace be offered to all "women at low risk of complications" (NICE 2017, 8).

In Canada, the reaction was very different. A *Canadian Medical Association Journal* (*CMAJ*) commentary that responded to the 2013 Cochrane review concluded that the evidence was not generalizable to Canada (Morgan et al. 2014, 1279). The authors called for collaborative models rather than midwife-led models of care for Canada, although they did not detail what collaboration would look like.

Access to midwifery care in Canada is limited. As midwives who are involved in provincial and national policy discussions, we felt it was important to examine and understand the nature of the disputes over the MLCM evidence. Based on interviews with Canadian health professional leaders, this chapter analyses how the Cochrane evidence has been received in the Canadian context and explores differing interpretations of the evidence. The themes that emerge from our research help make visible how knowledge produced through RCTs and systematic reviews is received, disputed, and debated in the real-life context of health care systems and interprofessional relationships.

A number of chapters in this volume use social science to critique how authoritative forms of knowledge neglect or objectify people's experiences of health care problems. This chapter uses social science insights about knowledge in a different way. Rather than focusing on what gets missed by established evidence-based discourses, we explore how authoritative forms of evidence are differently interpreted and mobilized by social actors. Many of the chapters in this volume address the social uses of evidence in ways that focus on how evidence is assimilated into managerial forms of reasoning. By contrast, we are concerned with how research evidence is enlisted by providers in the context of professional and interprofessional debates over models of care and the use of health care resources. We explore how midwifery provides an example of how RCTs, the benchmarks of evidence-based decision making, can be used to support midwifery models of care, even though such gold-standard forms of evidence do not guarantee acceptance and adoption. Rather than critique the evidence, we explore the contours of its reception by strategic actors in health care in Canada, showing how evidence – or lack of evidence – is far from the only factor at play. We seek to understand the policy issues and social dynamics that underlie resistance to evidence about a model of care that is an alternative to industrialized birth (Gawande 2006, 1).

Midwifery-Led Continuity of Care

Midwife-led care is care "where the midwife is the lead professional in the planning, organisation and delivery of care given to a woman from initial booking to the postnatal period" (Royal College of Obstetricians and Gynaecologists 2001, 6). "Midwife-led continuity models" describe models of care in which midwives autonomously provide on-call primary care to a defined caseload throughout pregnancy, birth, and early parenting. This contrasts with the most common model of care across both high- and low-income countries in which midwives work shifts in hospitals or clinics, often with physicians as the leaders of care.

Despite decades of attempts to humanize childbirth, the standard model of care in pregnancy and childbirth in most countries, whether provided mainly by midwives or by physicians, is fragmented and provided by a series of strangers in high-volume hospital settings designed for high-acuity care (Shah 2015, 2182). The RCTs included in the Cochrane review examine midwives' rather than physicians' use of the tools of evidence-based practice. They focus on the outcomes of care provided by non-physicians in a relational rather than an industrial model. The Cochrane review examined whether a model where midwives know the people they care for and take the lead role in the care improves outcomes. The goal of the studies was to provide evidence to guide health care policy. One of the Australian trials noted that "the evidence that this trial can provide is long overdue for maternity policy makers and service providers who are responsible for the effective design, delivery and costs of services that are the most frequent cause of hospitalization in Australia today" (Tracy et al. 2011, 7).

Although the norm internationally, midwifery is a recent innovation in Canada. Ontario regulated midwifery in 1994 and British Columbia in 1996. Two decades later all provinces and territories except the Yukon and Prince Edward Island have passed midwifery legislation, although New Brunswick and Newfoundland are at early stages of implementation. Midwifery has grown quickly in some provinces, with 385 midwives in British Columbia attending over 23 per cent of births in 2018 and 968 Ontario midwives attending 18 per cent of births (Canadian Association of Midwives 2019, 20). There are six undergraduate midwifery education programs in the country. All Canadian midwives currently work in systems that would be defined as midwife-led continuity models.

On the surface, midwifery care appears to be well aligned with Canadian health policy priorities. Provincial and national health policies call for primary care reform, a shift to community-based care, and the "right care at the right time in the right place" (Ontario Ministry of Health and Long-Term Care 2012, 7). Governments and professional bodies are committed to evidence-based health care, and governments and midwifery organizations alike maintain that midwifery care is an example of evidence-based health innovation and person-centred care. The national body of Canadian obstetricians officially supports the growth of midwifery and choice of care provider (Society of Obstetricians and Gynaecologists of Canada 2009, 662). However, plans to scale up access to midwifery care remain modest in scope, and health systems have restricted the growth of midwifery, particularly in jurisdictions where the profession has grown the fastest (Bourgeault 2014).

At the heart of this debate are policy questions about "who does what" in the health care system, about service design and health human resources planning. Globally, many publicly funded health systems use obstetricians as consultants rather than as primary attendants for the majority of low-risk births (Shaw et al. 2016, 2289). However, much of Canada depends on specialist care for healthy pregnancy and birth. For example, in Ontario just under 80 per cent of births are attended by specialists (Better Outcomes Registry Network Ontario 2018, 54). This high reliance on specialists has not gone unnoticed. A Canadian report on sustainability in maternity care recommended shifting to a system of primary care, which would depend more on care provided by family physicians and midwives (Reynolds 2000). A 2006 Ontario expert panel report recommended a target of 60 per cent of births attended by midwives and family physicians (Ontario Maternity Care Expert Panel 2006, 81). But Canada lacks transparent health human resources policies at national and provincial/territorial levels. The supply of care providers, according to family physician and health policy scholar Ruth Wilson (2013, 28), "swings reactively between over and undersupply," leaving health planning authorities, hospitals, and professions without guidance about provider mix. In the context of this policy gap, the system has tended to default to physician-led care for childbirth.

Our Approach

Canadian feminist scholars have been drawn to the study of midwifery. It is a health care practice dominated by women, and Canadian midwifery offers a model of care that is based in feminism, integrating social and medical approaches to childbirth. Much of the work has focused on the political and other obstacles to the historical shift in midwifery from social movement to profession, while emphasizing Canadian midwifery's model of care that integrates relational care, continuity, choice, and respect for physiologic childbirth (Bourgeault 2006; MacDonald 2017). Like Bourgeault and MacDonald (2000), we identify ourselves as "interested researchers," whose motivation and approach come from commitment to the field of study. As midwives and researchers with the goal of understanding barriers to the growth of midwifery, we use a critical social science approach.

We used a two-stage approach to examine Canadian discourse about the MLCM evidence. The first stage was a documentary analysis. We searched both the professional and lay literature for responses to the Cochrane review. We then analysed the documents we found to identify key arguments and themes. The second stage involved individual interviews with opinion leaders. We invited the authors of the *CMAJ* commentary and individuals in leadership positions in national professional organizations to participate. Those who agreed were sent the interview guide and a link to both the Cochrane review and the *CMAJ* commentary. We conducted semi-structured telephone interviews with six professional leaders in Canada (two midwives, two family physicians, and two obstetricians). We also interviewed a midwifery leader from the United Kingdom with many years of experience in Canada. Our questions focused on the relevance of the Cochrane findings, barriers and facilitators related to scaling up MLCM, other potentially appropriate models, and health human resources policy implications. Interviews were audio-recorded and transcribed. Interview transcripts were reviewed and coded to identify themes. Ethics approval was obtained at both Ryerson and Laurentian universities.

The MLCM Findings

The most recent version of the Cochrane review of MLCM includes fifteen RCTs with results for 17,762 births. MLCM was compared with standard care in the various research settings, with participants randomized to either MLCM or to the usual care that would be offered during pregnancy and birth. The care in the comparator groups might be provided by midwives working autonomously, by midwives working under medical supervision, or by nurses and physicians. Because midwifery care is the norm in most health systems, the comparator group in most trials received care from midwives working in non-continuity models (i.e., midwives doing shift work rather than being on call for a caseload of clients as in MLCM). In a few settings, the comparator group involved care provided by obstetricians or family physicians working with nurses, or care provided by different professionals at different points in the care. The midwife-led models all included consultation with physicians as needed, and some also included routine visits to a physician.

Both the 2013 and the 2016 Cochrane reviews focused on whether MLCMs made a difference in a set of defined primary and secondary outcomes. The review found that recipients of MLCM care were less likely to have epidural pain relief, an amniotomy, an episiotomy, or a birth with forceps or vacuum. They were less likely to have a preterm baby or experience loss of their pregnancy before twenty-four weeks. They were more likely to have a spontaneous vaginal birth, a longer labour, and a known midwife at their birth. There were no differences between recipients of MLCM and those in the comparator groups in terms of intact perineum, induction of labour, caesarean birth, pregnancy loss over twenty-four weeks plus neonatal death, or the many other measures of care for birth or newborn care. Studies included in the review showed high rates of satisfaction with MLCM. Seven of the studies looked at cost effectiveness and showed a trend towards overall cost savings using MLCM, particularly for intrapartum care. Because the studies used different methods of economic analyses, the reviewers suggest that more research is needed to confirm these findings.

The 2013 review concludes that "most women should be offered midwife-led continuity models of care, although caution should be exercised in applying this advice to women with substantial medical or obstetric complications" (Sandall et al. 2013, 2). In 2016, the summary adds that MLCM "provides benefits for women and babies and we have identified no adverse effects" (Sandall et al. 2016, 3). In the discussion, the authors state that "policy makers who wish to achieve clinically important improvements in maternity care, particularly around normalizing and humanizing birth, and preventing preterm birth should consider midwife-led continuity models of care and consider how financing of midwife-led services can be reviewed to support this" (24). The authors have presented a challenge to health policy planners to find ways to fund and support MLCMs. Canadian health policy planners have a different challenge. Canadian health systems have already integrated MLMC into a variety of funding models in different provinces and territories. Some use bundled-care models in which midwives are contracted by government or health agencies to provide care; others use salaried employment models. The challenge in Canada is not how to support MLMC but rather whether to scale up these models.

Canadian Responses to the Cochrane Review of MLCM

The Society of Obstetricians and Gynaecologists of Canada (SOGC) published a response which is included as a comment in the 2013 and 2016 Cochrane reviews. The SOGC indicated support for collaborative models of care and choice of care provider. But after acknowledging some of the benefits associated with MLCM, the author said that it does not follow from the findings that "most women should be offered midwifery-led continuity models and women should be encouraged to ask for this option" (Blake 2013a, comment on Sandall et al. 2016, 114). The author noted that the many outcomes where no difference was observed between MLCM and standard care were not listed in the abstract and argued that this omission failed to provide reassurance about the equal outcomes of the various models of care for most of the outcomes studied. Although the findings of fewer preterm births and fewer fetal deaths less than twenty-four weeks are noted as "interesting," the commentary states these findings are unexplained and unlikely to be related to the type of care provider.

In response to the SOGC's comments, the Cochrane review authors reformatted the abstract and conclusions to include reference to all outcomes, including those that show no difference. The authors noted that they agree with the SOGC that they could not identify a causal mechanism for the finding of fewer preterm births and fewer fetal deaths less than twenty-four weeks in the intervention group. They note, however, that midwife-led continuity of care is a complex intervention and that it may not be possible to measure the impact of philosophy of care or continuity of care on outcomes.

Many of the same concerns were raised by the SOGC in a 2013 editorial in its newsletter. The authors noted that the organization had to do "a lot of damage control to try and correct the erroneous impression" in the Cochrane recommendation that "most women should be offered midwife-led continuity models of care." The editorial states that the Cochrane review recommends midwifery care "over other care providers" and that the Cochrane reviewers appear "self-serving and misleading." The editorial references the SOGC "Policy Statement on Midwifery" (SOGC 2009) and reiterates its commitment to "a woman's right to choose" her care provider (Blake 2013b, 1).

A 2014 commentary in the *Canadian Medical Association Journal* by an interprofessional team of authors (including a family physician, a midwife, and two obstetricians) discussed similar issues and posed collaborative practice as better suited to Canada than midwife-led care (Morgan et al. 2014, 1279). The commentary summarizes the Cochrane findings by noting that although MLCM decreased the rate of several interventions, most outcomes did not differ by type of health care provider. The article expressed concern that fewer family physicians were doing obstetrics and predicted a shortage of obstetricians, highlighting challenges particularly in "rural and remote, inner city and Aboriginal communities" (1279).

The *CMAJ* authors question whether training more midwives in Canada is the appropriate response to the Cochrane review findings and recommendations. Acknowledging that midwife-led care may be part of the answer, they argue that the Cochrane evidence may not be applicable in Canada. They maintain that the Cochrane review goes "beyond the evidence" in suggesting midwifery care in most cases, and they are concerned that media attention to midwifery (Glanz 2013) may not help "public and professional understanding of what Canada needs to do to improve maternity services." Collaborative care, although not defined, is proposed as an approach to increase quality and "optimize and respect the skill set of each provider" (Morgan et al. 2014, 1279). Like SOGC, they recommend a national strategy to promote care coordinated across regions and professions and set out the priorities for a national birthing initiative. They cite resistance to change, payment models, professional cultures, and regulatory and medico-legal issues as barriers to collaborative care, and offer examples of successful collaborative maternity care practice and resources. Overall, the commentary focuses on the benefits of working well together across the professions. Our interviews explore these reactions to the Cochrane Review of MLCM in more depth.

Interview Findings

Most of the care providers (i.e., midwives, family physicians, and obstetricians) we interviewed accepted the Cochrane findings of the benefits of MLCM but raised concerns that there are not enough midwives to make the evidence applicable to Canada. Most of our interviewees pointed out that Canada's geography means that no single approach will work across urban, rural, and remote communities, but agreed that creativity and collaboration, including midwife-led models within other teams of providers, were key. Many noted that an important difference in the Canadian health system is that family physicians provide intrapartum care. This is not common in most of the health systems where the RCTs were being conducted. One obstetric leader worried that press coverage of the findings would undermine current care providers and models of care, even though the findings could be interpreted to reassure the public that all models were safe and had similar outcomes.

The midwives we interviewed emphasized that the evidence in the Cochrane review should not be dismissed because of current human resources; rather, human resource planning should be informed by the evidence. They pointed to barriers to the growth of midwifery, such as restrictions on midwives' hospital privileges and scope of practice, as a contradiction between statements of support from medical societies for interprofessional collaborative care and choice of care provider, and what appears to be medical control over access to practice in hospitals.

All informants acknowledged that MLCMs appeared to decrease rates of intervention. One of the family practice leaders noted that non-interventive care was increasingly valued across the professions: "everyone agrees ... [that in] the normal pregnancy, the low risk pregnancy ... where the labour is going well, we do not need to do anything." One obstetrician even stated that "somebody who is low risk ... quite frankly does not need an obstetrician and probably has more interventions because she's seeing an obstetrician."

The informants also agreed that physician responses to the Cochrane evidence would inevitably reflect concern that an expansion of midwifery would affect a physician's ability to earn a living and maintain a sustainable call group to allow adequate time off. Many noted that a shift to implement the review recommendations would require relationship building, because in many parts of the country there are misunderstandings about midwives and mistrust of midwifery skills and outcomes. This is true even in provinces with several decades of regulated midwifery integrated into health systems. One obstetrician disputed the potential for cost savings discussed in the Cochrane review, seeing the low-volume caseloads associated with MLCM as inefficient. Midwives cautioned against making a direct comparison between MLCM and physician care in terms of volume and cost, noting this not only devalues midwives' work but makes invisible the large cadre of nurses who staff Canadian hospital labour floors.

Improving relationships and increasing understanding of midwifery were major factors for informants who favoured a collaborative model rather than a midwife-led model as a next step for many parts of Canada. To explain their support for collaborative models, one family physician stated, "I personally think that sometimes slow shift is far more effective than wholesale change." One midwife pointed to a lack of clarity in the term "collaborative care" and preferred to use the term "interprofessional care" for the type of model where different providers share care, given that it is a professional expectation that all care providers be collaborative no matter what model they work in. Many noted the irony of repeated calls for collaborative care at the national and provincial levels but a lack of pragmatic government strategies to support new approaches.

None of our informants were aware of evidence supporting collaborative approaches. One obstetrician worried that some of the examples held up as models of collaboration in the *CMAJ* article required "add-on" funding to establish and maintain the service, and would therefore not be sustainable on a large scale across the country. One midwife noted that collaborative interprofessional models from other fields often promote care by low-risk and non-physician providers unless specialist care is necessary, a model that would support the growth of midwifery-led models.

One obstetrician concurred with the SOGC position that the Cochrane evidence gave the impression of being "self-serving" and "going beyond the evidence." This had created a negative interprofessional response, the informant believed, worrying that press coverage of the evidence increased rather than reduced barriers to the integration of midwifery into the health system. Several of the midwives we interviewed responded to the SOGC's concerns by noting that the Cochrane authors are leading midwifery scholars and academics trained in critical appraisal of RCT evidence, using a systematic approach that was unlikely to be biased. The United Kingdom midwifery expert said, "this is very high-quality evidence." Several midwives observed that if the authors were physicians writing about medical care it would be unlikely for them to be labelled as self-serving.

For midwifery leaders and for one of the obstetricians, the differences found in rates of preterm birth, lower rates of fetal death prior to twenty-four weeks, and several common interventions were important. These clear advantages of MLCM show the potential of not only improving care but reducing cost. One midwife questioned why these findings were not received by all care provider groups as relevant in the same way that evidence of other beneficial health care practices is normally received. The United Kingdom midwifery expert noted that lowering preterm birth by nearly 25 per cent is a very significant finding and that if this were a medical intervention being studied, it would likely be greeted with a great deal of interest and advocacy.

Why Is This Evidence in Dispute?

Although scientific evidence, and especially evidence from RCTs, is often considered to be neutral and objective, the health care and social science literature is rich with analysis of how evidence is created and interpreted within existing systems, hierarchical relationships, and professional interests and worldviews. Some evidence is applied quickly and almost universally, while other evidence is almost impossible to implement (de Melo-Martín and Intemann 2012; Enkin et al. 2006; Melnyk et al. 2012; Mykhalovskiy and Weir 2004; Van Wagner 2013).

Responses to the Cochrane review of MLCMs fit with many patterns described in research about the application of evidence in maternity care. Evidence that reinforces current systems is more easily adopted than evidence that demands systems change. Evidence that promotes intervention is taken up more readily than evidence for low-intervention approaches. Evidence that fits with pre-existing beliefs and practices has greater uptake (Van Wagner 2013). Responses to evidence may reveal more about values than about science, and discussion of values may be more supportive of change than debate about methods and outcomes (de Melo-Martín and Intemann 2012). The response of Canadian health care providers to the Cochrane review of MLCMs is an example of how disputes about evidence may reveal more about underlying health care system politics than about the methods or outcomes of the research.

Although some of our physician informants saw the MLCM review as being about midwifery care compared to physician care, this is not what the research focused on. The majority of studies in the review were conducted in the United Kingdom, Ireland, and Australia, where the comparison model is predominantly a different model of midwifery care in a system where midwives rather than nurses and physicians provide care for labour and birth. Despite this being well described in the Cochrane review, the reaction to the evidence often revealed discomfort with the idea of comparing outcomes achieved by different care provider groups. Reluctance to look at the possible benefits of care provided by different care provider groups creates a challenge for those who need to make health policy decisions about health human resources. The sensitivity of this topic for all involved is exacerbated by the perceived need to reassure the public that the current system is functioning well, and the need for health care providers to maintain collegial relationships.

We found grounds of agreement about the importance of collaborative interprofessional relationships and choice of care provider, but our findings flag important debates about these common grounds. The call for collaborative models of health care provision is now more than a decade old and our findings reinforce the critiques of collaboration that have emerged. Proponents of collaboration often assume that it will encourage a level playing field between the professions. In fact, research shows that although collaboration can work to challenge hierarchy and support change (Downe, Findlayson, and Fleming 2010; McIntyre, Francis, and Chapman 2012), it does not necessarily have this impact. Collaborative care may reinforce existing hierarchies and tensions between health care professions (Downe, Findlayson, and Fleming 2010; Lane 2006; Peterson et al. 2007; Reiger 2008; Reiger and Lane 2009). Leape and colleagues (2012, 849) describe a constellation of factors that can work against a culture of respect in health care, including hierarchical relationships, threats to self-esteem, and overwork. Barriers to collaboration, such as concerns about income and professional territory (Peterson et al. 2007; Hunter and Segrott 2014), are, as our informants noted, often the same barriers to increasing access to midwifery-led care.

Any move towards either well-integrated MLCMs or interprofessional models that include midwives clearly needs to engage providers from all groups in a discussion of best practices and underlying interests and values. For some informants concerned about a negative reaction to an overt call to increase access to midwifery care, the concept of collaborative care offers a way of promoting midwifery without causing offence to other professions. They advocated for collaborative interprofessional models of care to address problematic interprofessional attitudes and to build relationships of trust. Other informants looked to collaboration to avoid problems of competition. It is interesting to note that in the current era of evidence-based practice and policymaking, the proposals for collaboration coming from this group of health care leaders were largely based on hopes for building relationships rather than on evidence about outcomes. In other words, collaborative interprofessional models were posed as politically rather than clinically necessary.

Our findings reveal the need for open discussion of shared and differing goals and values between care provider groups. This dialogue is a precondition for the mutual recognition and respect across differences that defines collaboration and is necessary for both interprofessional models and integrated midwifery-led models. Our informants note that if underlying structural issues, hierarchies, and values are not addressed, collaboration seems unlikely to flourish. This perspective is reinforced by policy reports (Ontario Maternity Care Expert Panel 2006) and research findings (Munro, Kornelsen, and Grzybowski 2012; Peterson et al. 2007).

Some of our informants expressed concerns that midwife-led care bolsters silos and "separate professional identities" that need to be broken down. Critiques of interprofessionalism and collaboration have problematized demands to break down silos, boundaries, and professional identities without examining hierarchical relationships, status, and marginalization (Lane 2005, 2006, 2012; Reiger 2008). Reiger (2008, 469) warns midwives and physicians alike about "othering" colleagues in other professions but argues that it is asymmetrical power relationships rather than identities that feed negative stereotypes and undermine relationships. Lane (2012, 29) describes an Australian approach to collaboration between midwives and obstetricians that required midwives to have care plans approved by obstetricians, thus "negat[ing] all that genuine collaboration stands for – equality, mutual trust and reciprocal respect."

Our interviews revealed widely varying interpretations of the Cochrane recommendation that "most women should be offered MLCM." The debate is taking place in Canada in the context of midwifery as a new and growing profession that is beginning to have implications for health human resources planning. Our informants frankly addressed the financial and job satisfaction challenges that the growing midwifery profession may pose to other professionals. In keeping with the evidence about change in health care, informants saw strong leadership (Antwi and Mruganka 2014) to be key. Incremental and opportunistic change was identified as an effective strategy to overcome resistance to further growth of midwifery or to creative approaches to interprofessional collaboration. This need for leadership and uptake of strategic opportunities for change is consistent with recommendations about moving towards a primary maternity care system with midwives and family physicians as care providers for normal birth (British Columbia Ministry of Health 2016; Ontario Maternity Care Expert Panel 2006; Peterson et al. 2007).

Both the descriptors "led" and "continuity" are important to the MLCM, and both concepts were challenged by some of our physician informants. Concerns that midwife-led care contributes to silos, rather than being seen as a beneficial health care innovation that could be incorporated into a well-integrated system, need to be addressed in interprofessional and policy forums. Misunderstandings about the cost and the feasibility of continuity models also need to be addressed, and further research is critical to taking up issues of cost.

We found support for a more flexible use of midwives throughout the system, whether by expanding their scope of practice, participating in collaborative teams, or working in new midwife-led models. We also found interest in exploring whether the findings of the Cochrane review could apply to family physicians or to teams of midwives and family physicians providing care in similar models. We found support across all of the professions that MLCMs are a viable or even optimal model in urban settings, tempered by a strong desire to also support family physician-led care. There was broad agreement that in rural or remote settings the viability of the whole health care team may require variations that could include midwife-led care, family physician-led care, or teams of interprofessional providers.

One of the key questions underlying the debate about the Cochrane evidence is the policy question about who should attend low-risk birth. Canada has a notable lack of policy on this question. Informants were reluctant to quantify the ideal provider mix, although many looked to a policy of low-risk providers for low-risk births as an ideal to strive for. Although one of the family physician leaders cited policy changes moving in this direction in Quebec, policy papers in Ontario (Health Quality Ontario 2016) and British Columbia (British Columbia Ministry of Health 2016) focus on setting standards and defining quality care for low-risk birth rather than on an analysis of provider mix.

Calls for systems change aimed at achieving lower intervention rates are not coming only from midwives. George Carson, then president of the SOGC, wrote an editorial in September 2016 outlining the harms of the overuse of intervention and asking members to "choose wisely" and "do everything that matters and nothing else." Carson notes that "by doing less, not more, we will spare patients harm and can free up resources for what is really helpful" (791). This discussion about how to avoid the overuse of obstetrical intervention is happening on the global level as high-income countries struggle to control rates of intervention that have been characterized as "too much too soon" while low-income countries face care that is often "too little too late" (Shaw et al. 2016). In the 2016 *Lancet* series on maternal health, obstetricians from Canada, the United States, and Sweden co-authored a review of drivers of care in high-income countries. They recommend that

> different models of care by providers should continue to be explored and evaluated in terms of their ability to meet women's needs, and reduce interventions, and costs, while outcomes are improved ... With evolving evidence and guidelines to support low-risk women planning birth at home or in hospital birth centres ... and resurgence of midwife-led care by licensed midwives in [high-income countries] where it had disappeared or waned, the tide of intervention-oriented birthing might be turning. (Shaw et al. 2016, 2295)

The Cochrane findings and the growing body of evidence that shows excellent outcomes for midwifery care fits with this move to low-intervention approaches and challenges the system of care for low-risk birth and current health human resources distribution in Canada. Our findings suggest that the conversation about who should attend low-risk births can be difficult but not impossible to have across professions and at policy tables. Choice of care provider cannot be a reality without both short-term and long-term planning about the appropriate mix of care providers.

Conclusion

Debates in Canada about the Cochrane review of midwife-led care illustrate the many professional and health systems issues that influence the application of evidence. The Cochrane review of MLCM focused on clinical outcomes of a relational model of care led by midwives. The debates about the Cochrane review in Canada are not focused on outcomes but rather on interprofessional relationships, scopes of practice, provider demographics, health care provider remuneration, and system sustainability. Our conversations with leaders in family medicine, midwifery, and obstetrics reveal willingness to have an open but challenging discussion about how to continue to integrate midwifery into Canada's health care system. They also illuminate how concepts such as collaboration are understood and used in divergent ways. Calls for collaborative care models are offered as a relationship-building strategy but tend to obscure other crucial issues such as hierarchies, status, and marginalization.

The response of health professionals to evidence about midwife-led care provides an example of how evidence is interpreted within the context of interprofessional interests and relationships and complex systems. Understanding the policy issues and social dynamics underlying disputes about the MLCM evidence helps makes visible the politics that policymakers and advocates for the growth of midwifery and for low-intervention models of care for childbirth need to address. It illustrates the reality that interests can shape how evidence is received and applied to practice, even when evidence is presented by the esteemed Cochrane review process.

REFERENCES

Antwi, M., and K. Mruganka. 2014. *Change Management in Health Care: A Literature Review.* Queen's School of Business, Kingston. https://smith.queensu.ca/centres/monieson/knowledge_articles/files/Change%20Management%20in%20Healthcare%20-%20Lit%20Review%20-%20AP%20FINAL.pdf.

Better Outcomes Registry Network (BORN). 2018. One in a Million: BORN Ontario Biennial Report 2016–2018. Ottawa: BORN Ontario. https://www.bornontario.ca/en/publications/resources/Documents/BORN-Biennial-Report-2016-18.pdf.

Blake, J. 2013a. "Comment on Midwife-Led Continuity Models versus Other Models of Care for Childbearing Women." *The Cochrane Database of Systematic Reviews* 4, art. no. CD004667, by J. Sandall, H. Soltani, S. Gates, A. Shennan, and D. Devane. https://www.cochranelibrary.com/cdsr/doi/10.1002/14651858.CD004667.pub5/read-comments.

Blake, J. 2013b. "SOGC Responds to The Cochrane Review 'Midwife-Led Continuity Models vs Other Models of Care for Childbearing Women.'" *SOGC Newsletter,* n.p.

Bourgeault, I.L. 2006. *Push! The Struggle for Midwifery in Canada.* Montreal: McGill-Queen's University Press.

Bourgeault, I.L. 2014. "Why Do We Have So Few Midwives in Canada?" *EvidenceNetwork.ca.* https://evidencenetwork.ca/why-do-we-have-so-few-midwives-in-canada/.

Bourgeault, I.L., and M. MacDonald. 2000. "The Politics of Representation: Doing and Writing 'Interested' Research on Midwifery." *Resources for Feminist Research* 28 (1): 151–68.

British Columbia Ministry of Health. 2016. *Primary Maternity Care: Moving Forward Together.* Victoria: Government of British Columbia. http://www.deslibris.ca/ID/248084.

Brocklehurst, P., P. Hardy, J. Hollowell, L. Linsell, A. Macfarlane, C. McCourt, N. Marlow, A. Miller, M. Newburn, and R. Rowe. 2011. "Perinatal and Maternal Outcomes by Planned Place of Birth for Healthy Women with Low Risk Pregnancies: The Birthplace in England National Prospective Cohort Study." *BMJ* 344 (November): 1–13. https://doi.org/10.1136/bmj.d7400.

Canadian Association of Midwives. 2019. *Annual Report 2018–19.* Montreal: CAM. https://canadianmidwives.org/wp-content/uploads/2019/11/ACSF-Rapport_Annuel_EN_v5-1.pdf.

Carson, G. 2016. "Don't Just Do Something, Stand There." *Journal of Obstetrics and Gynecology Canada* 38 (9): 791–2. https://doi.org/10.1016/j.jogc.2016.06.004.

Chalmers, I., M. Enkin, and M. Keirse. 1989. *Effective Care in Pregnancy and Childbirth.* Oxford: Oxford University Press.

de Melo-Martín, I., and K. Intemann. 2012. "Interpreting Evidence: Why Values Can Matter as Much as Science." *Perspectives in Biology and Medicine* 55 (1): 59–70. https://doi.org/10.1353/pbm.2012.0007.

Downe, S., K. Findlayson, and A. Fleming. 2010. "Creating a Collaborative Culture in Maternity Care." *Journal of Midwifery and Women's Health* 55 (3): 250–4. https://doi.org/10.1016/j.jmwh.2010.01.004.

Enkin, M.W., S. Glouberman, P. Groff, A.R. Jadad, A. Stern, and Clinamen Collaboration. 2006. "Beyond Evidence: The Complexity of Maternity Care." *Birth* 33 (4): 265–9. https://doi.org/10.1111/j.1523-536X.2006.00117.x.

Gawande, A. 2006. "The Score: How Childbirth Went Industrial." Annals of Medicine. *The New Yorker*, 1 October. https://www.newyorker.com/magazine/2006/10/09/the-score.

Glanz, M. 2013. "Midwife-Led Care Best for Babies and Moms, Researchers Say." CBC News, 20 August. http://www.cbc.ca/news/health/midwife-led-care-best-for-babies-and-moms-researchers-say-1.1368417.

Godlee, F. 2012. "Obstetrics and the Wooden Spoon." *BMJ* 345 (1): e7017. https://doi.org/10.1136/bmj.e7017.

Hatem, M., J. Sandall, D. Devane, H. Soltani, and S. Gates. 2008. "Midwife-Led versus Other Models of Care for Childbearing Women." *The Cochrane Database of Systematic Reviews* 4, art. no. CD004667: 1–71. https://doi.org/10.1002/14651858.CD004667.pub2.

Health Quality Ontario. 2016. *Quality-Based Procedure for Low Risk Birth.* Toronto: Ontario Ministry of Health and Long-Term Care. http://www.health.gov.on.ca/en/pro/programs/ecfa/docs/hb_low_risk_birth.pdf.

Hunter, B., and J. Segrott. 2014. "Renegotiating Inter-Professional Boundaries in Maternity Care: Implementing a Clinical Pathway for Normal Labour." *Sociology of Health & Illness* 36 (5): 719–37. https://doi.org/10.1111/1467-9566.12096.

Lane, K. 2005. "Still Suffering from the 'Silo Effect': Lingering Cultural Barriers to Collaborative Care." *Canadian Journal of Midwifery Research and Practice* 4 (1): 8–16. https://www.cjmrp.com/files/v4n1_lane_cultural-barriers.pdf.

Lane, K. 2006. "The Plasticity of Professional Boundaries: A Case Study of Collaborative Care in Maternity Services." *Health Sociology Review* 15 (4): 341–52. https://doi.org/10.5172/hesr.2006.15.4.341.

Lane, K. 2012. "When Is Collaboration Not Collaboration? When It's Militarized." *Women and Birth* 25 (1): 29–38. https://doi.org/10.1016/j.wombi.2011.03.003.

Leape, L.L., M.F. Shore, J.L. Dienstag, R.J. Mayer, S. Edgman-Levitan, G.S. Meyer, and G.B. Healy. 2012. "Perspective: A Culture of Respect, Part 1 and Part 2." *Academic Medicine* 87 (7): 845–58. https://doi.org/10.1097/ACM.0b013e318258338d.

MacDonald, M.E. 2017. "The Making of Informed Choice in Midwifery: A Feminist Experiment in Care." *Culture, Medicine and Psychiatry* 42 (2): 278–94. https://doi.org/10.1007/s11013-017-9560-9.

McIntyre, M., K. Francis, and Y. Chapman. 2012. "The Struggle for Contested Boundaries in the Move to Collaborative Care Teams in Australian Maternity Care." *Midwifery* 28 (3): 298–305. https://doi.org/10.1016/j.midw.2011.04.004.

Melnyk, B.M., E. Fineout-Overholt, L. Gallagher-Ford, and L. Kaplan. 2012. "The State of Evidence-Based Practice in US Nurses: Critical Implications for Nurse Leaders and Educators." *Journal of Nursing Administration* 42 (9): 410–17. https://doi.org/10.1097/NNA.0b013e3182664e0a.

Morgan, L., G. Carson, A. Gagnon, and J. Blake. 2014. "Collaborative Practice among Obstetricians, Family Physicians and Midwives. " *Canadian Medical Association Journal* 186 (17): 1279–80. https://doi.org/10.1503/cmaj.140537.

Munro, S., J. Kornelsen, and S. Grzybowski. 2012. "Models of Maternity Care in Rural Environments: Barriers and Attributes of Interprofessional Collaboration with Midwives." *Midwifery* 29 (6): 646–52. https://doi.org/10.1016/j.midw.2012.06.004.

Mykhalovskiy, E., and L. Weir. 2004. "The Problem of Evidence-Based Medicine: Directions for Social Science." *Social Science & Medicine* 59 (5): 1059–69. https://doi.org/10.1016/j.socscimed.2003.12.002.

NICE. 2017. *Intrapartum Care for Healthy Women and Babies: Clinical Guideline* (CG190). https://www.nice.org.uk/guidance/cg190 1–89.

Ontario Maternity Care Expert Panel. 2006. *Maternity Care in Ontario 2006: Emerging Crisis, Emerging Solutions.* Toronto: Ontario Women's Health Council.

Ontario Ministry of Health and Long-Term Care. 2012. *Ontario's Action Plan for Health Care.* Toronto: Government of Ontario.

Peterson, W.E., J. Medves, B. Davies, and I. Graham. 2007. "Multidisciplinary Collaborative Maternity Care in Canada: Easier Said than Done." *Journal of Obstetrics and Gynaecology Canada* 29 (11): 880–6. https://doi.org/10.1016/S1701-2163(16)32659-7.

Reiger, K. 2008. "Domination or Mutual Recognition? Professional Subjectivity in Midwifery and Obstetrics." *Social Theory & Health* 6 (2): 132–47. https://doi.org/10.1057/palgrave.sth.2007.12.

Reiger, K.M. 2001. *Our Bodies, Our Babies: The Forgotten Women's Movement,* 1st ed. Melbourne: Melbourne University Press.

Reiger, K., and L. Lane. 2009. "Working Together: Collaboration between Midwives and Doctors in Public Hospital Settings." *Australian Health Review* 33: 315–24. https://doi.org/10.1071/AH090315.

Reynolds, L. 2001. "Recommendations for a Sustainable Model of Maternity and Newborn Care in Canada." In *Proceedings of the Future of Maternity Care in Canada: Crisis and Opportunity,* edited by L. Reynolds and M.C. Klein. London, ON.

Royal College of Obstetricians and Gynaecologists (RCOG). 2001. "The National Sentinel Caesarean Section Audit Report." London: RCOG Clinical Effectiveness Support Unit.

Sandall, J., H. Soltani, S. Gates, A. Shennan, and D. Devane. 2013. "Midwife-Led Continuity Models versus Other Models of Care for Childbearing Women." *The Cochrane Database of Systematic Reviews* (8) CD004667: 1–107. https://doi.org/10.1002/14651858.CD004667.pub3.

Sandall, J., H. Soltani, S. Gates, A. Shennan, and D. Devane. 2016. "Midwife-Led Continuity Models versus Other Models of Care for Childbearing Women." *The Cochrane Database of Systematic Reviews* (4) CD004667: 1–118. https://doi.org/10.1002/14651858.CD004667.pub5.

Shah, N. 2015. "A NICE Delivery: The Cross-Atlantic Divide over Treatment Intensity in Childbirth." *New England Journal of Medicine* 372 (23): 2181–3. https://doi.org/10.1056/NEJMp1501461.

Shaw, D., J.-M. Guise, N. Shah, K. Gemzell-Danielsson, K.S. Joseph, B. Levy, F. Wong, S. Woodd, and E.K. Main. 2016. "Drivers of Maternity Care in High-Income Countries: Can Health Systems Support Woman-Centred Care?" *The Lancet* 388 (10057): 2282–95.

Society of Obstetricians and Gynaecologists of Canada (SOGC). 2009. "Policy Statement on Midwifery." *Journal of Obstetrics and Gynaecology Canada* 31 (7): 662. https://doi.org/10.1016/S1701-2163(16)34248-7.

Tracy, SK., D. Hartz, B. Hall, J. Allen, A. Forti, A. Lainchbury, J. White, A. Welsh, M. Tracy, and S. Kildea. 2011. "A Randomised Controlled Trial of Caseload Midwifery Care: M@NGO (Midwives @ New Group Practice Options)." *BMC Pregnancy and Childbirth* 11 (1): 82. https://doi.org/10.1186/1471-2393-11-82.

Van Wagner, V. 2013. "Reconsidering Evidence: Evidence-Based Practice and Maternity Care in Canada." PhD diss., York University, Toronto. https://yorkspace.library.yorku.ca/xmlui/handle/10315/31318.

White Ribbon Alliance. 2011. "Respectful Maternity Care." https://www.whiteribbonalliance.org/respectful-maternity-care-charter/.

Wilson, C.R. 2013. "Policy and Evidence in Canadian Health Human Resources Planning." *HealthcarePapers* 13 (2): 28–31. https://doi.org/10.12927/hcpap.2013.23523.

6 "Tell Me Where It Hurts": A Case Study of the Impacts of Structural Violence, Syndemic Suffering, and Intergenerational Trauma on Indigenous Peoples' Health

CHRISTIANNE V. STEPHENS

The measurement and interpretation of population health outcomes is based largely on faith in the objectivity, reliability, representativeness, and generalizability of biostatistics. Quantitative health studies that analyse data through numerical comparisons and statistical inferences remain the gold standard of evidence-based medicine. Yet for many social scientists working with marginalized populations an age-old question remains: Do conventional epidemiological methods always provide an accurate and holistic picture of health? Or are there occasions when statistical figures underestimate the social suffering, health disparities, and inequities endured by specific groups of people?

Epidemiological research about patterns of disease and health risks in Indigenous communities is important because it can provide useful information on the prevalence of chronic diseases and the impacts of social determinants on health. However, epidemiological research has its limits. Studies have revealed that the health of Indigenous peoples in reserve communities and urban centres in Canada is not only poor but often inappropriately measured. It is also the case that explanations of poor health that are expressed through statistical associations can fail to reveal the true structural processes of inequality and colonialism at the root of health inequalities affecting Indigenous peoples. As a social scientist and medical anthropologist, I recognize the tension between numbers and narratives in researching Indigenous health. While I acknowledge the valuable role that baseline statistical data can play in understanding broad health trends, this chapter commits to a close narrative analysis of three relations (structural violence, syndemic suffering, and intergenerational trauma) to more fully reveal the complex interplay of biological, behavioural, sociopolitical, and historical factors (Waldram, Herring, and Young 2006) that shape health profiles, as well as the multiple ways that health outcomes experienced by Indigenous peoples are amplified by a shared history of cumulative trauma.

There are many factors that compromise the integrity of statistical information collected on First Nations health, among them variable coverage and quality of data, inconsistent and problematic use of ethnic identifiers for designating Native status in official records, insufficient infrastructure and human resources to properly collect and manage health information, and low response rates of reserve communities to the Canadian census and other federally administered surveys (Minore, Katt, and Hill 2009). There is growing awareness of the Eurocentric assumptions that inform biomedical, epidemiological, and evidence-based perspectives. These perspectives are problematic because they are often incommensurable with Indigenous worldviews, epistemologies, and methodologies. Other practices, such as the uncritical use of generic "Pan-Indian" surveys, contribute to false and misleading constructions of Indigenous experiences as homogeneous, glossing over "profound differences in traditions, identity, and residency" (Minore, Katt, and Hill 2009, 93).

The ethnographic field site that is the focus of this study[1] has revealed a confluence of additional factors that can hinder attempts to study health outcomes by standard epidemiological methods at the community level. Incomplete on-reserve health records of band members, minimal communication and information sharing between on- and off-reserve health care providers, negative community perceptions of the research process, and residents' aversion to health questionnaires that are not community-specific or culturally appropriate are some of the barriers encountered when attempting to measure and assess the health of reserve communities (Stephens 2012). These findings raise fundamental questions about the capacity of bureaucratic mechanisms to represent the spectrum of local health risks and the complex determinants that shape the contours of community health profiles. The consequences arising from such challenges extend beyond the realms of academic theorizing and ethical debates. Failure to maintain accurate community health statistics can impede efforts to identify health needs and priorities, which hinders ability to secure the resources required to develop and implement effective policies, programs, and best practices in health care management.

To address these issues, this study uses ethically and culturally sensitive measures and indicators developed in collaboration with community partners to collect and interpret baseline health data that will help to inform community health policy and strategic planning. The preliminary findings provide a general overview of the state of community health and its social determinants, as well as the cumulative impacts of high disease burdens compounded by complex trauma histories. This chapter presents a case study based on the illness experiences of multiple members of a single family. This is a qualitative study relying mostly on narrative analysis. An iterative process of data analysis (Strauss and Corbin 1998) was employed to explore themes from data collected through one-on-one interviews with participants. The discourses serve as an exemplar of how health outcomes and health care experiences are organized by three distinct relations: structural violence, syndemic suffering, and intergenerational trauma. The study findings will be used to improve the health status of community members by enhancing community health policies, programs, and service delivery.

Research Context

My research collaboration with members of the Ontario First Nation spans seventeen years, during which time I have conducted archival research on historical health outcomes, explored the impacts of residential schools on community well-being, and studied environmental risk perception and communication. The First Nation shares a number of characteristics with other Indigenous communities in Canada, including a long residential school history.[2] Elders in the community struggle with memories of physical, sexual, mental, and emotional abuse. These are silent wounds that manifest as anxiety, depression, post-traumatic stress disorder, and, in some instances, unhealthy coping behaviours (alcoholism, substance abuse, and other forms of self-harm) (Stephens 2006).

Environmental health issues are of major concern, especially the contamination of water and local fish and wildlife. The community holds stewardship over a rich mosaic of natural areas that residents rely on for their subsistence and livelihoods. Decades of accidental chemical spills and legal discharges from Canadian and American industries have historically impaired water quality in the region, threatening the integrity and sustainability of the local natural resources and traditional economies. My previous research revealed that community constructions of environmental risk differ radically from science and media constructions of "chemophobia" – a pejorative concept used to discredit people's concerns about contamination from toxic exposure (Stephens 2009). Community members deploy what I call "toxic talk," a unique genre of discourse through which experiential, locally grounded, and culturally entrenched ways of understanding environmental health risks are expressed (Stephens 2009). The research illuminates how residents experience environmental crises and conceptualize community health and well-being. Environmental issues and their health outcomes are not viewed as evolving in isolation from broader sociopolitical processes, but are framed as concrete examples of colonial violence that must be understood within a historical framework of Indigenous-settler relations.

The absence of baseline community health data has led to substantial knowledge gaps, which in turn breed uncertainty and stoke long-standing fears among residents about the safety of the environment and the potential health outcomes associated with exposure to contaminated food sources (Stephens 2012). Community anxiety is manifested as publicly voiced concern over the perception that community members are experiencing disproportionately high rates of morbidity and mortality. The lack of standard epidemiological data has evoked a sense of powerlessness over health matters. It also stands as a barrier to understanding changes in community health through time. The frustration of community members is palpable, especially for those fighting for environmental protection and social justice, who view their efforts as significantly hindered by the absence of reliable health information. Without a clear baseline, it is exceedingly difficult to assess the degree to which community health has been compromised by colonial incursions (Stephens 2012).

The search for solutions to these long-standing issues set in motion what would become the basis for the present community-driven, grassroots comprehensive health study. In 2008, I began working closely with different community departments and groups, all of whom share an interest in human and environmental health issues. Our primary goal was to develop a study to collect baseline data on the health status of residents, and to document the degree to which community health and well-being may be influenced by local physical and social environments. An important component of this project involves depicting the health information in a visual format known as *body mapping* in order to identify disease clusters and to provide a picture of community health that transcends educational, cultural, and language barriers and is easily accessible to community members (Keith and Brophy 2004). Publication of the community body-mapping research findings is forthcoming.

Our health study was developed and designed through the support and contributions of several community partners[3] and was approved by the community's research committees, chief and band council, and York University's Research Ethics Board. Participants included band members (eighteen years of age and older) who reside on reserve. They were selected through chain-sampling, and active recruitment drives were held at several community events. We worked hard to include participants who varied in terms of age, education, socio-economic status, residential locations, spiritual beliefs, employment status, occupation, and subsistence strategies (e.g., including those who continued to subsist on local resources such as fish and wild game).We developed a research tool for collecting the health information that the community sought. We were mindful of the need to develop questions that would reflect the ecological, social, economic, and demographic characteristics of the First Nation, along with the health needs and concerns of its residents. The product was an in-depth and comprehensive interview guide/questionnaire that applies a holistic lens and casts a wide net to capture the multiple variables that shape community health and well-being. The original intent was to train a community member from our research team to conduct the interviews. However, due to privacy concerns and to ensure that the confidentiality of participants was protected, I was asked by the team to conduct all of the study interviews. I completed 250 interviews over the course of two years (2015–16). Interviews were tape-recorded and averaged two hours in length. I also interviewed over thirty health care providers who work on and off reserve in nearby towns and cities including, for example, family physicians, addiction specialists, dentists, social workers, mental health workers, and traditional healers.

The case study draws on the oral histories and lived experiences of several members of the Wilson family – Rachel, her husband David, their adult children, and extended kin[4] whose lives are intimately connected and who share common experiences of illness and interactions with the health care system. My analysis involves "re-storying" and condensing the life histories and testimonies of family members into a cohesive narrative account in order to explore the multiple dimensions of their family health genealogy. I draw from the life histories to illustrate an important community-wide pattern that has emerged through the research. The narratives reveal both the obvious and the subtle ways that disease and trauma work their way through the bodies, minds, and spirits of multiple generations of community members.

What emerges from the data is that most health outcomes and health care experiences are shaped by three relations that are tied to the forces of colonialism, racism, and systemic discrimination. These are: *structural violence*, the social arrangements that put individuals and populations in harm's way, manifested in the sphere of health as health disparities and unequal access to health care experienced by the poor and marginalized (Farmer 1999, 2003, 2004, 2006); *syndemic suffering*, "situations in which adverse social conditions, such as poverty and oppressive social relationships stress a population, weaken its natural defenses, and expose it to a cluster of interacting diseases" (Mendenhall 2012; Singer and Clair 2003); and *intergenerational trauma*, the transmission of historical oppression and its negative consequences across generations (Brave Heart 2003; Brave Heart and De Bruyn 1998; Pember 2016).

Findings

Narratives of Structural Violence

For centuries, Indigenous populations have suffered from racism, classism, sexism, and discrimination operating within and perpetuated by social institutions that hinder people from fulfilling their basic needs. Structural violence alerts us to the distal causes of health disparities that foster the social conditions that allow certain diseases to thrive and hinder some people from accessing the health care services they require (Farmer 1999, 2003, 2004, 2006). The most blatant form of structural violence described by Rachel and members of her family is their experiences of the residential school system. These stories serve as powerful illustrations of the enduring impacts of residential school trauma on the health and well-being of the First Nation's community members.

Rachel was just four and a half years old when she and her older brother, John, were forcibly taken from their home and placed in the Shingwauk Indian Residential School in Sault Ste. Marie, Ontario, located approximately a six-and-a-half-hour drive north of her home community. The events of that day are seared into Rachel's memory. She recounts: "We were kidnapped from our homes and placed into the residential school. My brother and I, along with four other girls from our community, were taken from our community and sent to Shingwauk on the same day. When we arrived at the school, we were marched up a big set of stairs at the front of the building. It was very scary and intimidating."

Rachel talks a great deal about the food that was fed to students. She remembers the oatmeal or "mush" that was such a staple at residential schools that the institutions were referred to as "mush holes" by the students who attended them. Rachel describes how the mush and other foods in the school were foreign to her. She remembers the bland taste and occasions when the mush was inedible because it was spoiled or contaminated with maggots or mouse droppings. Despite the pressure to consume the mush, Rachel often refused to eat it. She shared other disturbing memories of children being forced to eat their own vomit after getting sick from consuming food that disagreed with them. She wonders whether abstaining from breakfast during her formative years and living with chronic daily stress, sadness, and separation anxiety have adversely affected her health. Rachel attributes the hypertension that she's managed since her early twenties and her macular degeneration to the difficult living conditions she endured while at Shingwauk. She recalls the time when she visited a dentist as an adult and was told that her teeth showed evidence of incomplete or underdeveloped tooth enamel – a marker that has been attributed to environmental stressors including, but not limited to, nutritional factors such as malnutrition or infection. Recent studies have sought to record and substantiate the potential long-term health effects of severe nutritional deficiencies on the health of residential school survivors (Galloway and Mosby 2017; Mosby 2013). Rachel remembers eating a poorly balanced diet with little in the way of proteins, fresh fruits, and vegetables. She attributes her current love of tomatoes to the deprivation that she experienced while at residential school. She remembers her chronic hunger and describes how the boys in particular were always "starving." She recalls how she would surreptitiously place her allotted portion of bread in the spot where her brother sat in the common dining room in an attempt to alleviate his hunger.

Rachel also talks about the rampant disease outbreaks that plagued the school and the inadequate health care that was provided to ailing students. She remembers being very sick with a bad fever at the age of five. She was taken to the school's infirmary but was not seen by a doctor. She explained that the school principal would need to write to Ottawa for permission to bring a doctor to examine the children, so students rarely if ever received the medical care they needed. Many children who contracted communicable diseases like tuberculosis or influenza were taken to the infirmary and were never seen again by their fellow students. The high mortality rates of students from disease and the related neglect have been documented by scholars (Milloy 1999) and identified by the Truth and Reconciliation Commission (2015) as an area requiring further investigation and redress.

The graves of children that populate Shingwauk's cemetery are a grim reminder of the young lives that were lost there. Rachel and her brother John were directly affected by death while at residential school. Their eldest brother, Steven, who was sent to Shingwauk years before Rachel and John's arrival, died there as a teenager from an untreated medical condition. Like many of the children who are buried in the school's cemetery, Steven's final resting place is not marked by a tombstone. Rachel's family visits the cemetery every year to clean the area where they believe Steven's grave is located. The cause of Steven's death was never disclosed to his family, and Rachel only learned the details of his passing from one of her brother's former classmates. Often the boys who attended Shingwauk would secretly abscond to the wooded areas surrounding the institution to hunt for small animals that they would use to supplement their meagre diet. During one such trip, Steven developed a sharp pain in his side. After he returned to the school seeking help, the staff placed him in the infirmary but failed to call a doctor to attend to him. Rachel and her family believe that the school staff were under the impression that Steven had tried to run away from the school and withheld treatment for his serious condition as a way of punishing him. He died a few days later from a ruptured appendix. The fact that her brother succumbed to a treatable condition, and no one was held accountable for his death, has left the family with little closure and an unrelenting emotional wound.

Rachel's younger brother, John, was burdened with an additional layer of sorrow. At the age of eight, John was summoned to sit with Steven in the infirmary where he was forced to watch his brother die and was warned by staff members: "this is what will happen to you if you run away." Bearing witness to his brother's painful death, along with the other traumas incurred while at residential school, took an immense toll on John. Rachel recounts how John became hypervigilant later in life; he always looked behind him when he walked and would sit with his back to the wall – a holdover from the residential school days when he lived in constant fear of being bullied or beaten by teachers and students. Rachel also remembers how quiet and withdrawn her brother was, how he never spoke up, and how easily he would "crumble under someone else's abuse." John abused alcohol and suffered from post-traumatic stress disorder (PTSD). Rachel strongly believes that her brother's drinking and mental distress were caused by the violence and trauma that were inflicted upon him at Shingwauk. She made a point of emphasizing that "John was only able to quit his drinking when he was able to give up his burdens."

John's negative residential school experiences not only tormented him psychologically; they also shaped his views of institutions and authority figures. His reluctance as an adult to seek medical attention for his degenerating health is a tangible behavioural outcome that is tied directly to this history. As one community health nurse who was familiar with John's health challenges confided to me: "John was terminally ill with brain cancer and my biggest challenge was to get him to talk to me, to tell me what his needs were, or tell me if he had pain or discomfort." She further explained that he was quiet, unassuming, proud, and kept his pain to himself, refusing to go to a doctor until his cancer had spread to other parts of his body and was too far gone to treat.

Rachel and her brothers were the second generation of their family to be sent to residential school. Their mother, Lily, a Potawatomi from Wisconsin, was sent to the Mt. Pleasant Residential School in the state of Michigan after her mother died. Residential school left Rachel's mother "dead inside," emotionally volatile, and lacking the ability to nurture her children. Rachel recounted the time when her mother tore up a new suit that Rachel had bought for herself with money she earned through a summer job. Rachel was perplexed by her mother's behaviour but surmised that it was likely due to her having "abdicated her role as a mother" when her children were taken away, and that this separation robbed her of the ability to bond with her children and develop the capacity to express emotions and parental love in a healthy way. Rachel believes that her mother felt guilty later in life:

> Before she died from a heart attack, my mother said: "I'm sorry, Rachel." My mother suffered from the effects of multiple strokes, so I didn't know if she meant that she was sorry for something that she said or did five minutes ago, or if it went further back, meaning that she was sorry for letting the Indian agent take me and my brothers away from our home and placing us in Shingwauk. My mother was a residential school survivor, so she was traumatized, and I guess she realized that she had hurt us. She also probably felt guilty for not being able to protect us. I guess the saying is true: hurt people *hurt* people.

Having their children taken away (or kidnapped, in the words of many survivors) and forcibly placed in the residential school system had devastating impacts on the parents who were unable to protect them. For many, the legacy of this history is expressed in guilt, anger, violence, regret, despair, denial, avoidance, and numbing or self-medicating behaviours. For children like Rachel, being torn away from her family led to deep abandonment issues that continue to affect her. She shared the following account: "I never say 'good-bye' to anyone. In our Native language it is common to say '*baamaapii,*' which means 'see you later,' but I think that my reason for not saying good-bye is rooted in being kidnapped from my family and from the fear of never seeing someone again if I ever speak that word."

Rachel's narratives also describe different forms of abuse, including bullying, physical violence, severe punishment, and forced acculturation to the ways of Western settler society, which contributed to the loss of her language and cultural identity. One particularly difficult memory is of her separation from her sibling upon arrival at Shingwauk and the unpleasant experience of having her hair cut and "de-loused":

> The school separated the boys from the girls so I was immediately separated from my brother, who I wasn't allowed to talk to for five years. They took us down to the playroom but it was not colourful like today's playrooms. It was an unfriendly place that was dark, cold, and dingy with exposed pipes. I remember it well because that's where they cut off our hair and doused us in kerosene because they thought we had bugs. They kept the kerosene on

> us for four days. It was just awful – the kerosene was greasy, smelled terrible, and was hard to wash off with the cold water they used to rinse out our hair.

Rachel speaks openly about how she coped with the stressors of life in the school, and how these experiences continue to shape her outlook and behaviours. The pressure to conform was instilled in students and persists in survivors. As she observes: "Living and dying by the bells, being always told to be quiet and sit still, not having permission to go to the bathroom when we needed to, finishing everything off of our plates – all these behaviours that were drilled into us affected my choices and I passed these rules and habits onto my kids." Conforming, avoiding conflict, fully assimilating, and always saying "yes" were the strategies that Rachel used to survive during her time in Shingwauk: "My coping mechanism was to obey the rules and fully assimilate. I didn't like to fight, or to be strapped, or be confined in a cupboard with water and bread. I gave up my individuality, my free will, and my freedom in order to survive."

Rachel's narratives powerfully illustrate the scope and brutality of structural violence perpetrated in residential schools, and echo experiences shared by many of the Elders interviewed as part of the study. An important part of Rachel's healing journey has been her heightened self-awareness and capacity "to connect the dots" between her past experiences and present-day reality.

Narratives of Syndemic Suffering

When structural violence is at play, people are not only at greater risk of getting sick – they get sicker and are more vulnerable to contracting other diseases, or developing more severe complications, an outcome known as syndemic suffering. Emily Mendenhall (2012) gives an excellent example of syndemic suffering in her research on the feedback loop of depression and chronic disease experienced by Mexican immigrant women. Her analysis focuses on a causal web of five core elements of health and well-being that she names syndemic VIDDA: Violence, Immigration, Depression, type II Diabetes, and Abuse. Scholars studying Indigenous health are beginning to recognize the value of syndemic theory as a model for understanding patterns of infectious disease outbreaks historically (Herring and Sattenspiel 2007; Stephens 2008a, 2008b, 2009) and developing effective responses to contemporary public health threats (Andermann 2017).

Rachel's husband, David, has a complex health history that reads like a textbook case of syndemic suffering. His experiences paint a vivid picture of the health outcomes associated with enduring a lifetime of biosocial stressors. David's life was shaped significantly by his time in residential school, the military, and prison. Life in total institutions (Goffman 1961) such as these is not only separated from the wider society but includes a lack of freedom, enforced conformity, and a transformation in identity through resocialization. After his time at Shingwauk (he and his brother decided not to go back to the school after returning home one summer and went to live in Detroit to be away from the authorities), David served fourteen years in the United States Marines and Air Force. He married Rachel (whom he knew as a toddler and became reacquainted with later on in life) and moved frequently across the United States, residing at a number of US military bases. Life in the military took David to different places around the world, including Greenland, Vietnam, Korea, Thailand, Japan, and the Philippines. Although David speaks proudly of certain aspects of his tours of duty, he recognizes that many of his military experiences have had a negative impact on his health. He sustained serious injuries: he was stabbed in the back in Korea by the first man he ever shot; in Vietnam he was shot by a sniper. He was also exposed to Agent Orange (a defoliant and known carcinogen) during his tour in Vietnam and strongly believes that his diabetes is the result of this exposure:

> When I was tested for diabetes at the age of fifty-five, the doctor at the veteran's hospital asked me whether I had served in Vietnam. When I confirmed that I had, he told me that a lot of Vietnam veterans with no family history of diabetes developed the condition as the result of exposure to Agent Orange, along with developing additional health problems.[5]

David also contracted malaria while he was stationed in the jungle during the Korean War. He was sick for at least a decade (1954–64) and wasn't diagnosed until he returned home and developed heart problems.

David admits to having a hard time adjusting to life when he returned from the military. He quotes his wife as saying that "he had an agenda all his own." David's life took a sudden turn when he was sentenced to a lengthy prison sentence for committing a serious crime. When he was released from prison, he felt further isolated and disconnected from his family and society at large. He had difficulty holding down a job, which was financially challenging for his family. At one point, he tried to return to military service but, as he explained, they wouldn't take him because he had already started a family. David also talked about the racism he experienced in the military: "There was lots of racism. I thought they'd be able to overcome racism in the Forces, but even the higher-ranking sergeants couldn't rise above it."

I asked David about whether his lengthy time in institutions affected him emotionally or psychologically. David did not speak directly about having PTSD. His response was simply: "Ask my wife about it, she knows better." When I did, she confirmed that David exhibits many of the symptoms associated with PTSD. What David did choose to disclose about his time in institutions is very telling:

> I went from residential school to the military and then also did time in prison. We lived and died by bells. I never got enough to eat or time to sleep. My time in residential school and prison taught me to be a fighter. My years in the military taught me to be a killer. They teach you how to do something as well as they can teach you and you can learn it, but they don't "untrain" you.

David compared his experiences in residential school to those in the military. He'd been in two wars, and despite "sleeping in foxholes full of mud, being shot at and at risk of being killed at any moment," he confesses that he "had a better time in Vietnam and Korea than the two years spent in Shingwauk."

Although David's emotional scars may not be visible to those who do not know him intimately, his multiple physical afflictions represent a "laundry list" of syndemic suffering. He has had ulcers and acid reflux since the age of twenty-five due to stress. He suffered from undiagnosed angina for years and experienced a heart attack at age fifty-one, which led to a quadruple bypass in his mid-fifties. He has a history of strokes, hypertension, and high cholesterol. His left leg was amputated on his seventieth birthday because of complications from diabetes. David has been diagnosed with four different types of cancers. He had cancer of the lower bowel, which was removed during surgery. He was diagnosed with prostate cancer at the age of sixty-eight, which was initially treated with surgery but later recurred. David was diagnosed with skin cancer at the age of seventy-seven and again underwent surgery. He was diagnosed with bone cancer at seventy-nine but has not received treatment because it is slow growing. David died in June 2017 after a devastating series of heart attacks and strokes. It was the second major loss experienced by the family in as many years. The Wilson's daughter, Deborah, had tragically died of cancer the previous year.

David's narratives reveal how co-occurring disease events, within the context of a family unit already stressed by collective trauma, grief, loss, and discrimination, are amplified, and how health crises pose significant challenges to those who are most vulnerable.

Narratives of Intergenerational Trauma

Intergenerational trauma is described as "a collective, complex, trauma inflicted on a group of people who share a specific group identity or affiliation (ethnicity, nationality, and religious affiliation) that has been experienced by a community over generations and encompasses the psychological and social responses to such events" (Evans Campbell 2008, 320). Researchers have studied the biological basis of trauma and its potential intergenerational transmission. Advances in the field of epigenetics are shedding light on the capacity of genes to carry inherited memories that can influence how we react to trauma and stress, while studies on adverse childhood experiences reveal that high rates of addiction, suicide, mental illness, sexual violence, and other social conditions may be influenced by historical and intergenerational trauma (Pember 2016, 3). Indigenous scholar Bonnie Durand notes that "many present-day health disparities can be traced back through epigenetics to a 'colonial health deficit,' the result of colonization and its aftermath" (quoted in Pember 2016, 3). Although the idea that memories can be embodied is relatively new for Western science, it is well known among Indigenous healers and Elders, who refer to it as "blood memory."

In my research, the most concrete examples of the psychosocial outcomes of intergenerational trauma were provided by Rachel and David's son, Paul. Despite being outgoing and financially successful, Paul describes himself as a "survivor of intergenerational trauma." Reflecting on the sheer magnitude of the residential school legacy, he notes:

> There were 150,000 children who were taken and put in these schools. They were robbed of a big chunk of their lives. These kids missed out on being nurtured or taught things in the Native culture by their grandparents, who'd teach their grandkids how to hunt, fish, and gather. I have two generations that went to residential school on my mom's side and three generations that went on my dad's side. My mom didn't know her grandmother, I hardly knew my grandparents. I don't have any recollection of grandparents. Although I've lived a normal life, I still have residential school stuff trickling down.

One of the most widely studied by-products of the residential school legacy is its impact on the parent-child relationship. Paul's narratives highlight how the absence of love, nurturing, and parental guidance has left an indelible mark on the children, grandchildren, and great-grandchildren of residential school survivors. He notes: "the most valuable component of families – love, care, and nurturing – were gone. What happens to the generations of those children it affects downstream? Some of the stuff that happened to them is what they do to their kids." There were no positive role models for healthy relationships. As Rachel informed me, residential school teachers were mostly unwed women with little experience with children. There was no nurturing in the schools, no reference point for giving or receiving kindness or care. In addition, students were routinely abused, which perpetuated later cycles of abuse within families. Paul speaks to the ripple effects of this history in terms of the pain and dysfunction he has experienced and witnessed in the lives of community residents. Although Paul admires his parents and is grateful for the life they have given him and his siblings, he is aware of how the rigid, authoritarian structure of his childhood, coupled with his "fragmented identity," which he attributes to the disconnection he feels from his ancestors, culture, and traditional territory, have affected his identity, self-worth, and belonging.

Paul discusses his proclivity for internalizing feelings of shame, guilt, anger, fear, and grief. He notes that "just like their parents who feel shame in discussing their residential school experiences, the children of survivors are unable to openly express their emotions." He also believes that this trait has been passed down to his own son, Joel (a young man in his twenties), who was unable to grieve the death of his maternal grandmother. Paul reflects on how Joel handled the pain "in the residential school way": he "kept it in" – a coping mechanism that Joel learned from his father, who learned it from his parents. Paul also describes another symptom that he attributes to intergenerational trauma: self-sabotaging and risk-taking behaviours that can lead to injury and death. Paul sees this trait in himself, especially in some of the risks that he takes in his personal life. Other traits and behaviours that Paul attributes to his parents' traumatic histories include his struggle to maintain fulfilling relationships and his inability to handle conflict in a healthy way. Paul also describes his deep scepticism and lack of trust of people, especially those who are non-Native. He sees this trait as a product of both intergenerational trauma and his recognition of the many broken promises and abuses perpetrated against Indigenous peoples in the areas of land and treaty rights, political autonomy, sovereignty, and self-governance. This distrust has influenced many areas of his life, shaped his day-to-day interactions, and negatively affected his mental health and personal and professional growth.

Rachel casts light on the interpersonal and wider social impacts of historical trauma and its intergenerational effects on female and male survivors and their children. Children at residential school were told "You're no good, you're going to hell." They carry this belief into adulthood and feel that they're not deserving of good health. The toxic residential school environment shaped how girls were socialized and how they viewed themselves. Male authority figures exercised control over the young girls, who felt powerless. These formative experiences greatly influenced their life choices: "society told females that we needed to get married and have children. A woman couldn't say 'no.' In residential school we had no voice, and this extended into our lives after we left the school." Young girls were thrust into the role of protectors, which Rachel identifies as traditionally a male role. Many girls took on a parenting role as they protected younger siblings and other vulnerable children. This has resulted in women who attend to everyone's needs except their own. Rachel explains how this ethos seeps into other areas of women's lives and prevents them from "doing things that need to be done" beyond family commitments, such as taking on larger societal issues. She also sees connections between historical trauma and the legacy of the "absent male" in Indigenous families due to incarceration, military service, addiction, and divorce.

To understand the profound impacts of colonial violence, assimilation, and forced acculturation, it is necessary to study both the negative outcomes of abuse and trauma and also the factors that contribute to Indigenous peoples' resiliency, that allow them to overcome adversity. As Rachel explains: "My husband and I have been married for sixty-two years. To get my family through all of this, I've been dedicated to 'building togetherness.' It's also important to become a champion for a cause that you are passionate about, whether it be health, environmental issues, or language revitalization in your community. You need to contribute to these things – it's an essential part of growing and healing." Rachel died from a massive stroke in the summer of 2019. Her advocacy work for Indigenous rights and reconciliation serves as an inspiration and lasting legacy for those in her community and beyond.

Conclusion

Health discourses provide insights into how people's "biography becomes their biology" (Myss 1996). The illness narratives of community members, as demonstrated by the Wilson family, reveal how structural violence, syndemic suffering, and intergenerational trauma influence a wide range of experiences, including health worldviews, clinical encounters, and the severity of disease. Through qualitative research we can bear witness to the ways in which these relations manifest in people's daily lives and the phenomenological aspects of personal pain, suffering, and trauma. We can also observe the ways in which the past lives on in the lives of residential school survivors and their descendants to shape contemporary eating patterns, parenting styles, disease outcomes, health-seeking behaviours, notions of self-worth, personal relationships, and strategies for managing stress, loss, and everyday hardships.

If poor health can be understood as the biological manifestation of poverty, injustice, inequities, and social suffering (Adelson 2005; Farmer 1999, 2003, 2004, 2006), then it behooves us to highlight the forces that give rise to inequity and injustice, and to engage in *pragmatic solidarity* with those who are marginalized by hearing, believing, and understanding their lived histories and using their experiences as a basis for all observations, judgments, and actions towards social justice (Farmer 2003, 146). The objectives of this research align with the principles of research-based advocacy. This study stands as a corrective to established, epidemiological, and survey-based research on Indigenous health and health care issues because of its ethnographic character, its move beyond "the numbers," its commitment to narrative and community engagement, and its explicit use of research for political change. The emphasis on informant discourses draws on the major strengths of qualitative research, including the insider's perspective that can reveal issues often missed by quantitative approaches, along with insights into relationships, causes, effects, dynamic processes, and forms of knowledge that might otherwise be inaccessible (Denscombe 2010; McLeod 2017). Focusing on structural violence, syndemic suffering, and intergenerational trauma helps to illuminate the historical, political, ideological, economic, and social factors that structure health disparities and inequities. As Charlotte Reading (2018, 5) explains: "Just as the maladies observed in the leaves are not generally the cause of unhealthy trees, inequities in human health frequently result from corruption or deficiencies in the unseen but critical root system."

Our research team's long-term goal for this study is to make the leap from listening, studying, and understanding to bringing forth positive change. The Truth and Reconciliation Commission (2015) and the National Inquiry into Missing and Murdered Indigenous Women and Girls (NIMMIWG) (2018) address the need to "expose hard truths about the devastating impacts of colonization, racism and sexism – aspects of Canada that many Canadians are reluctant to accept" (NIMMIWG 2018, para. 3). Part of the work of addressing and "bringing justice to injustice" includes the need for sustainable and culturally appropriate supports for healing and proactive measures that identify, reduce, and ultimately eliminate health disparities. Our research team sees the strategic use of our research findings as a first step towards reconciliation. The data will inform health policy through developing a strategic community health plan, enhancing existing health programs and creating new ones to fill service gaps, and educating on- and off-reserve health care providers on the structural and social barriers that compromise the delivery of high-quality and culturally appropriate health care to the First Nation community.

How we choose to respond to those who "tell us where and how it hurts" is as much an ethical decision as it is a logistical one. The biggest challenge for researchers and health care professionals is to restrain their impulse to administer temporary Band-Aid or magic-bullet biomedical solutions. Instead, we should strive to work collaboratively with Indigenous partners to conceptualize and co-create well-informed and sustainable interventions, while continuing to lend our voice to calls for accountability, reparation, and social justice for Indigenous peoples in Canada and abroad.

NOTES

1 The name of the First Nation community is withheld to protect the confidentiality of study participants.

2 Residential schools were government-sponsored religious educational institutions that were established in the early 1800s to forcibly assimilate Indigenous children into Euro-Canadian culture. The last residential school in Canada closed in 1996.

3 The research team consists of representatives from the community's health centre, First Nations and Inuit Home and Community Care (FNIHCC), the community's cultural research centre, and two community advocacy groups.

4 With the family's consent, I have used pseudonyms when referring to the study participants in order to protect their privacy and maintain confidentiality. At the time of the interviews, Rachel and David Wilson were in their early eighties and had been married for over sixty years. The couple's children are in their mid-fifties and early sixties. Rachel and David have several grandchildren and great-grandchildren.

5 Studies that have examined lipophilic chemical exposure as a cause of type 2 diabetes provide evidence that supports David's claim (Zeliger 2013).

REFERENCES

Adelson, N. 2005. "The Embodiment of Inequity: Health Disparities in Aboriginal Canada." *Canadian Journal of Public Health* 96 (2): 45–61. https://doi.org/10.1007/BF03403702.

Andermann, A. 2017. "Outbreaks in the Age of Syndemics: New Insights for Improving Indigenous Health." *Canadian Communicable Disease Report* 43 (6): 125–32.https://doi.org/10.14745/ccdr.v43i06a02.

Brave Heart, M.Y. 2003. "The Historical Trauma Response among Natives and Its Relationship with Substance Abuse: A Lakota Illustration." *Journal of Psychoactive Drugs* 35 (1): 7–13. https://doi.org/10.1080/02791072.2003.10399988.

Brave Heart, M.Y, and L.M. DeBruyn. 1998. "The American Indian Holocaust: Healing Historical Unresolved Grief." *American Indian and Alaska Native Mental Health Research Journal of the National Center* 8 (2): 56–78. http://www.ucdenver.edu/academics/colleges/PublicHealth/research/centers/CAIANH/journal/Documents/Volume%208/8(2)_YellowHorseBraveHeart_American_Indian_Holocaust_60-82.pdf.

Denscombe, M. 2010. *The Good Research Guide: For Small-Scale Social Research Projects.* 4th ed. Maidenhead, UK: Open University Press.

Evans Campbell, T. 2008. "Historical Trauma in American Indian/Native Alaska Communities: A Multilevel Framework for Exploring Impacts on Individuals, Families, and Communities." *Journal of Interpersonal Violence* 23 (3): 316–38. https://doi.org/10.1177/0886260507312290.

Farmer, P. 1999. *Infections and Inequalities: The Modern Plagues.* Berkeley: University of California Press.

Farmer, P. 2003. *Pathologies of Power: Health, Human Rights, and the New War on the Poor.* Berkeley: University of California Press.

Farmer, P. 2004. "An Anthropology of Structural Violence." *Current Anthropology* 45 (3): 305–17. https://doi.org/10.1086/382250.

Farmer, P. 2006. *AIDS and Accusation: Haiti and the Geography of Blame.* Updated with a new preface. Berkeley: University of California Press.

Galloway, T., and I. Mosby. 2017. "'Hunger was never absent': How Residential School Diets Shaped Current Patterns of Diabetes among Indigenous Peoples in Canada." *Canadian Medical Association Journal* 189 (2): E1043–5. https://doi.org/10.1503/cmaj.170448.

Goffman, E. 1961. *Asylums: Essays on the Social Situation of Mental Patients and Other Inmates.* New York: Doubleday Anchor, 1961.

Herring, D.A., and L. Sattenspiel. 2007. "Social Contexts, Syndemics, and Infectious Disease in Northern Aboriginal Populations." *American Journal of Human Biology* 19 (2): 190–202. https://doi.org/10.1002/ajhb.20618.

Keith, M.M., and J.T. Brophy. 2004. "Participatory Mapping and Occupational Hazards of Disease among Asbestos-Exposed Workers in a Foundry and Insulation Complex in Canada." *International Journal of Occupational Environmental Health* 10 (2): 144–53. https://doi.org/10.1179/oeh.2004.10.2.144.

McLeod, S.A. 2017. "Qualitative vs. Quantitative Research." https://www.simplypsychology.org/qualitative-quantitative.html.

Mendenhall, E. 2012. *Syndemic Suffering: Social Distress, Depression and Diabetes among Mexican Immigrant Women.* Walnut Creek, CA: Left Coast Press.

Milloy, J.S. 1999. *A National Crime: The Canadian Government and the Residential School System, 1879–1986.* Winnipeg: University of Manitoba Press.

Minore, B., M. Katt, and M.E. Hill. 2009. "Planning without Facts: Ontario's Aboriginal Health Information Challenge." *Journal of Agromedicine* 14 (2): 90–6. https://doi.org/10.1080/10599240902739802.

Mosby, I. 2013. "Administering Colonial Science: Nutrition Research and Human Biomedical Experimentation in Aboriginal Communities and Residential Schools, 1942–1952." *Histoire sociale/Social History* 46 (1): 145–72. https://www.muse.jhu.edu/article/512043.

Myss, C. 1996. *Anatomy of the Spirit: The Seven Stages of Power and Healing.* New York: Three Rivers Press.

National Inquiry into Missing and Murdered Indigenous Women and Girls (NIMMIWG). 2018. https://www.mmiwg-ffada.ca/wp-content/uploads/2018/08/Contest-bid-for-Legacy-Archive.pdf.

Pember, M.A. 2016. "Intergenerational Trauma: Understanding Natives' Inherited Pain." Indian Country Today Media Network. https://amber-ic.org/wp-content/uploads/2017/01/ICMN-All-About-Generations-Trauma.pdf.

Reading, C. 2018. "Structural Determinants of Aboriginal Peoples' Health." In *Determinants of Indigenous Peoples' Health: Beyond the Social,* 2nd ed., edited by M. Greenwood, S. de Leeuw, and N.M. Lindsay, 4–17. Toronto: Canadian Scholars Press.

Singer, M., and S. Clair. 2003. "Syndemics and Public Health: Reconceptualizing Disease in Bio-social Context. *Medical Anthropological Quarterly* 17 (4): 423–41. https://doi.org/10.1525/maq.2003.17.4.423.

Stephens, C.V. 2006. "'Speaking the Pictures in my Head': Using Elders' Residential School Discourses as a Vehicle for Theorizing the Past." In *Proceedings of the 37th Annual Algonquian Conference,* vol. 37, edited by C. Wolfart and A. Oggs, 311–32. Winnipeg: University of Manitoba Press.

Stephens, C.V. 2008a. "'She Was Weakly for a Long Time and the Consumption Set In': Using Parish Records to Explore Disease Patterns and Causes of Death in a First Nations Community." In *Multiplying and Dividing: Tuberculosis in Canada and Aotearoa New Zealand,* edited by A. Herring, J. Littleton, J. Park, and T. Farmer, 134–48. Auckland: Department of Anthropology, University of Auckland.

Stephens, C.V. 2008b. "Syndemics, Structural Violence, and the Politics of Health: A Critical Biocultural Approach to the Study of Disease and Tuberculosis Mortality in a Parish Population (1850–1885)." In *Proceedings of the 39th Annual Algonquian Conference,* edited by K. Hele, 581–613. London: University of Western Ontario.

Stephens, C.V. 2009. *Toxic Talk: Narratives of Pollution, Loss and Resistance.* PhD diss., McMaster University, Hamilton.

Stephens, C.V. 2012. "Challenges to Collecting Health Data in Reserve Communities." Unpublished report. McMaster University, Hamilton.

Strauss, A., and J. Corbin. 1998. *Basics of Qualitative Research: Techniques and Procedures for Developing Grounded Theory*. 2nd ed. Thousand Oaks, CA: Sage.

Truth and Reconciliation Commission of Canada. 2015. *Truth and Reconciliation Commission of Canada: Calls to Action*. Winnipeg: TRCC. http://trc.ca/assets/pdf/Calls_to_Action_English2.pdf

Waldram, J.B., D.A. Herring, and T. K. Young. 2006. *Aboriginal Health in Canada: Historical, Cultural, and Epidemiological Perspectives*. 2nd ed. Toronto: University of Toronto Press.

Zeliger, H.I. 2013. "Lipophilic Chemical Exposure as a Cause of Type 2 Diabetes (T2D)." *Reviews on Environmental Health* 28 (1): 9–20. https://doi.org/10.1515/reveh-2012-0031.

7 Satisfaction Not Guaranteed: Broadening the Discourse on Quality Improvement in the Home Care System

ALISA GRIGOROVICH

The last three decades of economic restructuring and health care reforms under neoliberal logics have fundamentally changed the nature of the care that is provided both within and outside the Canadian health care system (Armstrong and Armstrong 2010; England et al. 2007). A key aspect of this change has been the relocation of long-term care (e.g., non-acute, chronic) from public institutions to private homes and communities (Aronson and Neysmith 1997; Fuller 1998; Grant, Amaratunga, and Armstrong 2004). This relocation has, however, not been accompanied by sufficient reinvestment in community care, which has led to increased rationing and restriction of entitlements to publicly funded medical and supportive long-term care services (Aronson 2004; Daly 2007; Williams et al. 2001). The justification provided in dominant political discourse for moving care from institutions to homes and communities has been twofold. First, it is argued that this makes the health care system more "economically efficient," and second, it is suggested that moving services closer to home improves the quality of the care provided by making it more "patient-centred" (Armstrong and Armstrong 2001; Baranek, Deber, and Williams 2004).

To provide evidence for these claims, as part of the broader move towards the adoption of evidence-based medicine in Canada, industrial quality control techniques have been introduced into health care as a mechanism for measuring and regulating its quality (e.g., total quality management or continuous quality improvement). Rooted in positivism and market-based capitalist ideology, this quality assurance mechanism assumes that care is a commodity product, and that the quality of the care is a static phenomenon that can be disarticulated into abstracted and discrete units (e.g., numbers, indicators) that can be statistically measured and controlled (Emmerich et al. 2015; Mykhalovskiy et al. 2008; Swinglehurst et al. 2015). Furthermore, the managerial and rational logic underlying this type of evaluation reflects the belief that quality is enhanced through increased standardization of services and technical practices: that quality can be brought about through homogenizing services and their delivery to ensure that all individuals have access to the same type of care (McLaughlin and Kaluzny 2004).

This market-based accounting of quality is, however, at odds with the "logic of care" that holds that care is an essentially normative concept that has relational, interpersonal, and affective dimensions (Emmerich et al. 2015; Mol 2008; Tronto 1993). According to this type of logic, the meaning of good care is a local phenomenon; it is specific to the lived reality in which care receivers and caregivers are located in both time and place. The outcomes of care are thus not considered static, but unpredictable and contingent. As a result, such logic holds that evaluations of care cannot be abstracted from the context within which care is situated or made wholly subject to a quantitative performance audit (Emmerich et al. 2015; Jackson et al. 2006; Mol 2008; Mykhalovskiy et al. 2008). Building on this logic, a feminist political economy approach begins with the perspectives of care receivers and caregivers and attends to the political and economic structures and ideologies that influence their relations (Armstrong 2001; Sevenhuijsen 1998; Tronto 1993). Used as a means for redressing inequity and achieving social change, this approach necessitates a critical questioning of how well existing evidence on health care quality reflects the social reality of care (Armstrong 2001, 135).

Adopting this approach to exploring the quality of home care services, in this chapter I focus on the experiences of older lesbian and bisexual women who receive these services in Ontario. Specifically, I contrast the perspectives of these care receivers on what supports experiences of good (and not good) care, with how quality of care is conceptualized and evaluated by official quality improvement mechanisms, as reflected in the recent annual public performance report *Measuring Up* (Health Quality Ontario 2015). This group of women is under-represented in current research on home care and may be particularly vulnerable to experiencing restricted access to good care as a result of intersecting structural inequalities (e.g., heterosexism and homophobia, ageism, and sexism). Further, the current cohort of older lesbian and bisexual women have lived most of their lives in environments where homosexuality was pathologized and criminalized. As such, many have spent their lives socially isolated, concealing their sexuality and relationships in an attempt to protect themselves from rejection and victimization. In privileging the perspectives of these care recipients, this chapter seeks to contribute to an alternative counter-discursive account of quality based on care logics (Mol 2008) that resists and disrupts the rhetorical authority of evidence-based-medicine in current debates about how to improve health care systems (Armstrong, Armstrong, and Coburn 2001; Goldenberg 2012; Mykhalovskiy et al. 2008).

Home Care in Canada

Home care services can include medical care (e.g., medication administration, wound care), social care (e.g., meal preparation, personal care, laundry), therapy, and end-of-life care that is provided by regulated and unregulated health care providers within private homes. In Canada, these are considered to be "extended health services" and are not publicly insured under the Canada Health Act (1985).[1] Thus, although each province and territory has some form of publicly available care, the organization, payment structure, and types of services and level of support provided vary across Canada. In part the variability also results from the lack of provincial or federal resource allocation guidelines for long-term care. In Ontario, at the time of this study, the management and delivery of these services were coordinated by Community Care Access Centres (CCACs), who determined eligibility and decided what kind and how much service will be provided.[2] The actual work of care was contracted out to private not-for-profit and for-profit companies, through a competitive bidding process, where companies bid for the right to offer home care services. To remain competitive, companies typically seek to decrease the cost of care through a reduction in either the number of workers or paid work time. Overall, competitive bidding along with cutbacks in home care funding have led to widespread rationing of care in Ontario, which has had negative consequences for both providers and clients (Armstrong 2007; Aronson 2004; Aronson, Denton, and Zeytinoglu 2004; Daly 2007; Denton et al. 2006; England et al. 2007; Randall and Williams 2006).

Measuring Quality of Home Care in Ontario

Health Quality Ontario (HQO) is a provincial organization that measures and defines the indicators used for monitoring the quality of health care services (as well as setting the standards or targets for what these indicators should be). In its role as the provincial advisor on quality, the organization also uses this evidence to guide policy and health care reform. Its definition of quality is fairly broad (i.e., "achieving better health outcomes and experiences for every person living in Ontario") and quality is assessed based on six attributes: safety, effectiveness, patient-centred-ness, timeliness, efficiency, and equity

(HQO 2016). Each of these is evaluated using one (or more) quantitative indicator that measures the average for each region (e.g., Local Health Integration Network) and compares it to the average for the province, and in some cases to other jurisdictions. For example, the effectiveness of home care is evaluated by counting the number of readmissions to hospital, while efficiency is evaluated by counting the number of home care clients with "low to moderate care" needs who entered a long-term care home (HQO 2015). This approach to measuring quality reflects the widespread popularity of small-area-variation analysis in health services research that aims to influence health policy. This type of quantitative analysis is used to describe how rates of health service utilization vary across geographic areas, with the underlying assumption that such variations are meaningful (James 1989; Luft 2012). In particular, the underlying assumption of these studies is that if such variations cannot be explained by population-based differences (e.g., sex, age, morbidity) and do not statistically significantly influence patients' outcomes (e.g., survival, rehospitalization), then they reflect a misallocation of resources and an opportunity to cut costs (James 1989, 25). What this type of analysis misses is that variations may be the result of contextual factors that are "unmeasurable," or are impossible to plan for by looking "backwards" at past data (Ong et al. 2009).

Although the justification for HQO's existence includes ensuring that Ontario's health care system is more patient centred, transparent, and publicly accountable through objective evidence gathering (Ontario Ministry of Health and Long-Term Care 2011), there are multiple problems with how this organization collects, classifies, and publicly reports "evidence" on quality. For example, the 2015 annual public report (HQO 2015) offers only four indicators for home care and provides aggregate abstracted counts for each indicator (e.g., an average value), without linking these to sociodemographic or other context-specific details about the population of care recipients whose individual satisfaction ratings are aggregated to form the average rate reported for these indicators. Each indicator is a yearly average and does not capture variation across time. Many of the indicators lump data for multiple providers and/or types of home care services (e.g., medical and social supports). For example, the satisfaction indicator lumps together the ratings of both care clients and family members, and provides one score for all types of home care services received and across all of their care providers and case managers. There are also multiple exclusion criteria for each indicator. For example, for the satisfaction ratings respondents are excluded if they report not knowing their case manager or not seeing or speaking to their case manager prior to the time of the survey (HQO 2016). This indicator also reflects data from a survey of only ~4 per cent of all home care recipients/families who received home care (e.g., 29,000 recipients/caregivers surveyed in 2013/2014 versus ~700,000 people who received home care in 2014/2015) (OACCAC 2015). Finally, the report does not include any indicators for equity of home care, or any other types of care; although in 2016 HQO published a separate public report on equity (defined as the same rate of access to care across income groups), it focused on access to primary care and to cancer screening tests. As a consequence, while the public outputs of HQO quality assurance mechanisms offer rhetorically persuasive "evidence" of quality measurement and improvement, a closer examination of their content suggests that the evidence produced is far from neutral. Instead, these mechanisms are "*productive* and *world-making* ... [and bring] something new into existence, namely a declaration regarding the [meaning of] *quality* of the care being delivered" (Emmerich et al. 2015, 7).

Lesbian and Bisexual Women and Care

Research on health care experiences of lesbian and bisexual women has primarily focused on younger women accessing primary care, and has shown that they often receive prejudicial, improper, or poor-quality care (Barbara, Quandt, and Anderson 2001; Bjorkman and Malterud 2009; Jackson et al. 2006; Solarz 1999). For example, lesbian and bisexual women often receive inappropriate guidance regarding sexual health and reproductive care, as well as limited access to preventative screening tests (e.g., pap smears, mammograms). Disclosure of their sexual identity to providers can result in their being subjected to homophobia (e.g., demeaning comments, avoidance of physical contact) and even breaches of confidentiality (Barbara, Quandt, and Anderson 2001; Bjorkman and Malterud 2009; Jackson et al. 2006; Solarz 1999). Studies of providers' beliefs and attitudes consistently show that many report discomfort with providing care to lesbian and gay people (Chapman et al. 2012; Eliason and Raheim 2000; Hinchliff, Gott, and Galena 2005; Institute of Medicine 2011; Téllez et al. 1999).

While home care provision is an important concern for many older people, older lesbian and bisexual women face unique barriers to accessing needed medical and social support (e.g., a lifetime of reduced health-seeking behaviours, experiences of homophobic discrimination and social exclusion, and limited access to social determinants of health) (Grigorovich 2013; Solarz 1999; Stein, Beckerman, and Sherman 2010). They may also be more likely to rely on publicly funded long-term care in older ages than gay and bisexual men or heterosexual women (Barker

2004; Grigorovich 2013). For example, they been found to have higher rates of psychological distress and physical disability than older gay and bisexual men (Fredriksen-Goldsen, Kim, and Barkan 2012; Wallace et al. 2011). They have also been shown to experience poor health and disability at younger ages than heterosexual adults (Fredriksen-Goldsen, Kim, and Barkan 2012). Finally, they have been found to be on average poorer than older heterosexual women, with lesbian couples being poorer than heterosexual or gay couples (Albeda et al. 2009; Wallace et al. 2011).

The Study

This chapter draws on interview data that I collected for my thesis research, which was a qualitative case study of older lesbian and bisexual women's experiences with publicly funded home care services in Ontario (Grigorovich 2015a, 2015b, 2016). This population of women is rarely represented in health services research, and previous analyses of the impact of health care reforms on the home care system have not considered how sexuality may influence women's care needs and the quality of care they receive. Although it was known that many older lesbian and bisexual women harbour fears about encountering prejudice when accessing long-term care services (Brotman et al. 2007; Grant 2010; Stein, Beckerman, and Sherman 2010), at the outset of my investigation no Canadian research existed on their experiences of receiving home care. The purpose of my research was thus to obtain a rich and thick description of older lesbian and bisexual women's experiences of receiving home care, to examine barriers and enablers to access (within the context of neoliberal restructuring of health care in Ontario), and to identify recommendations for policy and training to improve access and equity. I took an intersectional and multiscalar approach in this research, drawing on feminist political economy and critical sexuality scholarship, and collected multiple types of data, including qualitative interviews, document and literature review (e.g., health and social care policy in Ontario and Canada, previous research), and contextual information (e.g., demographic questionnaires and field memos).

A detailed description of the methods used in this research has been provided elsewhere (Grigorovich 2015a, 2015b, 2016). In brief, to participate, individuals had to self-identify as a lesbian or bisexual woman (or a related term, such as "gay"), be at least fifty-five years old at the time of the study, have lived in Ontario while receiving home care, and have attempted to access or received these services sometime in the five years prior to their interview. I defined "publicly funded home care services" as any type of care service that was provided in the home to participants by a formal care provider (rather than by friends or family) and was not paid for privately. As part of the interviews, I asked participants to comment on whether they felt that they in fact received home care that was of good quality, and to comment on what they felt enabled (or hindered) the quality of care in the home care setting.

I interviewed sixteen women from across Ontario, who (at the time of the interview) ranged from fifty-five to seventy-two years of age. Most (n=9) were married or in a common-law relationship and lived with a female partner or spouse. However, irrespective of their relationship status, participants reported that they had minimal (if any) resources to draw on to supplement publicly funded home care services (i.e., informal caregivers, money for private care), as they are expected to do per Ontario's policy on home care. Most reported dual or multiple chronic conditions that limited their ability to perform activities of daily living (e.g., dressing, grooming, bathing, eating), instrumental activities (grocery shopping, meal preparation, housekeeping), and participation in valued activities outside their homes. All received medical home care (e.g., wound dressing, medication) from nurses and/or social care (e.g., bathing, dressing, meal preparation) from personal support workers.

Quality Is Variable and Unmodifiable

When I asked my participants whether they felt that the overall home care service that they received was of good quality, most participants responded that this was difficult for them to evaluate as they received care from multiple providers and had very different experiences across them. When describing aspects of good-quality care, they focused on their interactions with specific care providers, and the actions and attitudes of those care providers, rather than on the technical outcomes of receiving care. Their assessment of quality was thus contingent on their experiences with a particular provider, rather than reflecting an idealized or abstracted notion of what constituted good-quality care. Participants also reported that the quality of the care they received over time was variable, and unpredictable overall. As a consequence, when asked to describe what the concept of "quality of care" meant to them, participants described the meaning of "good" quality by juxtaposing their experiences with one provider with their experiences with another. This contingency is captured in their narratives below, where they describe the characteristics of home care provision that they felt enabled quality or were significant to their evaluation of the care that they received from a particular provider.

Although many participants expressed gratitude for having received home care and could speak to at least one example of good care, overall they were disappointed with the inconsistency in the quality of care. Negative experiences were particularly upsetting as they added to participants' overall discomfort with receiving home care and impinged on their ability to cope with symptoms of their illness or injury such as pain, fatigue, and depression. Participants expressed frustration with their inability to control the quality of care, or to modify the conditions of care that they felt could improve their experiences. As a result, many indicated they had low expectations of receiving good care in the future. For example, consider the account of one participant, who was no longer receiving care and who expressed concerns about needing home care again in the future:

> Depending on the services I would need, based on my experience, and hearing about [my friend's experience with home care], I don't have any confidence that the CCAC ... has my interests at heart. I don't have any confidence that I'm going to get a competent caregiver, whatever their type of care is, but certainly not nursing care. I mean in the end I had somebody who was really competent, but I went through a lot of people before that. And I don't have any confidence that any of this care will be set up to meet my needs [*laughs*]. (P1)

What Matters for Enabling Good Quality of Care?

To understand what the concept of quality of care meant to my participants, and to distill the characteristics of "good" and "not good" care, I asked them to describe what they felt mattered for enabling quality of care. In line with feminist research (Aronson 2004; Jackson et al. 2006) and ethics of theorizing (Sherwin 1998; Tronto 1993), the women I interviewed stated that quality of care was good when the care they received was both relational and responsive: when they felt that they established a good relationship with their care provider and when the provider demonstrated attentiveness and receptivity to understanding and responding to what participants wanted assistance with (Aronson 2004; Mol 2008). They emphasized that good-quality care was delivered in a manner responsive to the daily rhythm and organization of their lives and supported their relational autonomy (Aronson 2004; Sherwin 1998). Their accounts also highlighted the contextual importance of sexuality, as a social location and axis of structural inequality, for evaluations of quality. In particular, past and present experiences with discrimination, invisibility, and prejudice heightened older lesbian and bisexual women's feelings of being vulnerable and intensified the importance of having a good relationship with providers and remaining in control. To illustrate how these aspects of care provided the necessary conditions for good care experiences to happen, below I focus on two themes from my research: time and interpersonal and affective aspects of care. I then compare participants' perspectives to the way in which quality is imagined and assessed by HQO.

Time

Participants' accounts suggest that having enough time with providers was important for good quality. For example, they wanted providers to come on time, take necessary time to do all of the aspects of the required care tasks, and to stay the entire time that they were supposed to. Many described having received poor-quality care from providers who came late (or hours early), who did not want to stay the whole hour, or who were generally unreliable in terms of care scheduling and attendance. This was especially distressing because, as participants reported, the organization and planning of the home care provider's visit was already a time-consuming and exhausting process for which they had limited energy and resources. Receiving care from care providers who were not reliable or punctual was particularly frustrating for participants who needed assistance with basic self-care activities, as they felt trapped waiting for a provider to come and give them a bath or help them get dressed so that they could start their day. For example, the following participant explained why she was frustrated with the quality of the care she received from one provider:

> [My second care provider] was amazing. She was efficient. She was pleasant. She was reliable, like you knew when she was coming and she would ... yeah, she was excellent. I mean it was a godsend because until ... that was the problem with that other woman [that came before her]. She never showed up on time. And basically when [my spouse] left in the morning I'd sort of be sitting in my pajamas and until somebody came I couldn't get washed or dressed or anything. (P3)

Participants also expressed that having sufficient time was important for enabling good-quality care because it allowed providers and recipients to get to know each other, and to develop a mutually beneficial relationship so that care could be personalized. In particular, spending time together was important for ensuring that care providers had sufficient knowledge of the home space (e.g., layout and storage of items) and of participants' capacities and support needs. As one participant explained, getting to know each other was also bidirectional; this further demonstrates the interdependence between care receivers' and caregivers' actions and intents for enabling quality of care:

> Quality [is] developed by getting to know each other ... you develop that over time. You as a client have to have a little bit of patience. You have to be willing to be nice to the person. You have to be willing to be flexible with them as well ... You treat them like an equal and they treat you honestly ... and you end up with what you need. (P14)

Despite the importance participants accorded to the actions and intentions of individual providers, they also recognized that their interactions with providers were influenced by macro- and meso-level constraints, such as funding mechanisms and organizational care allocation policies. For example, participants reported that they were aware that both they and their care providers had limited power to modify the frequency of care provision due to budget cuts and rationing policies. They also understood that the timing of care was subject to organizational practices of inflexibility and overbooking (e.g., high caseloads, insufficient travel time for providers to attend to multiple care clients across the city). Reflecting on why the care she received from one nurse was of good quality, one participant made a connection between time and for-profit priorities that privilege cost-efficiency:

> [My second nurse] was reliable. She did everything she was supposed to do. She took all the time she needed. You know, I know she had other clients she had to go to, you know, but her bookings seemed to be paced out at an appropriate way. She wasn't racing off. She wasn't trying to maximize her income by racing off from my place to another. I guess that's another thing I would say, that high-quality care is not-for-profit care. For-profit care, by its very nature, has problems being high quality because, you know, the bottom line is money. (P1)

Finally, having enough time with a provider was also important for enabling trust in providers, and reducing care recipients' fears around experiencing homophobic prejudice or violence. Participants wanted to receive care from providers who were affirming and respectful of their sexuality and familial arrangements. This was particularly important in the context of home care, as care was of a personal nature and was provided in isolation in their private home. Many participants reported experiencing physical and verbal homophobia (or heterosexist invisibility) from primary care providers, natal families, and others. As a result, most typically did not explicitly disclose their sexuality to home care providers. Further, although many stated that they thought that providers would assume they were heterosexual, they nonetheless worried about managing providers' reactions to disclosure, and what could happen to them as a result. Consequently, participants who did disclose waited to first establish a good relationship with a particular provider, and attempted to gauge their potential reaction as they got to know them. Consider the example of one participant who explained that she gradually mentions her wife in conversation as a strategy that helps her assess whether a care provider may be homophobic:

> I just tell them that my *wife* should be coming home in a little while or that my *wife* and I just went on a vacation or my *wife* likes this. Just mentioning it and [seeing] if they have any questions [or if] they'll talk to me about it. Or maybe they're like, "Oh god, I didn't know she was gay" [*says in dismissive tone under her breath*]. (P15)

Similarly, another participant who lived alone explained that while her regular provider knew of her sexuality, she did not come out to temporary fill-ins, as the brief amount of time she spent with them was not enough to be sure they would not be homophobic:

> I have an established relationship with my ongoing caregiver. With the others, I don't want to jeopardize [my safety by coming out] ... I don't want to have somebody who is filling in for my regular caregiver be homophobic with me and then I am stuck with that person. So, I just have not said anything to the others. (P5)

Although passing as heterosexual or delaying coming out may be self-protective in the short term, engaging in such coping strategies may increase social isolation. The lack of disclosure may also reflect a broader lack of trust or confidence in providers that might prevent lesbian and bisexual women from openly sharing their values and preferences for care and establishing a caring relationship with providers. Consequently, having sufficient time with care providers to get to know them and to establish mutual trust is crucial for reducing older lesbian and bisexual women's vulnerability and fear of discrimination, thereby fostering quality of care.

Interpersonal and Affective Aspects of Care

Participants reported that they felt they received good-quality home care from providers who attended to the interpersonal and affective aspects of care. Specifically, they described having good experiences when providers actively enabled their comfort with receiving care by demonstrating positive affect and allowing them to direct the care. This was important for participants, as it made them feel less like a burden and enhanced their level of comfort with receiving support with intimate and personal tasks such as bathing. As one participant explained, good-quality care characterized care encounters after which she felt good:

> I feel good when that person is leaving my house. I feel good when they're entering my house. That they've made me feel good about the two of us interacting with each other ... Just really a good relationship and an uplifting relationship between the two of you. (P15)

Participants also emphasized the importance of having enough control or autonomy over what happened in their interactions with care providers. Their narratives emphasized a relational understanding of autonomy (Nedelsky 1989; Sherwin 1998), rather than the procedural and atomistic view of autonomy that is privileged in the neoliberal health discourse (Mol 2008; Rose and Miller 1992). That is, participants emphasized the importance of negotiating decision making with providers rather than making independent choices, and recognized that their capacity to direct care was enabled through their relationship with supportive providers. As an example of this, one participant described an experience with a provider that she felt was an example of receiving good-quality care: "She just treats you as an equal, like regardless of ability, I'm part of the team" (P6). Similarly, another participant said:

> Quality is if the ... [provider] listens to us ... And that they obviously respect you, that they don't talk down to you, that they don't talk to you like you're retarded and that they don't, I hate to use the word, but that they don't talk to you like you're feeble, right? You're not. Well, even if you are feeble, that they talk to you with respect. (P2)

Ensuring that they felt their provider respected them and that they had some autonomy over their care was important for participants because they felt vulnerable and disempowered as a result of being dependent on the assistance of formal care providers to do tasks they previously did on their own. Participants were also unused to accessing formal supports in general, and some were explicitly wary of accessing formal supports for fear of experiencing homophobia. One participant reflected on her experiences with two providers and described how quality of care is enabled through attending not only to technical needs but also to emotional ones:

> Quality home care means [that] the home care person actually takes care of the person's physical and ... I'd call it emotional ... yes, emotional needs. That's what makes you feel good. And that's quality care. And I don't know if they can always do that. Maybe they can't. But I think that's quality care. You don't have to make me feel wonderful, but you have to not make me feel bad. The second nurse made me ... well she didn't make me ... she pissed me off. But if I were not a stronger person she could have made me feel bad. (P13)

These non-technical components of care may be particularly important in enabling quality of care for older lesbian and bisexual women, given their history of social isolation and deep-seated mistrust of care providers. Failure to demonstrate such skill may also be interpreted by lesbian and bisexual women as evidence of providers' unconscious bias or stigma, which may make them even more reluctant to trust providers in future encounters, or to delay accessing home care altogether.

Opposing Concepts of Quality

Participants' relational and situated understanding of the importance of time and good interpersonal interactions with care providers can be contrasted with how these aspects of quality are evaluated within the *Measuring Up* report (HQO 2015). The report measures timeliness of care based on one indicator: the waiting times for receipt of home care services. Specifically, this indicator measures the percentage of clients who received care within five days from the time a case manager authorized the start of care. Focusing on this time period is problematic as it doesn't capture how long clients had to wait to receive authorization; this is significant because the Ontario Auditor General's report (2015) showed that authorization assessments were not being completed within the prescribed provincial timelines. It also prioritizes evaluation of timeliness at the system level rather than at the level of the individual receiving care, and thus fails to capture home care clients' experiences of waiting, as well as whether they themselves perceived these wait times as being "timely" (or as relevant to the quality of care they received). Finally, such measurements prioritize linear "clock time" of care while ignoring the importance of "process time," or the subjective and relational understanding of the time of doing the actual work of care (Davies 1994). As a consequence, this indicator fails to attend to aspects of time that my participants understood as being important for enabling quality, including having the time that they needed to develop trust in their care provider.

In terms of evaluating recipients' experiences of care, *Measuring Up* offers only one indicator: the percentage of clients surveyed who reported a positive experience with the services they received from both care coordinators and service providers. This information is collected using a phone survey that asks respondents to rate their experience with care on a quantitative five-point Likert scale (e.g., poor to excellent). As with timeliness, positive care experiences are reduced to one overall score that collapses experiences across time and across types of providers. Although my participants emphasized the importance of caring attitudes and providers' interpersonal skills for enabling quality, these aspects of care are not captured in this (or in any other) HQO indicator. Further, the report provides no demographic details about who was surveyed and what types of care they received or for how long, nor does it offer any explanation as to why recipients rated their service as they did.

Measuring Up offers evidence that the quality of home care needs no improvement by stating that "more than nine out of 10 Ontario patients surveyed continue to report having a positive experience with their home care" (HQO 2015, 6). However, this evidence becomes suspect if we consider how accurately existing indicators capture aspects of quality that are important to care receivers, and what they leave out. Reliance on one satisfaction indicator for information about patients' experiences of care is problematic for several reasons. First, this crude approach is insensitive to variation across providers and across time and cannot capture both positive and negative experiences of care. Second, it lumps the ratings of both care receivers and family members, incorrectly assuming that the two groups have similar expectations of home care. Satisfaction measures also often yield more positive results than qualitative evaluations of care, even in cases of marked dissatisfaction with provided care, because recipients often dismiss or excuse poor care (Evans 2010; Pollock et al. 2011; Sinding 2003; Williams 1994). Finally, it is questionable whether such instruments are even reliable and accurate quantitative measures, as respondents' ratings have been shown to be influenced by personal factors beyond the care itself, such as an individual's self-efficacy, social desirability, and their belief that reporting dissatisfaction will have a useful effect on the outcome of care (Worthington 2005).

The market-based logic underlying the use of satisfaction surveys incorrectly assumes that care receivers will act as "empowered consumers" who will critically and rationally evaluate receipt of care as they would a commercial good. Care receivers, however, do not evaluate care experiences critically and abstractly, divorced from embodied and affective forms of reasoning and power relations. They typically defer to providers' expertise and look to them to shape care relations and direct care choices (Mol 2008; Pollock et al. 2011; Sinding 2003). They also trust providers to provide good care, and may lack the professional knowledge needed to accurately evaluate care (Rankin 2003); their expectation of satisfaction with their services is thus in a sense "built into" their interactions with providers. Consequently, even when they receive poor-quality care, they often suppress their complaint because they feel dependent on providers' goodwill, are grateful for having received (any) care, and because suppressing a complaint makes them feel better (Evans 2010; Grigorovich 2015b; Pollock et al. 2011; Sinding 2003). For all these reasons, Pollock et al. (2011) have suggested that high satisfaction ratings are simply "an artefact" of the method of data collection. Given that my participants reported that they could not provide an overall rating of quality, and felt that they could not modify the conditions of care, they likely wouldn't have expressed dissatisfaction with the quality of their care even if they were surveyed. This makes the evidence on the quality of home care produced by HQO not only an inadequate representation of patients' experiences, but also misleading.

Conclusion

In this chapter I challenge taken-for-granted and normative understandings of the meaning of quality as it is conceptualized and measured within official quality assurance mechanisms by exploring the experiences of older lesbian and bisexual women who receive home care. Attending to their narratives demonstrates that quality is a complex and contingent social phenomenon that is affected through temporal and interactional aspects of care that give it meaning in practice. Further, it highlights how structural and social inequalities, in this case homophobia and heterosexism, influence personal histories and current care relations, and thus conceptions of good care. Contrasting my participants' understandings with existing indicators of quality shows the limitations of relying on numerical population-level counts to assess the quality of the home care system. Given that current measures do not reflect aspects of quality that are important to care recipients, and actively act to obscure their experiences of poor quality, my analysis raises questions about the ethics of continuing to rely on such measures for generating evidence to guide decision making.

NOTES

1 In Ontario (and Canada) publicly paid for home care services are assumed to be an "add-on" to the unpaid care that family members and friends are

expected to provide, and this assumption is stated within federal and provincial documents (see Armstrong 2007; Grigorovich 2013).

2 As of June 2017, the CCACs (and their staff) were absorbed into the Local Health Integration Networks (LHINs). The LHINs are crown agencies that plan and fund local health services and are now responsible for home and community care services operations, including the assessment of eligibility and case management.

REFERENCES

Albeda, R., M.V. Lee Badgett, G.J. Gates, and A. Schneebaum. 2009. "Poverty in the Lesbian, Gay, and Bisexual Community." Report. Los Angeles: Williams Institute. http://williamsinstitute.law.ucla.edu/research/census-lgbt-demographics-studies/poverty-in-the-lesbian-gay-and-bisexual-community/.

Armstrong, P. 2001. "Evidence-Based Health-Care Reform: Women's Issues." In *Unhealthy Times: The Political Economy of Health and Care in Canada*, edited by P. Armstrong, H. Armstrong, and D. Coburn, 121–45. Toronto: Oxford University Press.

Armstrong, P. 2007. "Relocating Care: Home Care in Ontario." In *Women's Health in Canada: Critical Perspectives on Theory and Policy*, edited by M. Morrow, O. Hankivsky, and C. Varcoe, 528–53. Toronto: University of Toronto Press.

Armstrong, P., and H. Armstrong. 2001. "Women, Privatization and Health Care Reform: The Ontario Case." In *Exposing Privatization: Women and Health Care Reform in Canada*, edited by P. Armstrong, C. Amaratunga, J. Bernier, K. Grant, A. Pederson, and K. Willson, 163–215. Aurora: Garamond.

Armstrong, P., and H. Armstrong. 2010. *Wasting Away: The Undermining of Canadian Health Care.* Toronto: Oxford University Press.

Armstrong, P., H. Armstrong, and D. Coburn. 2001. *Unhealthy Times: The Political Economy of Health and Care in Canada.* Toronto: Oxford University Press.

Aronson, J. 2004. "'Just Fed and Watered': Women's Experiences of the Gutting of Home Care in Ontario." In *Caring Possibilities: Women's Work, Women's Care*, edited by K. Grant, C. Amaratunga, P. Armstrong, et al., 167–84. Aurora: Garamond.

Aronson, J., M. Denton, and I. Zeytinoglu. 2004. "Market-Modelled Home Care in Ontario: Deteriorating Working Conditions and Dwindling Community Capacity." *Canadian Public Policy/Analyse de Politiques* 30 (1): 111–25. https://doi.org/10.2307/3552583.

Aronson, J., and S.M. Neysmith. 1997. "The Retreat of the State and Long-Term Care Provision: Implications for Frail Elderly People, Unpaid Family Carers and Paid Home Care Workers." *Studies in Political Economy* 53: 37–66. https://doi.org/10.1080/19187033.1997.11675315.

Baranek, P.M., R.B. Deber, and A.P. Williams. 2004. *Almost Home: Reforming Home and Community Care in Ontario.* Toronto: University of Toronto Press.

Barbara, A.M., S.A. Quandt, and R.T. Anderson. 2001. "Experiences of Lesbians in the Health Care Environment." *Women & Health* 34 (1): 45–62. https://doi.org/10.1300/J013v34n01_04.

Barker, J. 2004. "Lesbian Aging: An Agenda for Future Research." In *Gay and Lesbian Aging: Research and Future Directions,* edited by G. Herdt and B. De Vries, 29–72. New York: Springer.

Bjorkman, M., and K. Malterud. 2009. "Lesbian Women's Experiences with Health Care: A Qualitative Study." *Scandinavian Journal of Primary Health Care* 27 (4): 238–43. https://doi.org/10.3109/02813430903226548.

Brotman, S., B. Ryan, S. Collins, L. Chamberland, R. Cormier, D. Julien, E. Meyer, A. Peterkin, and B. Richard. 2007. "Coming Out to Care: Caregivers of Gay and Lesbian Seniors in Canada." *The Gerontologist* 47 (4): 490–503. https://doi.org/10.1093/geront/47.4.490.

Chapman, R., R. Watkins, T. Zappia, P. Nicol, and L. Shields. 2012. "Nursing and Medical Students' Attitude, Knowledge and Beliefs Regarding Lesbian, Gay, Bisexual and Transgender Parents Seeking Health Care for Their Children." *Journal of Clinical Nursing* 21 (7–8): 938–45. https://doi.org/10.1111/j.1365-2702.2011.03892.x.

Daly, T. 2007. "Out of Place: Mediating Health and Social Care at Ontario's State–Voluntary Sector Divide." *Canadian Journal on Aging* Suppl. 1: 63–75. https://doi.org/10.3138/cja.26.suppl_1.063.

Davies, K. 1994. "The Tensions between Process Time and Clock Time in Care-Work: The Example of Day Nurseries." *Time & Society* 3 (3): 277–303. https://doi.org/10.1177/0961463X94003003002.

Denton, M., I.U. Zeytinoglu, S. Davies, and D. Hunter. 2006. "The Impact of Implementing Managed Competition on Home Care Workers' Turnover Decisions." *Healthcare Policy* 1 (4): 106–23. https://www.hhr-rhs.ca/index.php?option=com_mtree&task=visit&link_id=6759&Itemid=64&lang=en.

Eliason, M.J., and S. Raheim. 2000. "Experiences and Comfort with Culturally Diverse Groups in Undergraduate Pre-nursing Students." *Journal of Nursing Education* 39 (4): 161–5. https://doi.org/10.3928/0148-4834-20000401-06.

Emmerich, N., D. Swinglehurst, J. Maybin, S. Park, and S. Quilligan. 2015. "Caring for Quality of Care: Symbolic Violence and the Bureaucracies of Audit." *BMC Medical Ethics* 16: 23. https://doi.org/10.1186/s12910-015-0006-z.

England, K., J. Eakin, D. Gastaldo, and P. McKeever. 2007. "Neoliberalizing Home Care: Managed Competition and Restructuring Home Care in

Ontario." In *Neoliberalization: Networks, States, Peoples,* edited by K. England and K. Ward, 169–94. Oxford: Blackwell.

Evans, A. 2010. "Governing Post-operative Pain: The Construction of 'Good and Active' Patients, 'Good and Busy' Nurses and the Production of Docile Bodies." *Aporia* 2 (3): 24–31. https://doi.org/10.18192/aporia.v2i3.2987.

Fredriksen-Goldsen, K.I., H.J. Kim, and S.E. Barkan. 2012. "Disability among Lesbian, Gay, and Bisexual Adults: Disparities in Prevalence and Risk." *American Journal of Public Health* 102 (1): e16–21. https://doi.org/10.2105/AJPH.2011.300379.

Fuller, C. 1998. *Caring for Profit: How Corporations Are Taking Over Canada's Health Care System.* Vancouver: New Star.

Goldenberg, M.J. 2012. "Defining Quality of Care Persuasively." *Theoretical Medicine and Bioethics* 33 (4): 243–61. https://doi.org/10.1007/s11017-012-9230-4.

Grant, J.M. 2010. *Outing Age: Public Policy Issues Affecting Gay, Lesbian, Bisexual and Transgender Elders.* Washington, DC: National Gay and Lesbian Task Force Policy Institute. https://www.thetaskforce.org/outing-age-2010/.

Grant, K., C. Amaratunga, and P. Armstrong. 2004. *Caring For/Caring About: Women, Home Care and Unpaid Caregiving.* Aurora: Garamond.

Grigorovich, A. 2013. "Long-Term Care for Older Lesbian and Bisexual Women: An Analysis of Current Research and Policy." *Social Work in Public Health* 28 (6): 596–606. https://doi.org/10.1080/19371918.2011.593468.

Grigorovich, A. 2015a. "Negotiating Sexuality in Home Care Settings: Older Lesbian and Bisexual Women's Experiences." *Culture, Health & Sexuality* 17 (8): 947–61. https://doi.org/10.1080/13691058.2015.1011237.

Grigorovich, A. 2015b. "Restricted Access: Older Lesbian and Bisexual Women's Experiences with Home Care Services." *Research on Aging* 37 (7): 763–83. https://doi.org/10.1177%2F0164027514562650.

Grigorovich, A. 2016. "The Meaning of Quality of Care in Home Care Settings: Older Lesbian and Bisexual Women's Perspectives." *Scandinavian Journal of Caring Sciences* 30 (1): 1–9. https://doi.org/10.1111/scs.12228.

Health Quality Ontario (HQO). 2015. *Measuring Up.* Toronto: Queen's Printer. http://www.hqontario.ca/System-Performance/Yearly-Reports.

Health Quality Ontario (HQO). 2016. *Indicator Library.* Toronto: Queen's Printer. http://indicatorlibrary.hqontario.ca/Indicator/Search/EN?searchTerms=experience&kwsGrid-sort=Rank-asc&kwsGrid-page=3&kwsGrid-pageSize=5&kwsGrid-group=&kwsGrid-filter=.

Hinchliff, S., M. Gott, and E. Galena. 2005. "'I Daresay I Might Find It Embarrassing': General Practitioners' Perspectives on Discussing Sexual Health Issues with Lesbian and Gay Patients." *Health & Social Care in the Community* 13 (4): 345–53. https://doi.org/10.1111/j.1365-2524.2005.00566.x.

Institute of Medicine. 2011. *The Health of Lesbian, Gay, Bisexual, and Transgender People: Building a Foundation for Better Understanding.* Washington, DC: National Academies Press.

Jackson, B.E., A. Pederson, P. Armstrong, M. Boscoe, B. Clow, K.R. Grant, N. Guberman, and K. Willson. 2006. "'Quality Care Is Like a Carton of Eggs': Using a Gender-Based Diversity Analysis to Assess Quality of Health Care." *Canadian Woman Studies* 24 (1): 15–22. https://cws.journals.yorku.ca/index.php/cws/article/view/6171.

James, B.C. 1989. *Quality Management for Health Care Delivery.* Chicago: Hospital Research and Educational Trust.

Luft, H.S. 2012. "From Small Area Variations to Accountable Care Organizations: How Health Services Research Can Inform Policy." *Annual Review of Public Health* 33: 377–92. https://doi.org/10.1146/annurev-publhealth-031811-124701.

McLaughlin, C.P., and A.D. Kaluzny. 2004. *Continuous Quality Improvement in Health Care: Theory, Implementation, and Applications.* Mississauga: Jones & Bartlett Learning Canada.

Mol, A. 2008. *The Logic of Care: Health and the Problem of Patient Choice.* London: Routledge.

Mykhalovskiy, E., P. Armstrong, H. Armstrong, I. Bourgeault, J. Choiniere, J. Lexchin, S. Peters, and J. White. 2008. "Qualitative Research and the Politics of Knowledge in an Age of Evidence: The Possibilities and Perils of Immanent Critique." *Social Science & Medicine* 67 (1): 195–203. https://doi.org/10.1016/j.socscimed.2008.03.002.

Nedelsky, J. 1989. "Reconceiving Autonomy: Sources, Thoughts and Possibilities." *Yale Journal of Law and Feminism* 1 (7): 7–36. https://digitalcommons.law.yale.edu/yjlf/vol1/iss1/5.

Ong, M.K., C.M. Mangione, P.S. Romano, Q. Zhou, A.D. Auerbach, A. Chun, B. Davidson, et al. 2009. "Looking Forward, Looking Back: Assessing Variations in Hospital Resource Use and Outcomes for Elderly Patients with Heart Failure." *Circulation Cardiovascular Quality and Outcomes* 2 (6): 548–57. https://doi.org/10.1161/CIRCOUTCOMES.108.825612.

Ontario Association of Community Care Access Centres (OACCAC). 2015. *CCAC Fast Facts.* http://oaccac.com/Quality-And-Transparency/Fast-Facts.

Ontario Auditor General. 2015. *Annual Report.* Toronto: Queen's Printer.

Ontario Ministry of Health and Long-Term Care. 2011. "Health Bulletin: Health Quality Ontario to Promote Evidence-Based Health Care." http://www.health.gov.on.ca/en/news/bulletin/2011/hb_20110404.aspx.

Pollock, K., N. Moghaddam, K. Cox, E. Wilson, and P. Howard. 2011. "Exploring Patients' Experience of Receiving Information about Cancer: A Comparison of Interview and Questionnaire Methods of Data Collection." *Health* 15 (2): 153–72. https://doi.org/10.1177/1363459309360789.

Randall, G.E., and P. Williams. 2006. "Exploring Limits to Market-Based Reform: Managed Competition and Rehabilitation Home Care Services in Ontario." *Social Science and Medicine* 62: 1594–604. https://doi.org/10.1016/j.socscimed.2005.08.042.

Rankin, J.M. 2003. "'Patient Satisfaction': Knowledge for Ruling Hospital Reform: An Institutional Ethnography." *Nursing Inquiry* 10 (1): 57–65. https://doi.org/10.1046/j.1440-1800.2003.00156.x.

Rose, N., and P. Miller. 1992. "Political Power beyond the State: Problematics of Government." *British Journal of Sociology* 43 (2): 173–205. https://doi.org/10.2307/591464.

Sevenhuijsen, S. 1998. *Citizenship and the Ethics of Care: Feminist Considerations on Justice, Morality and Politics.* London: Routledge.

Sherwin, S. 1998. *The Politics of Women's Health: Exploring Agency and Autonomy.* Philadelphia: Temple University Press.

Sinding, C. 2003. "Disarmed Complaints: Unpacking Satisfaction with End-of-Life Care." *Social Science & Medicine* 57 (8): 1375–85. https://doi.org/10.1016/S0277-9536(02)00512-9.

Solarz, A.L. 1999. *Lesbian Health: Current Assessment and Directions for the Future.* Washington DC: National Academies Press.

Stein, G.L., N.L. Beckerman, and P.A. Sherman. 2010. "Lesbian and Gay Elders and Long-Term Care: Identifying the Unique Psychosocial Perspectives and Challenges." *Journal of Gerontological Social Work* 53 (5): 421–35. https://doi.org/10.1080/01634372.2010.496478.

Swinglehurst, D., N. Emmerich, J. Maybin, S. Park, and S. Quilligan. 2015. "Confronting the Quality Paradox: Towards New Characterisations of 'Quality' in Contemporary Healthcare." *BMC Health Services Research* 15: 240. https://doi.org/10.1186/s12913-015-0851-y.

Téllez, C., M. Ramos, B. Umland, T. Palley, and B. Skipper. 1999. "Attitudes of Physicians in New Mexico toward Gay Men and Lesbians." *Journal of the Gay and Lesbian Medical Association* 3 (3): 83–9. https://doi.org/10.1023/A:1022287927588.

Tronto, J.C. 1993. *Moral Boundaries: A Political Argument for an Ethic of Care.* New York: Routledge.

Wallace, S.P., S.D. Cochran, E.M. Durazo, and C.L. Ford. 2011. "The Health of Aging Lesbian, Gay and Bisexual Adults in California." Policy brief, UCLA Center for Health Policy Research, 1–8. https://healthpolicy.ucla.edu/publications/search/pages/detail.aspx?PubID=27.

Williams, A.P., R. Deber, P. Baranek, and A. Gildiner. 2001. "From Medicare to Home Care: Globalization, State Retrenchment, and the Profitization of Canada's Healthcare System." In *Unhealthy Times: Political Economy Perspectives on Health and Care in Canada,* edited by P. Armstrong, H. Armstrong, and D. Coburn, 7–30. Toronto: Oxford University Press.

Williams, B. 1994. "Patient Satisfaction: A Valid Concept?" *Social Science & Medicine* 38 (4): 509–16. https://doi.org/10.1016/0277-9536(94)90247-X.

Worthington, C. 2005. "Patient Satisfaction with Health Care: Recent Theoretical Developments and Implications for Evaluation Practice." *The Canadian Journal of Program Evaluation* 20 (3): 41–63. https://evaluationcanada.ca/system/files/cjpe-entries/20-3-041.pdf.

PART TWO

Health Markets, Individualization, and Commodification

8 Cigarette-Packaging Legislation in Canada and the Smoking Subject

KIRSTEN BELL

In 2000, Canada became the first country in the world to legislate graphic warning labels on cigarette packets. This represented a key turning point in cigarette-packaging legislation because it explicitly recognized the potential of graphic warning labels to reduce cigarette consumption, as well as presenting factual information about the health effects of smoking (Health Canada 2000). In other words, warning labels were now conceptualized as an *intervention* into smoking – one seen to provide universal and repeated exposure to anti-smoking messages.

In 2012 the legislation was updated to significantly increase the size and intensity of the warnings, which now featured a series of highly confronting images: a needle skewering an eyeball; an open mouth revealing a tongue covered in revolting white growths; a man grimly displaying the stoma from his tracheotomy; a bald, emaciated woman on her death bed. In 2019 the legislation was updated again, with Canada following Australia's lead in implementing plain packaging legislation. As of November 2019, cigarette packets have been stripped of industry branding and are now a uniform brown colour, based on the assumption that this will reduce the attractiveness and appeal of tobacco products by removing distinctive features and increasing the prominence of the warning labels (Health Canada 2019a).

Although a primary goal of plain packaging initiatives is preventing the uptake of smoking (see Chapman and Freeman 2014; Health Canada 2019), a secondary target is current smokers themselves. The assumption underpinning this legislation is that "unbranded cigarette packets reduce the appeal of smoking, increase the salience of health warnings and correct misperceptions about the harms of tobacco use, thereby decreasing the number of young people who start smoking and increasing the number of people who quit" (Bell et al. 2015, 137). Reducing the prevalence of smoking is central to the logic of graphic warning labels, based on the assumption that the labels provide a forceful reminder of its dangers. According to Fong (2001, 2), "An individual who smokes one pack per day, for example, is potentially exposed to the health warning 7300 times in a single year."

As such legislation suggests, the cigarette packet is considered to be a powerful vehicle through which the tobacco industry seduces the public into a dangerous addiction; thus, the aim of plain packaging policies is to *disrupt* and *redirect* the power of the branded packet to serve public health rather than industry ends (Bell et al. 2015). Such views draw on a long-standing narrative about the power of marketing and advertising – a narrative that we take very much for granted today. However, Cronin (2004, 3) suggests that many of the claims made about advertising say as much about its importance as a trope for "rehearsing understandings of the social and social relations" as they do about the effects of advertising itself. Her key assertion is that such claims operate "as a form of currency that constitutes the social order in discursive, material and economic ways" (ibid.).

These insights form my starting point for this chapter, which explores the ways in which cigarette packaging has been conceptualized in tobacco control – a public health field of research, policy, and practice that aims to reduce the morbidity and mortality associated with tobacco use and its attendant burden on the health care system. Although I don't dispute the potential agency of branded cigarette packets, the claims that circulate about packaging in tobacco control and industry accounts tell us as much about how the social is understood – and thereby constituted – as they do about packaging itself. This is my interest in what follows: to consider what research and policy directions in cigarette packaging reveal about how smokers are legislatively imagined in public health and their material effects on how smoking is conceptualized and intervened into.

The general disposition of the chapter is storytelling rather than theorizing, although my orientation is broadly poststructuralist and informed by a critically engaged interest in dominant public health discourses on cigarette packaging. However, instead of treating these discourses as the end of the story (as some styles of discourse analysis are wont to do), I treat them as the beginning – by empirically investigating the ways that smokers have responded to these representations. Drawing on in-situ interviews with sixty people smoking in public spaces in Vancouver between 2013 and 2015, I discuss smokers' engagements with packages on their own terms, decoupled from the promotionist and cessationist agendas that have hitherto dominated research into this topic (see Haines-Saah and Bell 2016 for further details). By juxtaposing conceptions of cigarette packaging in tobacco control accounts with smokers' own narratives, I aim to illustrate the limitations of the ways in which the "smoking subject" has been constituted in public health and the need for a more critically engaged social science perspective on this topic.

The Logic of Cigarette Packaging Legislation

Several core assumptions underpin contemporary cigarette-packaging legislation as it has been promoted by the World Health Organization's (WHO) Framework Convention on Tobacco Control and enacted in Canada and elsewhere. First, the legislation assumes that smokers are not fully cognizant of the health effects of smoking and that informing them of these effects will encourage them to cease the habit. To quote the WHO report *Warning about the Dangers of Tobacco* (WHO 2011, 18), "Despite clear evidence about the dangers of tobacco use, many tobacco users worldwide underestimate the full extent of the risk to themselves and others." The underlying message is that education about the dangers of smoking will cause smokers to consciously *choose* not to partake.

Macnaughton, Carro-Ripalda, and Russell (2012, 458) have characterized this as the "rational agent" view, which assumes that smokers "need only be presented with the facts to respond appropriately." The figure of the rational, autonomous subject who reasons and makes choices is hardly unique to tobacco control. With us since the European Enlightenment, it today lies at the very heart of health care and public health (Mol 2008). Its influence is also evident in the concept of "health behaviour" and the various theories that have emerged to describe how behaviour change occurs (e.g., the "health belief" model, the "stages of change" model), which generally emphasize the cognitive and processing capacities of the individual (see Bell 2017).

Although the "rational human" model clearly underpins cigarette-packaging initiatives, Alemanno (2012) argues that such legislation relies to an even greater extent on "nudging" strategies, suggesting that this shift in emphasis has been a broader feature of recent directions in tobacco control policy. The concept of "nudging" was first systematically outlined by Thaler and Sunstein (2008). With its roots in the disciplines of psychology, behavioural economics, and marketing, nudging is based on the premise that environment largely dictates our behaviour, so people will make better decisions if their environments are rearranged to facilitate positive behaviour change. In essence, nudging shifts the focus away from a purely rational actor and posits, instead, an individual who makes imperfect choices based on a tension between short-term pleasure and long-term goals (Burgess 2012).

Macnaughton, Carro-Ripalda, and Russell (2012) describe this as the "non-agent" view of smokers, which understands them as "Pavlovian automatons" who are manipulated by the tobacco industry into enslavement by an addictive drug. Although the "rational agent" and "Pavlovian automaton" frameworks seem somewhat at odds, equally part of the Enlightenment vision is the assumption that humans are intellectually imperfect and subject to "tidal currents of passion and interest" that flow against, and distort operation of, their rational faculties (Shapin 2010, 48–9). Cigarette packaging legislation therefore aims to target both the "free, responsible, autonomous subject, capable of making the right choice insofar as she received the correct information" (Alemanno 2012, 38) and her emotional and impulse-driven self, who is swayed by environmental and affective cues.

In this framework, where smoking is positioned as an individual-level "health behaviour" that results from lifestyle choices and environmental cues, the social context and meaning of smoking become largely irrelevant (Frohlich et al. 2012; Haines et al. 2010; Poland et al. 2006). Thus, a linear, causal narrative about problem/solution and pathology/treatment can be established: that people smoke because they are addicted and can't stop; that they lack an awareness of the health consequences of smoking; and that they are deficient in the self-control or self-efficacy necessary to resist peer pressure and/or manipulation by the tobacco industry (Mair and Kierans 2007). Decreasing their ignorance via information and increasing their self-control via environmental cues that discourage smoking and encourage cessation therefore becomes the answer to reducing the incidence and prevalence of smoking. Viewed in this light, cigarette-packaging legislation becomes a model intervention. To quote Hammond (2011, 335), "In many ways, health warnings on tobacco packages are an ideal population-level intervention: they have broad reach, they cost little to implement and are sustainable over time."

The Evidence Base

The earliest research on cigarette packaging was conducted by the tobacco industry itself. As industry documents attest, the packet formed an intensive – and highly fetishized – feature of research throughout the twentieth century. A central impetus for such studies was the concept of "sensation transference" developed by the marketing pioneer and clinical psychologist Louis Cheskin, who was responsible for the iconic Marlboro packet. According to Cheskin, this effect occurred when "the auratic effects of the branded package are translated into innate qualities of the product" (quoted in Pottage 2013, 544). Thus, an extraordinary amount of attention was placed on the visual features of the cigarette packet, from its font to its colour and design motifs.

The industry's assumptions regarding the ways that pack design dictated smokers' responses to its content largely set the terms for subsequent health research into cigarette packaging. Indeed, today most public health researchers operate according to the same premise as the tobacco industry: that packaging *does* have an impact on smoking – a view that reaches its epitome in plain packaging initiatives. Questions therefore relate primarily to what degree it produces these effects and how they might be strengthened in the desired direction. In some respects, this very narrow gaze reflects the applied and instrumental turn in health research highlighted in this book's introductory chapter. However, it also relates to the specificities of tobacco research itself and concerns about the potential for industry appropriation, which increasingly dictate the ways that researchers engage with this topic.

Mair and Kierans (2007) have highlighted the growing alignment between tobacco research and tobacco control, noting that tobacco research is now expected to further the goals of tobacco control, with tobacco research "proper" defined by its commitment to ending the global tobacco "epidemic." As they point out, although this view of tobacco research stems from a desire to differentiate industry-funded and non-industry-funded research, defining legitimate tobacco research by its commitment to tobacco control renders it purely instrumental in function. In this respect, tobacco control research has, ironically, begun to mirror tobacco industry research.

The most influential tobacco control research is unquestionably the ongoing prospective cohort studies produced by the International Tobacco Control Policy Evaluation Project, which is headquartered in Canada. A product of the growing push for "evidence-based policy" (see Smith 2013), this project aims to evaluate the "psychosocial and behavioural impact of key national-level policies of the WHO Framework Convention on Tobacco Control" (http://www.itcproject.org/about) in order to facilitate its expanded implementation. It currently produces annual, nationally representative cohort surveys in more than twenty-five countries, although the evidence it has produced on the effectiveness of cigarette warning labels comes primarily from the International Tobacco Control Four Country Survey, which includes Canada, Australia, the United States, and the United Kingdom. Via comparisons between these countries, the research team has concluded that warnings that are graphic, larger, and stronger in content are more effective than small text-based labels (e.g., Borland et al. 2009; Hammond et al. 2007).

In the studies, "effectiveness" is measured in three ways: warning salience, that is, reading and noticing warnings; cognitive responses, or thoughts of harm and quitting; and behavioural responses, such as forgoing cigarettes, avoiding the warnings, and the like. Although quitting is an outcome of interest, the other measures are treated as proxies for changes in "smoking behaviour." In essence, the "elements" that constitute quitting are parsed into a series of discrete "variables" (noticing warning labels, thinking about quitting, responding strongly to labels, avoiding them, and so on) that are understood to be individually – and sequentially – linked to the desired outcome: quitting itself. These measures thus fundamentally rely on the rational agent and non-agent paradigms outlined above to make sense as meaningful "predictors" of behavioural change.

Challenging the Logic of Cigarette Packaging Legislation

The core assumptions that currently drive research on cigarette packaging are difficult to reconcile with research findings that step outside of this methodological and epistemological frame. As I have outlined elsewhere, the majority of people I interviewed in Vancouver insisted that such messages had no impact on their smoking (Haines-Saah and Bell 2016). The almost universal refrain was that the warning labels were not "telling me anything I don't already know." Although my research was conducted prior to the implementation of plain packaging legislation in Canada, exactly the same sorts of claims were made by smokers participating in the study at sites in Australia, the United States, and the United Kingdom, despite the marked differences in legislation between the four countries – from plain packaging in Australia to small textual labels in the United States (Bell et al. 2015).[1]

By highlighting this disjuncture, my aim isn't to adjudicate the truth of these claims but to illustrate the vast distance between the ways smokers often talk about cigarette packaging and its conceptualization in tobacco control research and policy. In essence, what we see are two radically different discourses on packaging that are largely incommensurable – something continuously borne out in the stories of smokers I encountered.

I met Jim in the fall of 2013 in Vancouver's central business district. A white fifty-six-year-old manager, Jim indicated that he smoked about three quarters of a pack a day and that he had been doing so for at least twenty years, "factoring in all the times I have quit and restarted." Like most people I interviewed, Jim couldn't identify the warning label on the packet of cigarettes he was currently smoking; he also struggled to recall any of the other labels, discussing one that is no longer in circulation (on impotence) and only two that are.

Specifically highlighting "the one with the woman skeleton," he volunteered that he knew people who transferred their cigarettes to another container when they got a packet bearing this label. When I queried him further, he clarified that *he* didn't do this but that "I know women who do because they find it terrifying." This led to a discussion of the potential impact of the labels, which Jim immediately disavowed: "no one ever expressed that they quit because of the labels." He continued: "they do make me think about considering quitting sometimes, but that's different from *actually* quitting." We both laughed at this observation, which he repeated for comedic effect: "yeah, they make me think about *considering* quitting."

Recall that in the International Tobacco Control Survey, thoughts of harm and quitting and avoiding the warning labels are both treated as measures of effectiveness.[2] But, for Jim, the notion that *thinking* about quitting actually *leads to* quitting was laughably simplistic – a view that makes sense in light of his lengthy history of relinquishing and restarting the habit. Quitting smoking, as Jim well knew, is not so easy. Likewise, he challenged the notion that avoiding the warnings was evidence of their effectiveness: if they bothered smokers that much, they merely transferred their cigarettes to another pack.

Bill, a sixty-year-old white smoker and out-of-work machinist, equally challenged the equation between avoidance and "impact." I met Bill in the fall of 2013 outside a YMCA where he was taking a break from his "how to look for work" class. Chatty and somewhat flirtatious, Bill informed me that he started smoking at the age of fifteen and had a pack-a-day habit – for the past five years he had mostly rolled his own cigarettes to try and save money. These he kept in a fake-crocodile-skin black case, which he handed to me for my perusal.

Bill characterized the images on the warning labels as "ugly" and "gross." "It's like looking at the blood-and-guts thing on *NC*[*IS*]-*CSI*." In his view, the labels showed "worst-case scenarios" and were an "exaggeration," although he was upfront in stating that he tried to avoid looking at them when purchasing loose tobacco or premade cigarettes. "We choose not to think about that [the health consequences of smoking]," Bill admitted.

In response to Bill's comments about avoiding the packs I asked him if he thought they therefore had an impact on his smoking. Evidently surprised by the suggestion, Bill immediately refuted it, leading to the following exchange:

BILL: Not at all. Not on *me*. But I already smoked.

KB: Right.

BILL: But I can see the point, when you show it to the kids that don't smoke.

KB: Right.

BILL: That's where it would have an effect.
KB: So you're basically say–
BILL: That's where it's of value.
KB: Right. So you're saying that you don't think the packets are aimed at smokers – people who are currently smoking? It's specifically aimed at –
BILL: – people who are about to start, like teenagers.

Contra the assumptions underpinning the International Tobacco Control Survey about the meaning of avoiding the warnings, Bill didn't see this as evidence that they were having an "impact" on smokers – quite the opposite. For Bill, the only group for whom the legislation might have any sort of effect was not-yet-smokers; he treated this as a kind of self-evident fact.

Non-smokers and Cigarette-Packaging Legislation

Many people I spoke with echoed Bill's assertion that the graphic warning labels weren't really aimed at them but at young people who hadn't started smoking yet. For example, in May of 2014 I interviewed Joe and Anna at a gazebo at a local college. One of only two designated smoking areas on campus, the gazebo had been created at the behest of the student union to protect smokers from inclement weather, and many friendships had been forged at the site, including Joe and Anna's. Joe was twenty-six, Korean born, and a psychology major; Anna was nineteen, majoring in criminology, and was born in the Philippines. Unlike Joe, who had been a pack-a-day smoker for seven or eight years, Anna informed me that over the past year she had transitioned from social to "regular" smoking. Although I was initially talking to Joe, it soon became a three-way conversation, with Anna often speaking up to counter or add to Joe's statements.

Like Bill, Joe characterized the warning labels as "extreme" and "exaggerated." He indicated that he didn't like the "moral crap" they contained, pointing specifically to the warnings about not smoking around children. He continued that he didn't like the ways the warning labels ended up "lecturing adults" – for Joe the government was "trying to destroy choice." Joe observed that "I already deal with enough shit for my smoking!" However, Anna interjected at this point, insisting that "the packaging is not directed to us." For her, it was really about the "anti-smoking lobby" and "pro-health people" trying to advocate their stance. Their target was therefore "not people who smoke, but people who don't."

In response to these observations, Joe speculated that the labels might have more of an impact on teenagers: "I guess it depends on how long they've been smoking." "Teens might be affected by all that image crap," he observed, "but it wouldn't impact someone who had been smoking longer." Anna added that although cigarette packets were now extremely "ugly," they didn't affect her personally because she carried a cigarette case. At this point she showed me the elegant black case she kept her smokes in and she and Joe reminisced about how Marlboros used to look before they were "filled with warnings and labels."

Joe and Anna's dialogue echoes many of the points made by Jim and Bill insofar as they each illustrate the dangers in reductive readings that treat actions (like avoiding the labels) as isolable from the context in which they are embedded. However, Anna's insistence that the labels were about the "anti-smoking lobby" and "pro-health people" trying to advocate their stance to people who *don't* smoke, and the implicit links Joe drew between the "moral crap" in the messages and the "shit" he got for his smoking from non-smokers, also suggest that they saw the legislation as reinforcing an environment of intolerance for smokers. This intolerance was something brought up by many informants, who frequently moved from a discussion of the labels to talking about the judgment they felt around their smoking, although few drew explicit links between the warning labels and this broader environment.

The primary exception was Luke, a down-on-his-luck sixty-three-year-old I met in the fall of 2013. I encountered Luke on a cold and foggy day when he was huddled with a bunch of other people smoking cigarettes near a side entrance of a local hospital that had officially implemented "smoke-free" grounds. Initially a little wary when I approached him for a chat, Luke queried, "You're not working for the cigarette companies, are you?"

Originally from Quebec, Luke informed me that he was "part French, part Scottish, part Huron Indian." When I asked about his occupation, he described himself as a "land developer"; however, as our conversation progressed it became clear that Luke was currently unemployed. Luke told me that he had lost everything in the market crash of 2008. Utterly broke, he had returned to Canada from the United States, where he had been living for the previous thirty years. Currently in poor health, Luke had spent time in and out of shelters – information he shared after a homeless guy approached us and asked him for a cigarette. Although Luke wasn't clear on what his health issues were, and I didn't want to push, my sense was that they were fairly serious. "It's my last vice," Luke joked of his smoking. "I don't want to go to heaven. I haven't got any friends up there."

When I asked Luke what he thought of the warning labels he responded, "it irritates me." He continued, "I know what the risks are. You know, it's like rubbing my nose in something that I'm already aware of. *Especially* if it's repetitive." In essence, the very repetition that is so valued in official public health discourse was precisely what he objected to. Dismissing the notion that the labels affected fellow smokers, Luke focused instead on their effect on *non*-smokers:

LUKE: I think they [the graphic warning labels] exacerbate the problem. I don't think they do any help, I think they exacerbate it.
KB: Okay, so how do they exacerbate the problem?
LUKE: By promoting negative behaviour on the part of non-smokers.
KB: Right.
LUKE: And by irritating the smokers.
KB: Right.
LUKE: And by propagating the bad behaviour.

Luke went on to observe that there were "more negative anti-smokers here in Canada than the US. I had one child who was maybe ten feet away from me go through this fake coughing routine. Okay, I can tell what's going on in *her* home."

The connections Luke drew between the warning labels and the promotion of a broader anti-smoking environment are unquestionably part of their intended function. For example, the WHO (2011, 23) asserts: "Warnings are also seen by non-smokers, affecting their perceptions of smoking and decisions about initiation, and ultimately helping to change the image of tobacco and 'denormalize' its use."

Tobacco Denormalization and Cigarette-Packaging Legislation

Although noticeably absent from Canada's newest tobacco control strategy (Health Canada 2019b), until recently, denormalization represented the fourth pillar of both the provincial and national tobacco control strategies (see BC Ministry of Health Services 2004). Pioneered in California, tobacco denormalization aims to utilize the power of social pressure to make smoking "less desirable, less acceptable and less accessible" (California Department of Health Services [CDHS] 1998, 3). In other words, it involves an ambitious attempt to transform social norms through "intentional human intervention" (3).

In many respects, the growing emphasis on tobacco denormalization strategies reflects Alemanno's (2012) observations about the newer generation of tobacco control policies relying more on nudging and less on cognitively based strategies that aim to intervene directly with the individual smoker. Indeed, tobacco control policies have been lauded for this approach and are increasingly being touted as a model for other so-called unhealthy behaviours such as high-fat/sugar diets and alcohol overconsumption. For example, comparing approaches to smoking and obesity, Kinmonth (2016, 170) argues that tobacco control policy has shifted over time from a focus on "individual behaviour, choice, and responsibility" to "the dangerous and addictive substance of tobacco, [and] the industry that profits from it." Accordingly, she argues that tobacco control measures since the 1970s have been more "social/systemic in nature" because of their focus on industry culpability.

Advocates of this perspective implicitly suggest that tobacco control policy runs counter to what has been termed the "neoliberalization" of health care and public health. Neoliberalism typically refers to the rise of deregulated and privatized solutions to health care based on the presumed efficiency and cost-effectiveness of market-driven models, and the emergence of forms of governmentality that promote new forms of subjectivity emphasizing individual responsibility for and ownership of health. Insofar as tobacco control aims to curb the movements of the tobacco industry via formal regulation, it appears to contradict these trends; however, it's questionable whether it represents a substantive shift in direction.

Recall the statement by Hammond (2011, 355) that "health warnings on tobacco packages are an ideal population-level intervention: they have broad reach, they cost little to implement and are sustainable over time." These sentiments are repeated in Borland et al.'s (2009, 358) observation that "such health warnings cost tax-payers nothing and potentially reach smokers every time they take a cigarette from a pack, buy a pack, or otherwise notice one." This assumption of cost-effectiveness is built into the logic of denormalization strategies more broadly. For example, in its original outline of tobacco denormalization, the California Department of Health Services (1998, 9) noted: "This population-based approach to cessation is far more cost effective and much less labor intensive than providing cessation assistance services to individuals."

Nudging strategies may shift the focus from individual cognition to environmental stimuli but, as I have already shown, they are based on an equally limited view of why people smoke that largely complements (rather than dislodging) the older emphasis on "individual responsibility." As Burgess (2012, 6) notes, nudging – identified as a form of "libertarian paternalism" by its authors – is intended to represent "a 'third way' between the regulation associated with the left and the 'leave it to the markets' approach of the right." For such reasons, Carter (2015) argues that libertarian paternalism is actually a *variant* of neoliberal governmentality insofar as it aims to affect how people perceive, problematize, and "govern" their own health.

As I have shown above, smokers I interviewed are well aware of this aspect of cigarette-packaging initiatives. Moreover, a consistently voiced view – especially amongst older smokers – was the ways in which the government actively profited from tobacco sales. In the spring of 2015, I met Dean, a white sixty-five-year-old man, outside a pub in one of Vancouver's most diverse eastside neighbourhoods. Now retired, Dean told me that he used to work in the logging industry and had been smoking since the age of twenty-seven. Currently a pack-a-day smoker, Dean had recently started using a "vape pipe" and was aiming to reduce his cigarette consumption to less than a pack a day. Gesturing to the pub we were standing in front of, he noted that there were nevertheless times when he preferred smoking to vaping – such as when he was having a beer.

When I asked to have a look at the label on his cigarette packet, he admitted that he'd purchased it on the black market, and it therefore didn't bear a regular label. "Who's gonna pay twelve dollars a pack when you can get cigarettes so much cheaper?" he asked, clearly feeling the need to justify himself. However, he indicated that even when he purchased "normal" packs, he didn't pay attention to the labels. "I've had two heart attacks," Dean said, "they're not telling me anything I don't know." He continued that this was a typical government tactic: they still sell cigarettes but give you a warning label on them. Dean concluded that "it's a two-sided deal" that benefited both groups.

These views were repeated almost verbatim by Gary, a white fifty-six-year-old Australian migrant I also met in the spring of 2015 in front of an expensive hotel in downtown Vancouver. Gary had been living in Toronto for the past thirteen years, but made frequent trips to both Vancouver and Australia – he was therefore familiar with the "plain" cigarette packs in Australia as well as the Canadian warning labels. Recently retired, Gary had previously been the CEO of a company and was probably the wealthiest person I interviewed, a substantial minority of whom were living on low incomes and/or struggling financially.

Like virtually everyone I talked with, Gary couldn't recall the warning label on the pack of cigarettes he was smoking. "They're a waste of money and time," he responded dismissively. Prefacing his following comments by saying "I don't like smoking" and "nicotine is more addictive than heroin," he observed that it was nevertheless "crazy for governments to make billions in taxes and then put up the warning labels."

During our conversation Gary observed that there have been a number of changes in the social acceptability of smoking over time. However, while smokers were now considered to be "socially inept," this shift had nothing to do with the warning labels themselves, which, he repeated, were "a waste of time." Encompassing both Canada and Australia's legislation, he expressed his struggle to understand the growing emphasis on the warning labels: "I can't get my head around selling the shit and making multi-billions on the one hand and then telling people not to do it on the other." He argued that if the government was really serious about smoking, they would ensure that cigarette taxes were put towards programs that provide smokers with medical and clinical assistance. The warning labels were thus a "facade": they didn't really *do* anything but merely provided the *appearance* of it. "You can't suck and blow at the same time," Gary concluded.

I don't think anyone who made such observations intended to suggest that the government should ban smoking; nor were they necessarily well informed about how much revenue the federal and provincial governments generate from tobacco sales – or the proportion of those monies diverted to smoking cessation services.[3] Instead, they were trying to express what they saw as the hypocrisy of cigarette warning labels as a facile intervention that pays lip service to discouraging smoking, but enables the government to benefit from tobacco sales and does nothing to actively support smokers to quit, while simultaneously placing the onus upon them to do so. Viewed in this light, such legislation seems to exemplify rather than override the neoliberalization of public health, despite its declared intent to rein in the tobacco industry via formal regulation.

Conclusion

In this chapter I have told a story about cigarette-packaging legislation that departs from how this subject matter is typically conceptualized in tobacco control and industry accounts. Rather than starting from the prima facie assumption that cigarette packaging (and advertising more generally) "works," I have instead suggested that the question itself is misplaced. Importantly, this isn't just a methodological issue – a matter of refining our approaches so that we can more efficiently isolate effects from outcomes – but an epistemological one.

Although the models of personhood underpinning tobacco control and public health clearly have a lengthy history, smoking is not a stable "behaviour" that can be isolated and intervened in but a complex bundle of practices that can't be divorced from its social context without seriously misapprehending it (Blue et al. 2016). It follows that cigarette packets themselves can't be intervened in to straightforwardly change smoking – something most people I interviewed were well aware of. In many respects this is an extremely obvious point, which is why it's a little surprising that so much effort is currently being invested in cigarette-packaging initiatives within tobacco control. However, as I have illustrated, this is largely a product of the very limited ways in which the smoking subject is conceptualized in the field.

That said, I don't intend to suggest that we merely take smokers' accounts at face value and conclude that cigarette packets don't matter. But *how* they matter is clearly not something that can be isolated or, arguably, legislated. Moreover, smokers' stories about cigarette packaging (much like tobacco control and industry accounts themselves) tell us something about how smokers are being imagined – albeit in this case it is *smokers themselves* doing the imagining. The resultant picture speaks to a growing sense of alienation on the part of smokers from legislation that ostensibly aims to support them but which many feel accomplishes the opposite of what it intends. In essence, the distance between tobacco control and tobacco industry perspectives is not so readily grasped by smokers themselves, given the ways that the former replicates the logic of the latter, albeit to an opposite intended effect.

While some readers might be tempted to dispute the specifics of these accounts (indeed, the underlying premise of nudging strategies is that the conscious responses of smokers are an unreliable means of ascertaining their effectiveness), it would be dangerous to dismiss them entirely. If tobacco control researchers are to seriously grapple with the social context and meaning of smoking, this must entail an openness to being transformed by the experience of engaging with smokers themselves and their own ways of seeing (Poland et al. 2006). Otherwise, researchers run the risk of endlessly reproducing their own received knowledge.

As Rebecca Haines-Saah (2012, 130) points out, "Unlike other health fields (e.g. mental health, HIV/AIDS) where so-called consumer/survivors are visible and have an active presence in research and policy forums, current and former tobacco users are virtually absent from tobacco control." Rather than positioning smokers as objects of intervention and control, what is needed are approaches that engage people who smoke as active subjects with critical insights to offer into the conditions of their own lives and the role of smoking within it (Haines-Saah 2012). Only by moving outside of established paradigms do we stand any chance of implementing strategies that smokers *themselves* see as improving public health.

NOTES

The study on which this chapter is based, titled "Confronting Cigarette Packaging," was funded by an operating grant from the Canadian Institutes of Health Research and the Canadian Cancer Society Research Institute. Rebecca Haines-Saah conducted six of the interviews with me in Vancouver, and my work with her on cigarette packaging, and that done in collaboration with my three co-investigators on the study (Simone Dennis, Jude Robinson, and Roland Moore), has unquestionably informed my thinking about this topic. I gratefully acknowledge their contributions here.

1 The study was specifically designed to speak back to the International Tobacco Control Four Country Survey.

2 In many respects, these assumptions echo the highly influential transtheoretical or "stages of change" model of smoking cessation, where smokers' readiness to quit is demarcated into six distinct stages, beginning with "precontemplation" (see Prochaska and Velicer 1997). However, despite the embrace of this model, it has been criticized for its simplistic view of human functioning (see Bunton et al. 2000).

3 According to statistics compiled by Physicians for a Smoke-Free Canada (2015), cigarette taxes amounted to over eight billion dollars in 2014–15, although a portion is actually earmarked for smoking cessation services or cancer research in some provinces.

REFERENCES

Alemanno, A. 2012. "Nudging Smokers: The Behavioural Turn of Tobacco Risk Regulation." *European Journal of Risk Regulation* 3 (3): 32–42. https://doi.org/10.1017/S1867299X00001781.

BC Ministry of Health Services. 2004. *BC's Tobacco Control Strategy: Targeting Our Efforts.* Victoria: BC Ministry of Health Services.

Bell, K. 2017. *Health and Other Unassailable Values: Reconfigurations of Health, Evidence and Ethics.* London: Routledge.

Bell, K., S. Dennis, J. Robinson, and R. Moore. 2015. "Does the Hand That Controls the Cigarette Packet Rule the Smoker? Findings from Ethnographic Interviews with Smokers in Canada, Australia, the United Kingdom and the USA." *Social Science and Medicine* 142: 136–44. https://doi.org/10.1016/j.socscimed.2015.08.021.

Blue, S., E. Shove, C. Carmona, and M.P. Kelly. 2016. "Theories of Practice and Public Health: Understanding (Un)healthy Practices." *Critical Public Health* 26 (1): 36–50. https://doi.org/10.1080/09581596.2014.980396.

Borland, R., N. Wilson, G.T. Fong, D. Hammond, K.M. Cummings, H-H. Yong, W. Hosking, G. Hastings, J. Thrasher, and A. McNeill. 2009. "Impact of Graphic and Text Warnings on Cigarette Packs: Findings from Four Countries over Five Years." *Tobacco Control* 18 (5): 358–64. https://doi.org/10.1136/tc.2008.028043.

Bunton, R., S. Baldwin, D. Flynn, and S. Whitelaw. 2000. "The 'Stages of Change' Model in Health Promotion: Science and Ideology." *Critical Public Health* 10 (1): 55–70. https://doi.org/10.1080/713658223.

Burgess, A. 2012. "'Nudging' Healthy Lifestyles: The UK Experiments with the Behavioural Alternative to Regulation and the Market." *European Journal of Risk Regulation* 3 (3): 3–16. https://doi.org/10.1017/S1867299X00001756.

California Department of Health Service (CDHS). 1998. *A Model for Change: The California Experience in Tobacco Control.* Sacramento: California Department of Health Services, Tobacco Control Section.

Carter, E. 2015. "Making the Blue Zones: Neoliberalism and Nudges in Public Health Promotion." *Social Science and Medicine* 133: 374–82. https://doi.org/10.1016/j.socscimed.2015.01.019.

Chapman, S., and B. Freeman. 2014. *Removing the Emperor's Clothes: Australia and Tobacco Plain Packaging.* Sydney: Sydney University Press.

Cronin, A.M. 2004. *Advertising Myths: The Strange Half-Lives of Images and Commodities.* Routledge: London.

Fong, G.T. 2001. *A Review of the Research on Tobacco Warning Labels, with Particular Emphasis on the New Canadian Warning Labels.* Waterloo: Tobacco Labelling Resource Centre.

Frohlich, K., E. Mykhalovskiy, B.D. Poland, R. Haines-Saah, and J. Johnson. 2012. "Creating the Socially Marginalised Youth Smoker: The Role of Tobacco Control." *Sociology of Health & Illness* 34 (7): 978–93. https://doi.org/10.1111/j.1467-9566.2011.01449.x.

Haines, R.J., J.L. Oliffe, J.L. Bottorff, and B.D. Poland. 2010. "'The Missing Picture': Tobacco Use through the Eyes of Smokers." *Tobacco Control* 19 (3): 206–12. https://doi.org/10.1136/tc.2008.027565.

Haines-Saah, R.J. 2012. "After the Smoke Has Cleared: Reflections from a Former Smoker and Tobacco Researcher." *Contemporary Drug Problems* 40: 129–53. https://doi.org/10.1177/009145091304000107.

Haines-Saah, R., and K. Bell. 2016. "Challenging Key Assumptions Embedded in Health Canada's Cigarette Packaging Legislation: Findings from In Situ Interviews with Smokers in Vancouver." *Canadian Journal of Public Health* 107 (6): e562–7. https://doi.org/10.17269/CJPH.107.5681.

Hammond, D. 2011. "Health Warning Messages on Tobacco Products: A Review." *Tobacco Control* 20 (5): 327–37. https://doi.org/10.1136/tc.2010.037630.

Hammond, D., G.T. Fong, R. Borland, K.M. Cummings, A. McNeill, and P. Driezen. 2007. "Text and Graphic Warnings on Cigarette Packages: Findings from the International Tobacco Control Four Country Study." *American Journal of Preventive Medicine* 32 (3): 202–9. https://doi.org/10.1016/j.amepre.2006.11.011.

Health Canada. 2000. *The Tobacco Act: History of Labelling.* Ottawa: Health Canada.

Health Canada. 2019a. "Plain and Standardized Appearance for Tobacco Packaging and Products". Government of Canada. https://www.canada.ca/en/health-canada/news/2019/05/plain-and-standardized-appearance-for-tobacco-packaging-and-products.html.

Health Canada. 2019b. "Canada's Tobacco Strategy". Government of Canada. https://www.canada.ca/en/health-canada/services/publications/healthy-living/canada-tobacco-strategy.html.

Kinmonth, H.A. 2016. *The Social Construction of Obesity in Australian Preventive Health Policy*. PhD diss., Australian National University, Canberra.

Macnaughton, J., S. Carro-Ripalda, and A. Russell. 2012. "'Risking Enchantment': How Are We to View the Smoking Person?" *Critical Public Health* 22 (4): 455–69. https://doi.org/10.1080/09581596.2012.706260.

Mair, M., and C. Kierans. 2007. "Critical Reflections on the Field of Tobacco Research: The Role of Tobacco Control in Defining the Tobacco Research Agenda." *Critical Public Health* 17 (2): 103–12. https://doi.org/10.1080/09581590601045204.

Mol, A. 2008. *The Logic of Care: Health and the Problem of Patient Choice*. London: Routledge.

Physicians for a Smoke-Free Canada. 2015. "Tax Revenues from Tobacco Sales." http://www.smoke-free.ca/pdf_1/totaltax.pdf.

Poland, B., K. Frohlich, R.J. Haines, E. Mykhalovskiy, M. Rock, and R. Sparks. 2006. "The Social Context of Smoking: The Next Frontier in Tobacco Control?" *Tobacco Control* 15: 59–63. https://doi.org/10.1136/tc.2004.009886.

Pottage, A. 2013. "No (More) Logo: Plain Packaging and Communicative Agency." *University of California Davis Law Review* 47: 101–31.

Prochaska, J.O., and W.F. Velicer. 1997. "The Transtheoretical Model of Health Behavior Change." *American Journal of Health Promotion* 12 (1): 38–48. https://doi.org/10.4278/0890-1171-12.1.38.

Shapin, S. 2010. *Never Pure: Historical Studies of Science As If It Was Produced by People with Bodies, Situated in Time, Space, Culture, and Society and Struggling for Credibility and Authority*. Baltimore: Johns Hopkins University Press.

Smith, K. 2013. *Beyond Evidence-Based Policy in Public Health: The Interplay of Ideas*. Basingstoke: Palgrave Macmillan.

Thaler, R., and C. Sunstein. 2008. *Nudge: Improving Decisions about Health, Wealth, and Happiness*. New Haven: Yale University Press.

World Health Organization. 2011. *Report on the Global Tobacco Epidemic 2011: Warning about the Dangers of Tobacco*. Geneva: World Health Organization. http://www.who.int/tobacco/global_report/2011/en/.

9 Public Good, or Goods for the Public: The Commercialization of Academic Health Research

KELLY HOLLOWAY AND MATTHEW HERDER

The commercialization of research has been a priority for the Canadian government since the 1970s, consistently motivated as an effort to harness knowledge production capacity in universities in the service of industries, publics, and ultimately the global "knowledge economy." The commercialization of research is "the conversion of research results into products, services, and processes that can be the object of commercial transactions" (Downie and Herder 2007). The notion that scientific research produced in the academy should be commercialized has been debated, resisted, and critiqued historically but, as we will argue, it is becoming the norm in biomedical research. Biomedical research is the basic research that supports knowledge in the field of medicine, informing health services. It is the way that scientific research (bench research) is translated into clinical practice. In the past forty years, this translation has come to be synonymous with commercialization. Increasingly, companies are playing a role in moving scientific discoveries from the university "from bench to bedside."

The research we report on in this chapter is motivated by a concern that if commercial interests are embedded in biomedical research, the questions that are pursued by researchers and the knowledge that is produced in Canadian universities will be skewed towards commercial application, and ultimately towards profit. We build on the work of scholars who have contemplated what could be lost when the university ceases to be the place where research is driven primarily by curiosity, or even by a drive to serve the public good (Atkinson-Grosjean 2006; Cooper 2009; Elliott and Hepting 2015; Krimsky 2004; Newson and Buchbinder 1988; Slaughter and Rhoades 2004). We also complicate this dynamic by indicating that researchers' motivations are complex, changing, and informed by context.

We present data from three parts of a broader investigation of the commercialization of academic research in Canada. The first part is a survey of over nine hundred Canadian academic scientists from biochemistry, molecular biology, microbiology and immunology, pharmacology and psychiatry, and physics and chemistry. The second part addresses academic health researchers' localized engagements with commercialization through a case study exploring how biomedical researchers understand the place of commercialization in their research at one Canadian university.[1] The third part is a reflection on our observational work attending an annual science policy conference in Canada over two years. We pay particular attention to emerging researchers because their employment is often precarious, which makes their status in academia more vulnerable, and because their experiences and values give us an indication of how the next generation of scientists could approach commercialization.

We argue that commercialization is being normalized in the transmission of science education to the next generation of researchers, in the daily interactions of the lab, and in the development of governmental science policy. There is no linear trajectory from the lab to the policy arena or vice versa. These phenomena exist dialectically, informing each other and giving each other meaning. There is an interplay between the rhetoric and the internalized notions of scientific responsibility. There are also disruptions to the normalization of commercialization within the laboratory and beyond. However, at this point, there does not seem to be any direct, organized challenge to commercialization in Canada, such as might occur through a public campaign or policy proposal, whether led by government, universities, research institutions, or civil society organizations. This absence has implications for the way that individuals within the biomedical research sector in the country can address public health matters. We end our chapter by raising concerns about the future of health research in Canada.

We understand commercialization in its historical context. We suggest that the policies and practices that came about with the move to a neoliberal economic model resulted in important changes within academic science. The emergence of neoliberalism meant a shift in thinking at the state level about the purpose of the university, from an institution devoted to strengthening the economy and encouraging an engaged citizenry through teaching and research, to the breeding ground for innovations that would become central to the success of the new knowledge economy (Mirowski 2011; Newstadt 2015; Noble 1979; Olssen and Peters 2005; Sears 2003). One fundamental piece of the transformation has involved the role of the academic scientist, from that of a scholar who might work with industry to that of an entrepreneur who initiates an industry derived from her or his research. This can have an impact on the kind of research that takes place at public institutions. For instance, Cooper's (2009) research addresses the direct and indirect influences on the choices academic scientists make about their scientific research. He argues that commercialization shifts the focus of the life scientist to "a greater interest in research that generates patents or commercializable findings and away from research based on scientific curiosity and potential contributions to scientific theory" (647). Proponents of the neoliberal model seek to create individuals that are enterprising and competitive (Olssen and Peters 2005). The responses from participants in our study point to the interplay of the daily work of researchers, their agency, and the structures that shape scientific research.

Since the 1970s, commercialization has been articulated as good for the economy and, therefore, the public through the Canadian government's science policy. Canada lacks legislation akin to the United States' Bayh-Dole Act,[2] which is frequently credited with motivating the shift towards more commercially oriented research (Aldridge and Audretsch 2011; Grimaldi et al. 2011; Mowery et al. 2001; Thursby and Thursby 2011). But through a multitude of policy measures, Canadian governments, research funding agencies, and academic research institutions have steadily embraced commercialization as well (Downie and Herder 2007; Fisher and Atkinson-Grosjean 2002; Polster 2007; Sá and Litwin 2011). The result is that the majority of Canadian universities and colleges have put into place mechanisms to facilitate the acquisition and management of intellectual property and to pursue the commercialization of academic research – ostensibly, in the name of serving the broader Canadian public.

The rationale for Bayh-Dole encompassed the idea that public goods from the university are a waste of public money if they cannot be used in the private sector (Glenna et al. 2007). Serving the public good or public interest was thus translated into producing knowledge that enhances economic performance. Grischa Metlay (2006) argues that notions of "intellectual property" in academic research did not change considerably over the past century, but the meaning of the public good or public interest changed dramatically. A similar process took place in Canada (Atkinson-Grosjean 2006). Seizing upon this shift, universities positioned themselves as an "innovative and publicly oriented organization uniquely capable of transforming federally funded public goods into commercially available consumer goods" (Atkinson-Grosjean 2006, 582). By the latter part of the twentieth century intellectual property became a way to smooth the division of labour into public-private partnerships, all in the name of ensuring university-generated knowledge did not go unused.

Our findings are a window into the effects of entrepreneurialism and commercialization on biomedical research at Canadian universities. We suggest there is an ongoing shift in the kind of scientific research that is being produced in the context of the neoliberal university.

Methods

We obtained a grant from the Canadian Institutes for Health Research in 2012 to study the commercialization of academic research. Our findings are based on three sets of data. First, we conducted a survey focusing on emerging (master's and PhD students as well as postdoctoral fellows) and established (assistant, associate, and full professors) researchers affiliated with nine (of the seventeen) Canadian academic institutions housing a medical school. Of the potential 6,575 graduate student, postdoctoral fellows, and faculty respondents, 995 completed the survey (response rate of 15 per cent), answering a variety of questions about their career stage, training, and levels of exposure to, and views about, commercialization. Second, we conducted interviews with thirty biomedical researchers at different career stages at Dalhousie University, where we focused on several aspects of academic research activity and the commercialization thereof, including patenting, presenting at conferences, creating a company, attending events that promote commercialization, applying for funding, and interacting with the university's Industry Liaison and Innovation Office. Third, we engaged in observational research at the Canadian Science Policy Centre (CSPC) conference in 2013 and 2014. The CSPC was founded in 2009 as a "grassroots" effort to bring the science policy community together. It comprises "a diverse group of young and passionate professionals from industry, academia, and science-based governmental departments."[3] "Science" is broadly conceived for these conferences, with session titles that are open and somewhat ambiguous, such as "Canadian Innovation: Understanding the Role of IR&D" and "Inspiring Excellence – Engaging Students in Meaningful Science Experiences." The conferences were a relevant ground for our study given the many speakers and sponsors from the biomedical and health sciences who attended. We focused specifically on sessions that addressed emerging researchers in the biomedical and health sciences in order to document the kind of messages conveyed to this particular demographic. While findings from these three studies are reported elsewhere (Holloway and Herder 2019), this chapter presents a cross-cutting analysis of the data sets in order to more fully consider their combined implications for the political economy of biomedical and health science.

Findings Overview

We found that key interlocking themes emerge from the three portions of our study. Our findings from the survey indicate that exposure to commercialization is becoming a normal part of the research culture for biomedical and health sciences researchers in Canadian universities. The volume of exposure to commercialization practices appears to be increasing over time, making commercialization a consistent and integral part of the education of emerging academic scientists across Canada. Our findings from the interviews with scientists suggest that while there are certainly tensions, senior researchers commercialize because it is expected by their institution, their profession, and the granting agencies that fund their work. When mentoring emerging researchers, they communicate that the commercialization of research is important in order to succeed as an academic scientist. What appears to be transmitted to practising scientists is that they should commercialize for their own good. And finally, our observations of the science policy conference in Canada indicate that there is a fairly well-honed message that commercialization is a public good; it is necessary for the economy. This theme emerged from the interviews as well. These interconnected, mutually reinforcing themes – that commercialization is the norm, it is for your own good, and it is a public good – are dispersed across our findings, but each investigation revealed the themes in unique and nuanced ways, from exposure to commercialization, to internalized ideas about what it means to be a scientist, to public events organized by government officials to craft a vision for the future of biomedical and health science.

Survey of Canadian Scientists: A Growing Norm of Commercialization

Findings from our survey examined exposure to commercialization across researchers' career stages. In general, the survey findings indicate that emerging researchers are subject to greater commercialization – whether formally or informally – than their more established forebears. When gender, current career stage, number of industry-funded grants, and faculty group are controlled for, three logit models revealed no significant relationships between graduation cohort and either exposure or timing of first exposure to commercialization. However, the model measuring volume of exposure revealed that compared to the earliest cohort, both the 1980–96 and 1997+ groups experience a significantly higher annual volume of exposure to commercialization ($p < 0.005$; Table 9.1). In real terms, over half of Canadian academic scientists who graduated

Table 9.1. Formal and informal exposure to commercialization by current career stage

	Formal exposure to commercialization during training and career to date: Yes/no (% Yes)	*Informal* exposure to commercialization at stage of training: Yes/no (% Yes)			
		Undergraduate student	Master's student	PhD student	Postdoctoral fellow
Current career stage					
Master's student	25/117 (17.6%)	77/47 (61.6%)	77/46 (62.6%)	X	X
PhD student	40/103 (28.0%)	66/28 (70.2%)	61/28 (68.5%)	86/38 (69.4%)	X
Postdoctoral fellow	28/57 (32.9%)	32/27 (55.6%)	20/16 (55.6%)	44/21 (67.7%)	32/23 (57.7%)
Assistant professor	19/25 (43.2%)	12/20 (37.5%)	6/14 (30.0%)	11/16 (40.7%)	15/10 (60.0%)
Associate professor	31/24 (56.4%)	14/26 (35.0%)	6/14 (30.0%)	15/24 (38.5%)	10/26 (27.8%)
Full professor	63/19 (76.8%)	23/38 (37.7%)	8/27 (22.9%)	23/49 (31.9%)	24/39 (38.1%)

after 1980 had a greater annual volume of formal exposures to commercialization than those who graduated prior to 1980 (Table 9.2). On average, they were exposed to a formal commercialization activity, such as filing a patent application, at least once and up to three times per year. By contrast, the majority (77 per cent) of those who graduated prior to 1980 were, on average, exposed to such activities less than once annually. This difference in exposure to formal commercialization activity is significant ($p < 0.005$; Table 9.2).

More recent graduates also have a significant amount of informal exposure to commercialization (see Table 9.1). The majority of emerging researcher participants attended brown bag lunches where they learned about intellectual property (IP) and its relevance for their scientific work; journal clubs; meetings with technology transfer offices and industry liaison officers, whose job is to help them commercialize their scientific discoveries; and meetings with and presentations from company representatives during their training, even at an undergraduate level (Table 9.1). The extent to which emerging researchers who graduated after 1980 may have a higher level of exposure than the generation

Table 9.2. Timing and volume of formal exposure to commercialization

	Exposure to IP		Timing of first exposure		Average annual volume of exposure		
Graduation cohort	% exposed formally	% not exposed	% first exposed pre-PhD	% exposed post-PhD	% < 1	% 1.01–3.0	% 3.01–13.5
Pre-1980	87.1	12.9	0	100	77.27	9.09	16.67
1980–96	66.15	33.85	9.3	90.7	37.14	54.29	8.57
1997+	42.54	57.46	32	68	11.43	54.29	34.29
Statistical association	$N = 230$, Chi2, df = 2, $p < 0.00$		$N = 120$, fishers exact, $p < 0.00$		$N = 92$, Chi2, df = 4, $p < 0.00$		

Note: Ordinal logistic regression model measuring the relationship between graduation cohort and average annual volume of intellectual property (IP) exposure, controlling for current career stage, number of public grants, number of industry grants, gender and faculty group, with the earliest graduation cohort used as a reference category (N = 73).

Table 9.3. Distribution of commercial interest score by career stage

	Interest in commercialization		
	Mean	Std. dev.	*N*
Master's students	2.3	0.98	144
PhD students	2.3	0.97	136
Postdoctoral fellows	2.4	1.1	83
Assistant/associate professors	1.82	0.91	92

Note: Distribution calculated by taking the mean responses to "Rate the importance of each of the following reasons from your perspective for pursuing a research project": (1) commercial potential; (2) patentable results; and (3) starting a company (higher score out of five indicates increased interest), and at least somewhat concerned about scooping

before them could have an impact on their motivations and concerns when it comes to research.

Our findings also indicate that emerging researchers were more likely to be interested in IP/commercialization than established researchers (Table 9.3). The majority of respondents, regardless of career stage, are concerned about being scooped (meaning that another scientist has published or patented an idea before they have had a chance to do so themselves) or uncomfortable discussing results (meaning that they do not want to share their scientific discoveries with peers because they could be publishable or patentable) (Tables 9.3, 9.4).

Table 9.4. Ordinal logistic regression results measuring the impact of career stage (X) on the level of safety discussing results (Y) and concern about scooping (Y), while controlling for age, gender, and faculty group

		Selecting for PhD students (*N* = 480)				Selecting for postdoctoral fellows (*N* = 480)			
		Level of safety discussing results		Concern about scooping		Level of safety discussing results		Concern about scooping	
		Coef	*p*	Coef	*p*	Coef	*p*	Coef	*p*
Career stage	Master's students	0.48	0.058*	–0.87	0.000**	0.71302	0.019**	–0.90267	0.001**
	PhD students								
	Postdoctoral fellows								
	Assistant/associate professors								
	Full professors								
	Faculty (med)	–0.61	0.080*	0.6	0.070*	–0.60854	0.08*	0.599431	0.063*
	Gender (women)								
	Age (continuous)			–0.02	0.088*			–0.0247	0.088*

Note: only significant results are reported
*significant at $\alpha = 0.05$
**significant at $\alpha = 0.01$

The growing exposure to IP/commercialization is likely linked to emerging researchers' interest in these matters. We wanted to develop a more in-depth understanding of how this interest develops among emerging researchers. Our interviews were able to further illuminate how commercialization has entered into scientific training.

Interviews with Academic Scientists: Your Own Good

Our findings from thirty qualitative interviews indicate that commercialization is not a fully accepted norm yet, but could become fully accepted through translation to the next generation of scientists, lack of debate and discussion about commercialization and, particularly, through the idea that commercialization is a scientist's responsibility to the wider public. We found that established researchers wrestled with the tensions of commercialization more than emerging researchers. Students and postdocs had a more limited range of opinions about commercialization and ultimately believed that they should be knowledgeable and experienced with commercialization if they were going to succeed (Holloway and Herder 2019). This was something that the established researchers actively conveyed to their students and trainees, even if they were conflicted about it. While some wholeheartedly endorsed commercialization, more were conflicted if not opposed; but despite this range of opinions, there was very little open discussion or criticism of commercialization with colleagues. While these established researchers had been privy to debates about commercialization earlier in their careers, most were not engaged in such a debate at the time of the interviews. Thus, the context in which emerging researchers enter into academia is one in which commercialization is fast becoming an accepted norm.

Researchers also indicated that there was a change in their understanding of responsibility as academic scientists. Some participants said that commercialization was a scientific responsibility (Holloway and Herder 2019). Researchers wanted their work to lead to something useful, and commercialization seemed like the most direct and practical route. These participants were concerned that if they did not patent, for instance, their innovations would be lost in the world of academic publication – that no one would take them up and translate them into practical applications. For example, one participant, a full professor, said, "I don't really have the time, the expertise or the desire to patent anything ... The conundrum is that if you don't patent it, does it get lost? Does it become completely useless so that nobody can use it? And that, I have to say, bothers me." Another related theme regarding responsibility was that researchers felt the need to justify the fact that they were doing useful work. They wanted to use the public money they received from research grants responsibly – which meant that they needed to commercialize. Researchers felt pressure to equate useful science with science that could be commercialized. Ultimately, they seemed to internalize the feeling that if their work is useful it can potentially be commercialized. Some were conflicted about this, but the tensions identified did not seem to translate into a debate or discussion about the merits of commercialization and, further, did not seem to be translated to emerging scientists. A student participant who was part of a training program at the university devoted to commercialization said, "I don't really know why we would debate it, pros and cons, if I have to do a project that has to be commercialized." While our qualitative findings come from a case study of Dalhousie University, we emphasize that Dalhousie follows a similar trajectory to other institutions in Canada – a formula of sorts. A comparison of responses to our survey questions across Canadian research institutions suggests that Dalhousie was not an atypical Canadian university context.

The processes by which commercialization has become the primary way to bring scientific discoveries to the public appear to our study participants to be outside of what scientists do in the laboratories. In short, with few exceptions, the community of biomedical researchers that is arguably best situated to speak to the tensions that commercialization presents does not appear to openly question this shift. Commercialization seems to have had a silencing effect, which may prove lasting in light of a host of new policies and programs that target researchers in training, coupled with dwindling opportunities for academic employment. Programs such as Mitacs, and Dalhousie's RADIANT Neurotechnology and NSERC CREATE: BioMedic, teach emerging researchers how to see their scientific work as potentially "commercializable" and offer them the practical skills they need to undertake the work of commercialization and move into industry when they are finished their training. Most of the emerging researchers in our sample saw commercialization as positive or at least inevitable and were pragmatic about the fact that, given the job market in academia, they would have to demonstrate that their work was commercializable in order to be an appealing candidate for industry. Both emerging and established researchers raised the challenges of obtaining academic employment in biomedical research as an issue that cannot change, and will probably worsen. Rather than precipitating a discussion about why there are fewer faculty positions in those fields, and how this has emerged as a trend in higher education, researchers regarded it as an inevitable feature of the job market and an impetus to commercialize. Demonstrating an openness to commercialization and IP were seen as integral to finding employment in industry.

Emerging researchers tended to accept that commercialization would have to be part of their work, even if it was not a natural fit with the kind of research that they were doing at the moment. It is possible that if these researchers become more familiar with the process of commercialization, they will register objections, but they have not been privy to a critical discussion about what the transformation has meant for science or the university – in some cases they will not be aware that there has been a transformation. Therefore, they lack a framework by which to understand that disgruntlement, and have nothing to compare it to; they enter a world already made.

Observational Analysis of the CSPC: The Public Good

Our observational analysis of two public meetings devoted to science policy in Canada indicates that at governmental and policy level, there is an effort to promote the commercialization of research and translate the importance of this mission to emerging scientists, all in service of the Canadian economy. The CSPC is the brainchild of Mehrdad Hariri, the CEO and president of CSPC and a scientist in the fields of veterinary medicine, cell biology, and functional genomes. In a 2011 promotional video for the conference, Hariri described the conference as a way for scientists, usually isolated with "little interaction with society at large," to have a say in the decision-making processes of governments and the private sector (CSPC 2011). In 2016, the CSPC had 200 speakers and 685 participants. The conference is sponsored by Canadian university research departments, pharmaceutical companies, and professional associations, granting agencies, and government representatives such as Industry Canada and the Canadian Foundation for Innovation. CSPC participants are described as an assortment of policymakers, government and industry representatives, university administrators, and academic scientists. Conference topics cover everything from international trade to R&D innovation to science mentorship. Focusing on sessions that were directed towards emerging researchers, we gathered evidence of a culture in which commercialization is strongly encouraged as a feature of scientific work but also as a career motivation.

In the 2013 conference, sessions with such titles as "Is a PhD Really a Waste of Time?," "From Pipeline to Network: Rethinking Graduate Training to Embrace Diversity and Promote Innovation," and "Student Entrepreneurs as a Knowledge Vehicle" encouraged emerging researchers to accept that there are very few jobs in the biomedical and health sciences, but that their expertise is becoming essential for the economy in the form of R&D. This general message was put to participants very concretely by senior policymakers and administrators at the conference, producing a pro-commercialization tenor to the event. In a panel called "Strategies to Enhance Productivity of Knowledge Workers," Wendy Cukier, vice-president of research and innovation at Ryerson University, said that in creating a talent pool for economic and social development from universities, we must recognize that foundational science is insufficient: "If you focus on science, technology, engineering and maths and don't provide other sets of skills that will allow people to understand end-users, to understand application, to understand broad context, or to work in teams with people who know those things, we're really missing the boat."

Greg Rickford, then minister of state (science and technology), gave the keynote presentation for the conference, called "Global Competitiveness and Innovation Policy." He discussed how to bridge the gap between ideas and the marketplace and celebrated funding that brings university and industry together. There was a consistent message from speakers from university administrations and government and industry representatives that research must be considered in terms of its commercial application. This message was conveyed very clearly to emerging researchers at the conference. These researchers were also told that they should be looking for jobs with industry. A session called "Student Entrepreneurs as a Knowledge Vehicle" explored how to break down the divide between academia and the private sector by introducing the "entrepreneurial mindset." Panellists included two speakers from the Rotman Research Institute at Baycrest Health Sciences; Bill Mantel, assistant deputy ministry, Research, Commercialization and Entrepreneurship Division, serving the Ministry of Research and Innovation and the Ministry of Economic Development, Trade and Employment; Wendy Cukier; and three PhD students who took part in science-based entrepreneurial programs during their graduate education. Many of them argued that universities must transform the "culture" of academia to be friendlier to the private sector and create better infrastructure in the academy to train emerging scientists in business skills. Some of these panellists lamented the lack of what they called "soft skills" amongst graduate students and postdocs in the sciences: leadership, communication, administration, creativity, and interpersonal ability. For example, Nana Lee, coordinator for graduate professional development at the University of Toronto, claimed she can help PhDs communicate, manage their time, learn entrepreneurial skills, understand and apply ethical practices, and work effectively in teams and as leaders.

This is not a ubiquitous message at the CSPC. The conference includes presentations by academic researchers, some of whom express frustration with elements of the push to commercialize. For instance, a presenter at the 2013 conference said she feels that she can no longer say she is interested in her grant applications to NSERC, but now uses the term "foundational science" to indicate that it can have commercial implications. If there were criticisms of commercialization they tended to be articulated at this level – as a frustration with a particular feature of the way that funding operates.

Similar themes arose at the CSPC in 2014. An example of how emerging researchers are encouraged to follow a particular direction was the celebration of one emerging researcher's accomplishments. In a panel entitled "Looking to 2020 and Beyond: Training the Next Generation of Innovation Leaders in Canada," panellist Andre Bezanson offered insights about how scientists who do not commercialize their findings can "get lost in the ether." At the time, Bezanson was a postdoctoral researcher at Dalhousie University in biomedical engineering. He related how, during his undergrad, where he was funded by Mitacs, he worked with Daxsonics Ultrasound Inc. to shrink ultrasound probe technology to the size of a pencil eraser. Bezanson was offered a position in the company. He encouraged his peers to think about how academia and industry are changing and how governments are changing too – then plan and strategize accordingly. Another panellist, Ross Laver, vice-president, policy and communications with the Canadian Council of Chief Executives, an association composed of the CEOs of 150 leading Canadian companies, celebrated Bezanson's story as one of adaptation and flexibility and noted Bezanson's next project to develop a technology that gets rid of wrinkles, because there is such a large market of ageing baby boomers.

The aim of the CSPC sessions devoted to emerging researchers, the character of advice offered by panellists to emerging researchers, and the emerging researchers selected as success stories at the conference suggest that there is a concerted effort, on the part of the conference organizers and their supporters, to promote and encourage the commercialization of research within the next generation of researchers. The fact that this is taking place at a policy level is an important piece of the analysis that we present.

Discussion

Our findings suggest that the understanding of university-generated knowledge as a public good needing, by definition, to be commercialized through intellectual property and industry partnership continues to be invoked to this day. It is certainly apparent in Canada, as evidenced by the activities of the CSPC and by the numerous federal and provincial programs aimed at commercializing university research.[4] In other words, the neoliberal program has enveloped the notion of the public good within the logic of the efficiency of the market, whereby the efficiency of the market is the public good. Further, it would seem that this notion is present in the way that the usefulness of academic science is currently conceived by governments, by university administrators (Glenna et al. 2007), and perhaps increasingly by scientists themselves.

Academic science and, for the purposes of this paper, the biomedical and health sciences are gradually being transformed to orient quite concertedly to a commercialization model. Our investigation offers a close analysis of how this is taking place. Our survey presents generalizable findings about how researchers are exposed to commercialization at different stages of education and career. Emerging researchers are exposed to far more commercialization activities than researchers that preceded them. In a context with little to no critical engagement in what commercialization is and its effects for the science community or the country, this increased exposure contributes to its ascendance as the norm. Our interviews offer in-depth insight into what is happening in researchers' laboratories and their thoughts, motivations, and struggles. While some researchers grapple with the idea that their work must be commercializable, it appears to be becoming an accepted norm simply out of a pragmatic necessity to secure funds – and that is what is conveyed to emerging researchers. Finally, our observational analysis of the CSPC is a window into how science policy in Canada engages certain members of the academic and policy community to present an impetus for commercialization. Organizers and panellists at this conference, who include key members of the Canadian government, suggest that commercialization is an essential move for the health of the Canadian economy. Through our interviews, we saw how this message was taken up by researchers – commercialization is their responsibility.

This gradual acceptance of commercialization will have an impact on health services defined broadly. We register a concern that the research will be guided by commercial priorities, and the ability to appropriate information, which may not correlate positively with improved health outcomes. Kapczynski and Syed (2013, 1908) explain that patents are supposed to encourage market innovation by permitting inventors to exclude others from the results of their investment and prevent them from appropriating its returns. However, exclusion is not always correlated with social value. Information that may be difficult to appropriate in the form of a patent, such as a surgical checklist to prevent operating room infections or the effectiveness of a new drug compared to an existing treatment, may nevertheless hold tremendous social value. But as Kapczynski and Syed note, the patent system does not encourage those kinds of innovations. In short, the idea that commercialization and the strategies it tends to encode will translate into more useful knowledge and better health care is an assumption worthy of question; yet most researchers in our study seem prepared to accept that assumption.

We have indicated that context of commercialization is integrated into the daily work of academic scientists and how processes of commercialization are related to researchers' understanding of their responsibilities, which are continually changing. Our findings resonate with Cooper's (2009) work, suggesting that academic scientists have internalized the idea that the usefulness of their work is tied to its commercial potential. Our research has also delved into the indirect influences, particularly through our attention to the transmission of ideas and practices to emerging researchers.

Our work has implications for how the privatization of knowledge is affecting the biomedical sciences in Canadian universities. Claire Polster (2015) uses the term "the privatization of knowledge" to refer to the dual process of converting publicly subsidized knowledge into intellectual property and research sponsors paying for the ability to shape research design. While there has been considerable attention paid to how clinical care has been privatized in terms of public and private ownership of hospitals and clinics, our work indicates how clinical care is privatized through the knowledge produced at universities. For biomedical research this means a focus on more profitable "lifestyle" concerns of the wealthy as opposed to widespread diseases of the poor (Mahood 2005). In an era where "knowledge translation" is emphasized as an essential element of research by universities and granting agencies, it is essential to take account of what kind of knowledge is being translated and for whom.

Those scientists, taxpayers, and even decision makers at the federal and provincial levels who argue that publicly funded university-based science should be useful for the public have a valid point – one that has been present historically, prior to Bayh-Dole and neoliberal state transformations. However, how that usefulness is defined is fundamentally important. The seemingly gradual disappearance of critical discussion of commercialization among academic biomedical scientists is concerning. We suggest that critical debate is necessary in order to fully consider whether commercialization is an appropriate way forward for the biomedical and health sciences. If this discussion is limited to a set of impressions based on experiences with commercialization, the trajectory in which emerging researchers increasingly normalize it as a part of their practice will likely continue. Discussions of commercialization must openly contend with those structural reconfigurations that affect the everyday work of science, such as the increasing casualization of academic labour (Brownlee 2015). Commercialization practices and the interests and imperatives that contribute to them, like the shifts in the supply and demand for academic scientists, are not simply "external" developments and thus outside of the responsibility of researchers. When they are conceived of in this way, however, researchers can limit the kind of science done in universities today and in the future.

NOTES

This research was funded by the Canadian Institutes of Health Research, grant #EOG 123678. Dr. Janice Graham, Dr. Brian Noble and Professor Tina Piper informed the survey's questions and design, and Professor Yoko Yoshida provided additional guidance for the statistical analysis.

1 Participants came from a variety of different departments, including pathology, hematopathology, paediatrics, neurosurgery, pharmacology, biochemistry, molecular biology, bioinformatics, genomics, biomedical engineering, epidemiology, microbiology, geriatric medicine, immunology, neuroscience, dentistry, psychology, and cancer immunotherapy.

2 The Bayh-Dole Act is United States legislation passed in 1980 permitting universities to use federal research funds to produce an invention and then retain the title on any patent issued for that invention, precipitating a massive increase in university patenting. Prior to this the federal government retained the licence for all university inventions using public funding for research.

3 CSPC website, "About the CSPC," https://www.sciencepolicy.ca/content/about-cspc.

4 For instance, the Centres of Excellence for Commercialization of Research, the Canadian Innovation Commercialization Program, the Centre for Commercialization of Regenerative Medicine, MaRS Innovation, the ONtrepreneurs (Ontario Neurotech Entrepreneurs) Program, the Collaborative Health Research Projects, the Ontario Centres of Excellence Collaborative Commercialization Programs.

REFERENCES

Aldridge, T.T., and D. Audretsch. 2011. "The Bayh-Dole Act and Scientist Entrepreneurship." *Research Policy* 40 (8): 1058–67. https://doi.org/10.1016/j.respol.2011.04.006.

Atkinson-Grosjean, J. 2006. *Public Science, Private Interests: Culture and Commerce in Canada's Networks of Centres of Excellence.* Toronto: University of Toronto Press.

Brownlee, J. 2015. *Academia, Inc: How Corporatization Is Transforming Canadian Universities.* Halifax: Fernwood.

Canadian Science Policy Centre (CSPC). 2012. "Mehrdad Hariri." YouTube, 25 November 2012. https://www.youtube.com/watch?v=xzB_apUOw2Q.

Cooper, M.H. 2009. "Commercialization of the University and Problem Choice by Academic Biological Scientists." *Science, Technology, & Human Values* 34 (5): 629–53. https://doi.org/10.1177/0162243908329379.

Downie, J., and M. Herder. 2007. "Reflections on the Commercialization of Research Conducted in Public Institutions in Canada." *McGill Journal of Law and Health* 1: 23–47. https://papers.ssrn.com/sol3/papers.cfm?abstract_id=2288646.

Elliott, P., and D.H. Hepting. 2015. *Free Knowledge: Confronting the Commodification of Human Discovery.* Regina: University of Regina Press.

Fisher, D., and J. Atkinson-Grosjean. 2002. "Brokers on the Boundary: Academy-Industry Liaison in Canadian Universities." *Higher Education* 44 (3–4): 449–67. https://doi.org/10.1023/A:1019842322513.

Glenna, L.L., W.B. Lacy, R. Welsh, and D. Biscotti. 2007. "University Administrators, Agricultural Biotechnology, and Academic Capitalism: Defining the Public Good to Promote University–Industry Relationships." *Sociological Quarterly* 48 (1): 141–63. https://doi.org/10.1111/j.1533-8525.2007.00074.x.

Grimaldi, R., M. Kenney, D.S. Siegel, and M. Wright. 2011. "30 Years after Bayh-Dole: Reassessing Academic Entrepreneurship." *Research Policy* 40 (8): 1045–57. https://doi.org/10.1016/j.respol.2011.04.005.

Holloway, K., and M. Herder. 2019. "A Responsibility to Commercialize? Tracing Academic Researchers' Evolving Engagement with the Commercialization of Biomedical Research." *Journal of Responsible Innovation* 6: 1–21. https://doi.org/10.1080/23299460.2019.1608615.

Kapczynski, A., and T. Syed. 2013. "The Continuum of Excludability and the Limits of Patents." *Yale Law Journal* 122 (7): 1900–63. https://papers.ssrn.com/sol3/papers.cfm?abstract_id=2280578.

Krimsky, S. 2004. *Science in the Private Interest: Has the Lure of Profits Corrupted Biomedical Research?* Lanham: Rowman & Littlefield.

Mahood, S. 2005. "Privatized Knowledge and the Pharmaceutical Industry." Paper presented at the conference Free Knowledge: Creating a Knowledge Commons in Saskatchewan, University of Regina, 15–18 November.

Metlay, G. 2006. "Reconsidering Renormalization: Stability and Change in 20th-Century Views on University Patents." *Social Studies of Science* 36 (4): 565–97. https://doi.org/10.1177/0306312706058581.

Mirowski, P. 2011. *Science-Mart: Privatizing American Science.* Cambridge, MA: Harvard University Press.

Mowery, D.C., R.R. Nelson, B.N. Sampat, and A.A. Ziedonis. 2001. "The Growth of Patenting and Licensing by U.S. Universities: An Assessment of the Effects of the Bayh-Dole Act of 1980." *Research Policy* 30 (1): 99–119. https://doi.org/10.1016/S0048-7333(99)00100-6.

Newson, J., and H. Buchbinder. 1988. *The University Means Business: Universities, Corporations and Academic Work.* Toronto: Garamond.

Newstadt, E. 2015. "From Being an Entrepreneur to Being Entrepreneurial: The Consolidation of Neoliberalism in Ontario's Universities." *Alternate Routes: A Journal of Critical Social Research* 26: 145–69. http://www.alternateroutes.ca/index.php/ar/article/view/22316.

Noble, D.F. 1979. *America by Design: Science, Technology, and the Rise of Corporate Capitalism.* New York: Oxford University Press.

Olssen, M., and M.A. Peters. 2005. "Neoliberalism, Higher Education and the Knowledge Economy: From the Free Market to Knowledge Capitalism." *Journal of Education Policy* 20 (3): 313–45. https://doi.org/10.1080/02680930500108718.

Polster, C. 2007. "The Nature and Implications of the Growing Importance of Research Grants to Canadian Universities and Academics." *Higher Education* 53 (5): 599–622. https://doi.org/10.1007/s10734-005-1118-z.

Polster, C. 2015. "The Privatization of Knowledge in Canada's Universities and What We Should Do about It." In *Free Knowledge: Confronting the Commodification of Human Discovery*, edited by P.W. Elliot and D.H. Hepting, 56–66. Regina: University of Regina Press.

Sá, C.M., and J. Litwin. 2011. "University-Industry Research Collaborations in Canada: The Role of Federal Policy Instruments." *Science and Public Policy* 38 (6): 425–35. https://doi.org/10.3152/030234211X12960315267732.

Sears, A. 2003. *Retooling the Mind Factory: Education in a Lean State.* Toronto: University of Toronto Press.

Slaughter, S., and G. Rhoades. 2004. *Academic Capitalism and the New Economy: Markets, State, and Higher Education.* Baltimore: Johns Hopkins University Press.

Thursby, J.G., and M.C. Thursby. 2011. "Has the Bayh-Dole Act Compromised Basic Research?" *Research Policy* 40 (8): 1077–83. https://doi.org/10.1016/j.respol.2011.05.009.

10 Making Sense of Vaginal Mesh

ARIEL DUCEY WITH BARRY HOFFMASTER,
MAGALI ROBERT, AND SUE ROSS

Vaginal mesh is now the subject of the largest mass-tort litigation in United States history, involving an estimated 100,000 plaintiffs in state and federal courts. Lawsuits against the manufacturers of these devices are also underway in Canada. From the early 2000s to about 2015, transvaginally placed synthetic mesh implants were widely used around the world to surgically treat some types of prolapse (descent of the pelvic organs) and urinary incontinence in women. Litigants in the court cases report debilitating complications, including irreversible chronic pain, and usually that they were not informed such complications were possible. Many women benefited from the less invasive surgical approach and more durable repair the new procedures entailed, but neither the numerator nor denominator are known: how many devices were implanted and how many resulted in complications.

My research, with colleagues in health services research, bioethics, and surgery – Sue Ross, Barry Hoffmaster, and Magali Robert, respectively – has focused on the surgeons who treat these disorders in women: their ways of thinking about their work and responsibilities, and when and how they should adopt new procedures or devices. In recent years, we have interviewed dozens of surgeons and stakeholders in pelvic floor surgery, observed consultations between patients and surgeons in one specialized treatment clinic, observed international and major European and North American medical conferences for physicians and allied health care professionals who treat pelvic floor disorders, and assembled and analysed documentary evidence such as print advertisements for mesh devices, commentaries and op-eds by clinicians concerning mesh kits, and the development of textbook descriptions of when and how to treat pelvic floor disorders.

This chapter draws upon interviews with clinicians who perform pelvic floor surgery. There are differences among these clinicians (for instance in terms of experience, training, surgical repertoire, and practice type), which are important to a more extended analysis of pelvic floor surgery. For reasons of confidentiality, here clinicians are identified by the initials of the pseudonyms our research team assigned them, and I have refrained from mentioning gender – also a difference that matters, but which needs to be handled with care because of how small this community of Canadian clinicians is and how readily some readers could use gender markers in combination with other details about practice preferences to identify particular respondents.

As a result of the collaborative nature of this research, some of the explanations for the widespread use of transvaginal mesh that would have once been sufficient to me are now less so. The purpose of this chapter is to illustrate how working with colleagues in other disciplines altered my way of approaching this research and understanding this case. I wish to describe a certain stance, which is simultaneously scholarly, emotional, and moral, in the sociological study of health care and medicine. It is a position from which I think there is no escaping the question of how to intervene. What might be done to change things? Transvaginal mesh should not have been so widely used. Yet many of the accepted ideas about what good medicine is entail explanations of medicine's failings that are arguably too removed from the messiness of practice to be the basis of effective intervention. Health care services research today is often oriented around good medicine as evidence based; much of bioethics still makes recourse to principles for practice, such as "first do no harm"; and critical medical sociology calls for medicine that is independent from the influence of corporate interests as well as social categories such as gender, class, and race that have been used to render some lives and bodies less valuable than others. Our research approach has not been to assess medical professionals on these terms, but to document the processes through which medical practitioners make sense of things and seek to demonstrate responsibility on the basis of actions and interactions that are always particular to a patient and case, but also always affected by extra-individual forces that make some ways of acting more possible. In the case of transvaginal mesh, action was not always taken with sufficient evidence for safety and effectiveness; medical professionals did not appear to adhere to ethical principles; and decisions were influenced by bias and self-interest – but even together, these factors do not fully illuminate the transvaginal mesh debacle. As a result, many typical ways of trying to prevent such debacles in the future are likely to fall short. The question that therefore shadows the following account of how transvaginal mesh came to be so widely used is: might this more ethnographic account produce better interventions?

Cowboys and Dinosaurs

The case of transvaginal mesh illustrates problems that have long been recognized by researchers in the traditions of critical medical sociology and health services research. Pelvic floor surgery was dramatically altered in the late 1990s by the development of the tension-free vaginal tape (TVT), a less-invasive surgical treatment for stress urinary incontinence (leakage of urine from coughing or jumping). It entails placing a strip of synthetic mesh under the urethra via an incision in the vagina, then pulling the tape into place through two small incisions in the lower abdomen. For many, it was a procedure *that made sense*:

> It was 1999 ... and I was at a conference in Cape Town. And I, it was an international conference and I walked down the hall and there's all these stations where the companies always show their wares, and their new stuff. And I remember stopping at a booth and looking at a video ... and I basically couldn't leave. I was watching this thing and I was thinking, my god, this makes so much sense. If this works it's going to change the world of what we do. And it did. It was the first TVT. (EE)

When the definitive paper introducing the TVT appeared in 1996 (Ulmsten et al. 1996), the device had already been sold to Johnson & Johnson as a kit bundling the procedure with the mesh tape and a set of customized tools, and it was rapidly and widely adopted.The advantages of the transvaginal rather than abdominal surgical approach and apparent physical tolerability of synthetic mesh then became the basis for the use of larger mesh pieces that wrapped around or above the vagina and the uterus to varying degrees, supporting pelvic floor organs. Many surgeons began to experiment with the transvaginal placement of mesh of varying shapes, sizes, and materials, the most entrepreneurial of whom developed viable commercial products – sold to or developed with device companies. Dozens of kit-devices made by competing companies were brought to the market in the 2000s, all of which were approved by regulators in Canada and the United States without requiring device-specific evidence of safety or effectiveness, because of their classification as moderate risk (until 2016) and as substantially equivalent to other devices on the market (see Hines et al. 2010; on similar regulatory issues in Europe see Kent and Faulkner 2002).

The TVT has now been extensively studied and is regarded by most (but not all) surgeons as at least as safe and effective as previous surgical treatments while resulting in more durable repairs with a less-invasive surgical approach. The more general group of "midurethral slings," based on the TVT, are considered the gold standard for surgically treating stress urinary incontinence. On the other hand, the use of transvaginal mesh kits to repair pelvic organ prolapse was always more contested.

> As soon as TVT came on the market, what it did is exploded the ability of companies to make money ... Before, there was nothing for them, a bunch of sutures. I mean, I'm sorry, that's not going to drive any market per se, or competition in any way. And so it allowed – kind of opened up the ability to use all this stuff, and bringing everything together, people became more – what's the word? I was going to say "cowboy," but that's not really the word – more inventive, let's say, and less traditional in how they were looking at things, and trying new things. (AK)

Extensive research and commentary have identified the shortcomings in the system of regulating medical drugs and devices in Canada and elsewhere. Health services researchers often emphasize the need for greater government funding of regulatory agencies, rather than systems that rely upon fees paid by manufacturers, to assure impartiality; or the creation of more transparent decision-making processes allowing for input from more stakeholders, including patients; or the creation of more rigorous standards for evidence at both the pre- and post-market stages. In the transvaginal mesh case, manufacturers and not regulators defined whether their devices were substantially equivalent to other devices on the market. Critical medical sociologists often raise larger issues usually taken to be external or a matter of context, but which in fact shape the production of "evidence" through and through. Such research shows how profit-making imperatives can contradict those of public health and patient well-being so that medical and scientific knowledge itself is arranged to reflect the aims and interests of drug and device manufacturers (Abraham and Ballinger 2012; Lexchin 2016). Medical devices do not have patent protections such as those granted to new pharmaceuticals, nor are the development costs as high, which encouraged the rapid proliferation of "me-too" device-procedures – variations on licenced devices sufficient to establish marketable differences but not so great as to draw extra scrutiny by regulators. The creation of these devices as "kits" additionally had the potential to create surgeon-customers bound to bundles of a manufacturer's products, and these kits were marketed, and apparently perceived, as making surgery for prolapse and urinary incontinence simpler and therefore possible for a wider range of clinicians and patients.

Did surgeons become "cowboys" or more "inventive" in this context? "Cowboys" – a term used several times by our respondents – seemed to be another way of referring to those clinicians usually called, in scales of innovativeness (Rogers 2003), innovators and early adopters – those physicians who try new approaches and products earlier than others. But "cowboy" connotes something irresponsible – a willingness to buck the rules, perhaps those of evidence and prudence. AK's shift to the adjective "inventive" captures the ambivalence with which some physicians may view colleagues farther along on a spectrum ending in "cowboys." Cowboys are understood to be necessary to surgical or medical advancement, daring what others will not. At the other end of the spectrum from a cowboy is a "dinosaur," which is what one surgeon, who to this day does not use the TVT, felt perceived as by colleagues:

> I have to say, in retrospect, I would not have had the guts to develop the TVT ... I wouldn't have been brave enough. I would have been – there's just too much potential for something to go wrong, I don't know if I could live with myself if it did. (CH)

Yet the adoption of transvaginal mesh is not only a matter of surgical dispositions or surgical decision-making styles – the descriptors "dinosaur" and "cowboy" both implausibly connote isolatable and immutable surgical types. The adoption of transvaginal mesh is just as much about a market-driven context that encouraged more clinicians to use devices for which they were inadequately trained or skilled, and to use them in patients for whom the risks could have been anticipated to outweigh the benefits.

> You know those kits are just cruel and unusual punishment, they're horrible. They were developed by equipment manufacturers who said it's easy, anybody could do it. They would take you to a weekend course in Miami and send you back with some free kits, and horrible things began to happen. (OG)

The kits were developed by companies often in collaboration with specific surgeons – between "cowboys" and companies – but they were rapidly absorbed into everyday practice. The adoption of transvaginal mesh might be characterized as the internationally synchronous and extensive, largely untracked and unmonitored beta-testing of device-procedures on patients. Analyses that focus on regulatory weakness and the dangers of mixing profit making with medical care are invaluable as diagnoses of problems in the current configuration of markets and innovation in health care, problems that made a situation like transvaginal mesh likely. However, they also gloss over what did and did not make sense and the possible permutations of responsible action to the people who implant(ed) synthetic mesh in women's pelvic floors. Making sense is not a matter of surgeons' dispositions interacting with context. The effects of the market context were mediated by communities of practice and by situated clinical activities. The mesh kits that were suddenly available to try and purchase, and the training gained on those trips to Miami, would only be widely used in practice if they also accorded with many physicians' learned judgment (Gordon 1988) about what makes sense.

Judgment

Sue Ross first approached me to contribute to the qualitative methods of a study of when and how stakeholders in pelvic floor surgery consider the ethical and economic dimensions of new devices and procedures. Dr. Ross, a health services researcher, was responsible for organizing clinical studies and trials of new device-procedures in an obstetrics and gynaecology department at an academic medical centre. In her role she had, for instance, led an industry-funded clinical trial comparing two mesh slings for the treatment of incontinence and then encountered difficulty getting the results published because of the "negative" finding – there was no statistically significant difference in outcomes between the slings. There is documented publication bias against studies with such findings (e.g., Easterbrook et al. 1991). Surgeons she worked with had also been among the first to adopt an early, significant variation of the TVT procedure as part of a clinical trial she led, and the trial was stopped early when they noticed an increase in post-operative complications. Soon it became known through their, and other, early studies and formal and informal reports at scientific meetings that the specific type of polypropylene material used to make the sling did not allow it to be incorporated into surrounding tissues, resulting in extrusions into the vagina. The device, ObTape, was removed from the market by its manufacturer, Mentor. It had been on the market in the United States for just three years (2003–6), during which time the *New York Times* estimated sixteen thousand American women had the tape implanted. Once another device-kit for the procedure using the emerging industry-standard for polypropylene was available, the surgical approach ObTape introduced was widely adopted. Such experiences led Dr. Ross and her colleagues to publish a commentary in the *Journal of Obstetrics and Gynecology Canada* titled "Ethical Issues Associated with Introduction of New Surgical Devices, or Just Because We Can, Doesn't Mean We Should" (Ross et al. 2008), and to undertake qualitative research to explore how surgical devices come to be used.

I brought to the research project the long-standing tradition of critical medical sociology that has documented non-clinical influences on medical and surgical decision making (e.g., Becker et al. 1967; Bloor 1976; Eisenberg 1979; McKinlay, Potter, and Feldman 1996; Silverman 1981; Waitzkin 1993), such as economic interests and bias and stereotypes. But through the experience of interviewing surgeons, regulators, administrators, and those involved in assessing new medical technologies, Dr. Ross and I developed a similar kind of unease with dominant strains in our respective disciplinary traditions: a tendency to see the world in technocratic terms, as awaiting better systems of organization and control to produce better outcomes. Better regulations, better guidelines, better information systems, better clinical trials – these are what James Scott (1998) called "seeing like a state": dreams of rationality and planning and objectivity and universality, a modernist way of seeing the world. Evidence-based medicine is arguably the most recent form of this way of seeing.

Dr. Ross persuaded a surgeon colleague, Dr. Magali Robert, to become involved with our burgeoning qualitative research, and we wrote a paper describing how the most recent elaboration of the TVT concept, a so-called mini-sling comprised of a shorter mesh strip with "self-affixing anchors" on each end and requiring only a single vaginal incision for placement, came and went from the market in the absence of good evidence. In this case clinical trials only appeared midway through the device's eight-year life on the market, and lacked meaning because the "standard" comparator treatment was being continually displaced, such that devices about which little is known by the criteria of evidence-based medicine were often compared to one another (Ross, Robert, and Ducey 2015). This trend in "evidence" for mesh kits more broadly made it difficult for the traditional purveyors of evidence-based medicine, who assess health technologies or compile meta-analyses of evidence (i.e., health technology assessment agencies or synthesizers of evidence such as the Cochrane review), to reach definite conclusions about when and how to use transvaginal mesh.

The point of our paper was not, however, to argue that only devices and procedures demonstrated as an improvement in high-quality clinical trials should be approved by regulators and adopted by hospitals and surgeons. The market for vaginal mesh products intensified the challenges to evidence-based surgery, but did not create them. Surgical procedures are not as readily studied and compared as pharmaceuticals or other types of medical interventions. No two patients are exactly alike in their clinical history or anatomy, as are no two surgeons in their training and experience. In assessing any new surgical device, the variability of surgeons and patients cannot be entirely eliminated or controlled for. In the situation of vaginal mesh, distinct components of the procedure – the device as such, the surgical approach or technique used with the device, and the skills and decisions of surgeons – are often impossible to separate for the purposes of forensic investigation or research. Together they are also the basis for continual and often subtle but consequential variation in surgical work. The culture of surgery has long supported continual tinkering with operations and instruments to improve results (Wilde 2004), such that the line between everyday adjustments in practice and innovations is often blurred (Riskin et al. 2006; Rogers et al. 2014). These observations do not mean, alternatively, that personal experience is the only viable basis of decision making in surgery, often positioned as the rival of evidence in the battle over principles of good doctoring (Armstrong 1977; Lambert 2006; Pope 2003).

I once suggested in a team meeting that it was irrational for surgeons to have ever used the mini-sling, which available evidence quickly suggested was less effective than previous versions. Dr. Robert responded by describing a case in which it made sense to use the device: the patient's life was disrupted by her incontinence but her clinical situation made more invasive forms of surgery, including the TVT, riskier, so Dr. Robert put in a mini-sling. As she told the story, it seemed Dr. Robert was and remained dubious about the clinical improvements promised by the makers of mini-slings; nevertheless, in this case the patient's incontinence was resolved. This decision was situated in practice, and was shaped by intersecting layers having to do with the patient, the surgeon, the health care system, and the market for surgical devices. And Dr. Robert's judgment was also grounded in painstakingly acquired experience and skill (Dreyfus 2004; Dreyfus & Dreyfus 2004). Exposure to the work of surgeons, through collaboration and qualitative interviews and observations, raised doubts about the value of idealized and abstracted depictions of medical practice, such as "art" and "science" – which are in addition themselves continually redefined and mobilized as part of various projects to improve medical practice (Berg 1995; Berkwits 1998; Gordon 1988; Lawrence 1985; Mykhalovskiy and Weir 2004; Schlich 2007; Whelan 2009). The more promising path appeared to be to document the processes and outcomes of situated judgments in conditions of contingency and uncertainty (Lutfey and Freese 2007; Pope 2002; Tanenbaum 1994). Mitigation of the dangers of the profit-driven, unregulated market for surgical implants and devices will come from medicine neither as a perfect science nor as a perfect art.

The tradition of critical medical sociology had prepared me to question, not to understand, clinical judgment, because the history of the medical profession's sanctioned and unsanctioned abuses of trust and authority warrants interrogation (e.g., described in Dixon-Woods, Yeung, and Bosk 2011; Rothman 1991). Understandably, critical medical sociology tends to treat actors in medicine and health care, especially those with power, as deficient: deficient in ethical principles, deficient in the production and use of clinical evidence, deficient in the capacity to see how their practice is subject to bias or conflicts of interest, deficient in their willingness to standardize their practices and to account for them. This image did not readily fit the physicians and researchers in pelvic floor surgery with whom I was engaged, as I intellectually processed their ways of working and talking about their work, but also came to gain a more emotional and personal sense of their feelings of responsibility. In an increasingly chaotic context of continual device changes, Drs. Ross and Robert, along with numerous colleagues, were working to make surgical procedures comparable and to measure their outcomes and report and publish their results. Such physicians and allied researchers were not mere relays in others' agendas, interests, or imperatives.

In another respect, I was well prepared for this encounter with the situated, complex work of surgeons by research from science and technology studies and the history of medicine that shows practices in medicine, and surgery, to necessarily intertwine elements of context, social categories, and clinical considerations (Berg 1992; Mol 2002; Moreira 2001; Pope 2002; Schubert 2007). The production of evidence itself is subject to this negotiation of scientific, social, and political considerations (Berg, van der Grinten, and Klazinga 2004; May 2006; Molewijk et al. 2003; Richards 1988). This does not mean medical decisions are arbitrary, only that routines for how to practise are created to manage multiple, and changing, considerations. What this type of research tends not to do, however, is attend to the moral and normative aspects of how physicians navigate this complexity – that their routines and actions are also bound up with their understanding of what it means to practice medicine responsibly (Ducey and Nikoo 2018; Halpern 2004; Kaufman 1997). Surgeons must not only determine what to do with given varied factors, but their determinations must coincide with their understanding of what is the right thing to do for their patients. This is the dimension of "making sense" that needs to be highlighted. Making sense is not a matter of straightforward evaluation, of asking and answering apparently unambiguous questions: Is there evidence to support this change of practice? Does the use of this device accord with ethical principles? Must this innovation be dismissed because it has been produced and pushed by people who stand to personally gain from its adoption? Such questions are not unambiguous, and answers to them will flex based upon moral and emotional considerations.

"Making Sense"

Synthetic mesh "made sense" in the particular path of pelvic floor surgery – as a concept in relation to physiology and anatomy – but also as a morally and emotionally responsible shift in practice. In the absence of mesh, the surgical techniques for supporting the urethra or pelvic floor organs rely on the patient's "native tissues" – creating supports out of fascia, ligaments, and muscles using incisions and sutures. If a woman has a pelvic floor disorder, it is already a sign that something about these tissues or structures is no longer functioning optimally. Therefore, surgeons had long been experimenting with graft materials from other parts of the body or animal donors to reinforce their repairs, and various synthetic grafts had been experimentally used for prolapse since the 1960s (Dwyer 2006). Synthetic mesh had also been widely and successfully used to repair abdominal hernias, an analogous "prolapse" in another part of the body:

> I think that the theory upon which the decision to proceed with mesh was founded was sound. We had placed mesh under the urethra, so transvaginal placement of mesh had been around for years. It was working well. Those slings stayed where you put them, ok? And then when I was researching this and deciding whether or not I would do this, most of the supporting data came from general surgery for the treatment of hernias. They have a huge literature on, mesh treatment of hernias is great ... They just put the mesh in primarily [as the first approach to treatment] – that's how good it is. So the expectation that the mesh would behave well was, I believe, quite well founded. (GS)

In addition, surgeons felt the high rate of "failure" of native tissue procedures was unacceptable. According to one surgeon, the failure rates were "up to fifty per cent ... which is the flip of a coin":

> If you have a procedure that has such a high failure rate, like a native tissue anterior repair, then the question is, what don't we understand that is leading to this? Because clearly we keep doing this procedure that we know doesn't work. It's like the definition of insanity ... You can easily see why people wanted to put mesh in, because it's almost unethical to offer them a native tissue repair. (EH)

So too, when surgeons did use synthetic mesh their experience was not only or primarily of complications from these new device-procedures, but of successes:

> The thing that they don't understand, I really don't think they understand, is that whatever percentage numbers you want to put on for a complication – let's just use the number 3 per cent, 5 per cent – whatever number you want to use. So 5 per cent as the complication, but they're ignoring the other 95 per cent, the thousands and thousands of women who have really, their quality of life has been remarkably improved, and having patient after patient coming into your office and thanking you for improving and changing their lives, they feel like a new woman and so forth – that's the fact they don't fully comprehend. (JH)

The experience of talking to women for whom the implantation of synthetic mesh "changed their lives" doubtless carried weight. The rationale for synthetic mesh was therefore comprised of elements of scientific reasoning, prior clinical experience with mesh and native tissue repairs, and the moral and emotional dimensions of interacting with and seeking to help patients.

On the other hand, surgeons' feelings about the failure of native tissue repair, and their ways of interpreting the research on failures, were not independent of the availability of a new surgical option. The new surgical option may have changed perceptions of what was a failure. Not all surgeons saw the mesh kits in the same way.

> I think that there were a group of people who felt that the rate of failure of our more traditional prolapse surgeries was too high and for that reason, we must have something that's going to reduce that failure rate and the mesh was likely to be that thing. So there was a lot of argument there about "we need to do something more about these failures, what we should be aiming for is 100 per cent success," which is crazy because that never happens no matter what you're doing or using. (BL)

Were surgeons who adopted mesh kits for prolapse aiming for 100 per cent success, or something better than the 50 per cent failure rate associated with native tissue repairs? Were the measures used to establish a 50 per cent failure rate scientifically and clinically valid? It depends on whom you talk to, and how they seek to present themselves and remember.

In addition, some surgeons did not experience success with the kits, or any success was overshadowed by complications or unexpected results.

> My big beef with it was it never stayed where I left it, and so I think that the conclusion is for me, is that the anchoring points weren't adequate. Like, you know, when the general surgeon is fixing a ventral hernia, they do it laparoscopically, they lay the mesh in there, and then they put multiple tacking points, ka-ching, ka-ching, ka-ching, ka-ching [the sound of a surgical stapler]. Whereas when we were doing these mesh vaginal repairs, we were anchoring them at the sacrospinous ligament and the obturator internus membrane, and underneath the pubourethral ligament, so they would ... the expectation was that it would granulate in just like the slings do. But the problem is, is that I found, and that's why I quit so quickly, I betcha I only did at the most ten, is that I'd come back and say, "Well, that's not where I left this bloody thing." (GS)

The appeal of the mesh kits must also be understood in the broader trajectory of surgical innovation and division of surgical labour (Zetka 2001). Some interview respondents said or suggested that because of the advent of laparoscopic surgery for incontinence and prolapse in the mid-1990s, surgeons may have felt they needed to be able to offer seemingly similar "minimally invasive" surgical options. Laparoscopy is not easy to learn and is often described as a time-consuming, complex technique. The transvaginal mesh kits therefore could have appealed to some surgeons, perhaps to generalist gynecologists and urologists more than subspecialists in pelvic floor disorders, because they could offer a "minimally invasive" procedure without needing to learn laparoscopy.

Though a full discussion of these issues is beyond the scope of this chapter, they make clear that considering what makes sense to surgeons does not thereby mean neglecting incompatibilities in their views, the possible influence of wanting to appear responsible on what they say as distinct from what they might do in practice, or the organizational, professional, and institutional trajectories that shaped what could and could not make sense.

From Wrong to Fallible

Such differences among surgeons in experiences, reasoning, emotions, arguments, and clinical decisions suggest that perhaps distinctions can and must be made between ways of "making sense" that allowed for better or worse treatment. Surely not all of these surgeons can be said to be right? Surely to intervene we must know who is right and who is wrong?

At one point, I circulated to the team Joan Cassell's (1991) ethnographic study of surgical work, in which she felt compelled to include in her analysis a provisional, nuanced, and careful categorization of "surgical sins." One chapter focused on the decision by an "old-time" and "prima donna" surgeon, known for his volatility, confidence, and technical facility – a cowboy? – to undertake a then still uncommon approach to colon surgery on a patient who died from infection a week later. The surgeon was criticized by his colleagues. He argued there were no mistakes in the surgery itself and it was not the source of the infection, but his colleagues pointed to aspects of the patient's clinical situation that elevated the risks of infection and which the standard procedure would have reduced. How does a researcher, particularly a non-surgeon, tease apart the elements of a surgeon's decision in order to evaluate it? "After almost three years of observing surgeons," writes Cassell (1991, 22), "I was still unable to evaluate judgment. I could observe *results* ... but I had to rely on [other surgeons] for evaluations of clinical skills." Results are not necessarily a measure of whether a surgeon was right or wrong, responsible or irresponsible. The procedure used by the prima donna surgeon has since become the standard approach to resection of the left colon. Is this also to be the course of the transvaginal use of synthetic mesh to treat prolapse – that once it is more apparent when and how to use it, and who should use it, it will be standard? Even today there are regional and national cultures around the procedure, such that it is widely used as a primary repair in France but largely as a secondary repair (only after a patient's first native tissue repair has failed) in Canada and England. How does one judge judgment?

This would seem to be the domain of clinical ethics, and early on in our work Dr. Ross suggested we needed a bioethicist on our team as an obvious complement to our expertise in health services research, surgery, and critical sociology. Yet a search of the literature showed the case of vaginal mesh had not registered with bioethicists, perhaps because devices for pelvic floor surgery do not raise typical bioethical concerns – those having to do with who shall live and who shall die, or breakthrough technologies that challenge widely and deeply held beliefs. Nor had ethics boards in hospitals or universities noticeably served to limit or control the adoption of transvaginal mesh kits. Bioethics has long been criticized by social scientists for failing to be relevant to specific, everyday moral decisions (DeVries and Subedi 1998; Fox and Swazey 1984; Zussman 1992) – but also by some ethicists, including Dr. Barry Hoffmaster (1994, 2001). In recent work (Hoffmaster 2011; Hoffmaster and Hooker 2009a, 2009b, 2018), he has used empirical research to identify four specific resources of rationality people use in morally complex situations – observation, creative construction, formal and non-formal reasoning methods, and systematic critical appraisal – to improve the capacity for moral judgment, while recognizing that both the resources and those using them are fallible as well as capable of development. The approach is related to that of ethics as design (Whitbeck 1996) – an agent-based perspective in which ethics is seen to be a practice of developing morally reasonable solutions in conditions where there are real constraints on resources and possible actions, as well as no perfect solutions. In this view, surgeons have to make rational judgments, and a judgment is rational if it emanates from a process of deliberation that is rational. And a process of deliberation is rational when it utilizes the four resources (Hoffmaster 2018).

This perspective recognizes that what is deemed moral and responsible practice can vary by situation, context, and moment, and is therefore quite compatible with social scientific understandings of the construction or negotiation of medical practice and knowledge. This work rejects forms of philosophy or bioethics that emphasize universal, decontextualized notions of morality, but it nevertheless retains an anticonstructionist quality in the notion of coherent, fundamental resources that can improve the process of judgment. Rather than resolve or ignore these epistemological tensions with some social science, I see this project as a way to explore what can happen in the space of these tensions (Mykhalovskiy et al. 2019).

For instance, attending to the processes and tools for improved rationality is a means of assessing some ways of defining and responding to clinical-moral issues as better than others on the basis of the processes through which such definitions and responses were arrived at. This allows for critique that is also oriented towards improving medical practice. Additionally, this shifts the focus away from individual decisions or practitioners as bad apples and individualized responsibility (see Goodwin 2014), towards a focus on whether and how systems and contexts foster or constrain the development of moral capacity. Rather than judge physicians' decisions as right or wrong, or gauge their behaviour by whether they apply abstract ethical principles and criteria, we might examine the processes by which physicians come to make decisions, and work to improve them. Generating and using better clinical evidence has become the primary means of identifying and weeding out bad practices or bad apples in medicine, but it can effectively suggest the only practices that are good and responsible are those known through evidence to be so (see Gordon 1988). Types of "intelligence" in addition to formal metrics and evidence (Martin, McKee, and Dixon-Woods 2015; Shojania and Dixon-Woods 2013) are needed to identify worse *and* better practices, enhancing the critical facility of those who provide and study health care services.

The challenge raised by the case of the adoption of transvaginal mesh was to engage in critique because there is a need for improvement – but without making recourse to an (impossible) objective, evidence-determined medicine governed by regulators, ethics review boards, and surveillance systems, and without making recourse to a (at best partial) depiction of those responsible for allocating and delivering medical care as deficient. In the effort to change medical practice it is essential to learn and collaborate with health care professionals on the project of making care better, a goal they share – in this case, reducing the likelihood of a repeat of the transvaginal mesh mess. Health care improvement is arguably more likely when it works from within the specificities of values and practices of a given setting (Zuiderent-Jerak 2007; Zuiderent-Jerak et al. 2009), rather than from a position of imposing values on practitioners who are assumed to lack them. Therefore, a better intervention would be to facilitate surgical judgment – to assist surgeons, and design conditions that assist surgeons, in recognizing and critically, reflexively navigating the trajectories and contexts in which they are situated: the trajectory of the profession in terms of how surgical skills and privileges are distributed and controlled; their personal history of training and experience and awareness of what works in their hands; the effects of collective norms on what they know and see as responsible; the context of a market and regulatory regime that does not and almost always cannot make determinations of whether and when to use any particular device; the nature of everyday decisions as inherently clinical and moral; and the emotional and personal ramifications of patients' expectations and surgical outcomes.

Extended, interdisciplinary engagement with the case of vaginal mesh shows the extent to which it escapes the typical ways of knowing and intervening in health services research, formal ethical review, bioethical analyses, and health technology assessment. In critical medical sociology, favoured explanations for medicine's wrongs – the undue influence of for-profit interests, the failures of government regulation for device safety, the long-standing problems of professional self-governance, the irresponsibility of surgeons who acted in the absence of good evidence – do not explain "what makes sense." That these devices could come to market with little to no data on their safety and effectiveness, and could additionally be sold and adopted at unprecedented speed and scale, requires interventions at the level of systems and regulations. But many apparent remedies to situations such as the transvaginal mesh case cannot affect important aspects of surgical practice, organization, and values. Most importantly, they do not affect surgical judgment, in which we must still place our trust and our bodies.

ACKNOWLEDGMENT

This project was supported by an Ethics Catalyst grant (139100) from the Population and Public Health Institute of the Canadian Institutes of Health Research (CIHR).

REFERENCES

Abraham, J., and R. Ballinger. 2012. "The Neoliberal Regulatory State, Industry Interests, and the Ideological Penetration of Scientific Knowledge: Deconstructing the Redefinition of Carcinogens in Pharmaceuticals." *Science, Technology and Human Values* 37 (5): 443–77. https://doi.org/10.1177/0162243911424914.

Armstrong, D. 1977. "Clinical Sense and Clinical Science." *Social Science and Medicine* 11: 599–601. https://doi.org/10.1016/0037-7856(77)90041-5.

Becker, H.S., B. Geer, E.C. Hughes, and A.L. Strauss. 1967. *Boys in White: Student Culture in Medical School.* Chicago: University of Chicago Press.

Berg, M. 1992. "The Construction of Medical Disposals: Medical Sociology and Medical Problem Solving in Clinical Practice." *Sociology of Health & Illness* 14 (2): 151–80. https://doi.org/10.1111/j.1467-9566.1992.tb00119.x.

Berg, M. 1995. "Turning a Practice into a Science: Reconceptualizing Postwar Medical Practice." *Social Studies of* Science 25: 437–76. https://doi.org/10.1177/030631295025003002.

Berg, M., T. van der Grinten, and N. Klazinga. 2004. "Technology Assessment, Priority Setting, and Appropriate Care in Dutch Health Care." *International Journal of Technology Assessment in Health Care* 20 (1): 35–43. https://doi.org/10.1017/S0266462304000765.

Berkwits, M. 1998. "From Practice to Research: The Case for Criticism in an Age of Evidence." *Social Science and Medicine* 47 (10): 1539–45. https://doi.org/10.1016/S0277-9536(98)00232-9.

Bloor, M. 1976. "Bishop Berkeley and the Adenotonsillectomy Enigma: An Exploration of Variation in the Social Construction of Medical Disposals." *Sociology* 10 (1): 43–61. https://doi.org/10.1177/003803857601000103.

Cassell, J. 1991. *Expected Miracles: Surgeons at Work.* Philadelphia: Temple University Press.

DeVries, R., and J. Subedi. 1998. *Bioethics and Society: Constructing the Ethical Enterprise.* Upper Saddle River, NJ: Prentice Hall.

Dixon-Woods, M., K. Yeung, and C. Bosk. 2011. "Why Is UK Medicine No Longer a Self-Regulating Profession? The Role of Scandals Involving 'Bad Apple' Doctors." *Social Science and Medicine* 73: 1452–9. https://doi.org/10.1016/j.socscimed.2011.08.031.

Dreyfus, H., and S. Dreyfus. 2004. "The Ethical Implications of the Five-Stage Skill-Acquisition Model." *Bulletin of Science, Technology and Society* 24 (3): 251–64. https://doi.org/10.1177/0270467604265023.

Dreyfus, S. 2004. "The Five-Stage Model of Adult Skill Acquisition." *Bulletin of Science, Technology and Society* 24 (3): 177–81. https://doi.org/10.1177/0270467604264992.

Ducey, A., and S. Nikoo. 2018. "Formats of Responsibility: Elective Surgery in the Era of Evidence-Based Medicine." *Sociology of Health and Illness* 40 (3): 494–507. https://doi.org/10.1111/1467-9566.12659

Dwyer, P. 2006. "Evolution of Biological and Synthetic Grafts in Reconstructive Pelvic Surgery." *International Urogynecology Journal* 17: S10–S15. https://doi.org/10.1007/s00192-006-0103-0.

Easterbrook, P., J. Berlin, R. Gopalan, and D. Matthews. 1991. "Publication Bias in Clinical Research." *The Lancet* 337 (8746): 867–72. https://doi.org/10.1016/0140-6736(91)90201-Y.

Eisenberg, J. 1979. "Sociologic Influences on Decision-Making by Clinicians." *Annals of Internal Medicine* 90: 957–64. https://doi.org/10.7326/0003-4819-90-6-957.

Fox, R., and J. Swazey. 1984. "Medical Morality Is Not Bioethics: Medical Ethics in China and the United States." *Perspectives in Biology and Medicine* 27: 336–60. https://doi.org/10.1353/pbm.1984.0060.

Goodwin, D. 2014. "Decision-Making and Accountability: Differences of Distribution." *Sociology of Health and Illness* 36 (1): 44–59. https://doi.org/10.1111/1467-9566.12042.

Gordon, D. 1988. "Clinical Science and Clinical Expertise: Changing Boundaries between Art and Science in Medicine." In *Biomedicine Examined*, edited by M. Lock and D. Gordon, 257–95. Dordrecht: Kluwer.

Halpern, S. 2004. *Lesser Harms: The Morality of Risk in Medical Research.* University of Chicago Press.

Hines, J.Z., P. Lurie, E. Yu, and S. Wolfe. 2010. "Left to Their Own Devices: Breakdowns in United States Medical Device Premarket Review." *PLoS Medicine* 7 (7): 1–8. https://doi.org/10.1371/journal.pmed.1000280.

Hoffmaster, B. 1994. "The Forms and Limits of Medical Ethics." *Social Science and Medicine* 39 (9): 1155–64. https://doi.org/10.1016/0277-9536(94)90348-4.

Hoffmaster, B. 2001. *Bioethics in Social Context.* Philadelphia: Temple University Press.

Hoffmaster, B. 2011. "The Rationality and Morality of Dying Children." *Hastings Center Report* 41 (6): 30–42. https://doi.org/10.1002/j.1552-146X.2011.tb00154.x.

Hoffmaster, B. 2018. "From Applied Ethics to Empirical Ethics to Contextual Ethics." *Bioethics* 32 (2): 119–25. https://doi.org/10.1111/bioe.12419.

Hoffmaster, B., and C. Hooker. 2009a. "How Experience Confronts Ethics." *Bioethics* 23 (4): 214–25. https://doi.org/10.1111/j.1467-8519.2009.01709.x.

Hoffmaster, B., and C. Hooker. 2009b. "What Empirical Research Can Do for Bioethics." *American Journal of Bioethics* 9 (6-7): 72–4. https://doi.org/10.1080/15265160902893940.

Hoffmaster, B., and C. Hooker. 2018. *Re-Reasoning Ethics: The Rationality of Deliberation and Judgment in Ethics.* Cambridge, MA: MIT Press.

Kaufman, S.R. 1997. "Construction and Practice of Medical Responsibility: Dilemmas and Narratives from Geriatrics." *Culture, Medicine and Psychiatry* 21: 1–26. https://doi.org/10.1023/A:1005345716123.

Kent, J., and A. Faulkner. 2002. "Regulating Human Implant Technologies in Europe – Understanding the New Era in Medical Device Regulation." *Health, Risk and Society* 4 (2): 189–209. https://doi.org/10.1080/13698570220137060.

Lambert, H. 2006. "Accounting for EBM: Notions of Evidence in Medicine." *Social Science and Medicine* 62: 2633–45. https://doi.org/10.1016/j.socscimed.2005.11.023.

Lawrence, C. 1985. "Incommunicable Knowledge: Science, Technology and the Clinical Art in Britain 1850–1914." *Journal of Contemporary History* 20 (4): 503–20. https://doi.org/10.1177/002200948502000402.

Lexchin, J. 2016. *Private Profits versus Public Policy: The Pharmaceutical Industry and the Canadian State.* Toronto: University of Toronto Press.

Lutfey, K., and J. Freese. 2007. "Ambiguities of Chronic Illness Management and Challenges to the Medical Error Paradigm." *Social Science and Medicine* 64: 314–25. https://doi.org/10.1016/j.socscimed.2006.08.037.

Martin, G., L. McKee, and M. Dixon-Woods. 2015. "Beyond Metrics? Utilizing 'Soft Intelligence' for Health Care Quality and Safety." *Social Science and Medicine* 142: 19–26. https://doi.org/10.1016/j.socscimed.2015.07.027.

May, C. 2006. "Mobilising Modern Facts: Health Technology Assessment and the Politics of Evidence." *Sociology of Health and Illness* 28 (5): 513–32. https://doi.org/10.1111/j.1467-9566.2006.00505.x.

McKinlay, J., D. Potter, and H. Feldman. 1996. "Non-medical Influences on Medical Decision-Making." *Social Science and Medicine* 42 (5): 769–76. https://doi.org/10.1016/0277-9536(95)00342-8.

Mol, A. 2002. *The Body Multiple.* Durham: Duke University Press.

Molewijk, B., A. Stiggelbout, W. Otten, H. Dupuis, and J. Kievit. 2003. "Implicit Normativity in Evidence-Based Medicine: A Plea for Integrated Empirical Ethics Research." *Health Care Analysis* 11 (1): 69–92. https://doi.org/10.1023/A:1025390030467.

Moreira, T. 2001. "Involvement and Constraint in a Surgical Consultation Room." *Bulletin Suisse de Linguistique Appliquée* 74: 13–32. https://doc.rero.ch/record/18352/files/05_Moreira.pdf.

Mykhalovskiy, E., K.L. Frohlich, B. Poland, E. Di Ruggiero, M.J. Rock, and L. Comer. 2019. "Critical Social Science with Public Health: Agonism, Critique, and Engagement." *Critical Public Health* 29 (5): 522–33. https://doi.org/10.1080/09581596.2018.1474174.

Mykhalovskiy, E., and L. Weir. 2004. "The Problem of Evidence-Based Medicine: Directions for Social Science." *Social Science and Medicine* 59 (5): 1059–69. https://doi.org/10.1016/j.socscimed.2003.12.002.

Pope, C. 2002. "Contingency in Everyday Surgical Work." *Sociology of Health and Illness* 24 (4): 369–84. https://doi.org/10.1111/1467-9566.00300.

Pope, C. 2003. "Resisting Evidence: The Study of Evidence-Based Medicine as a Contemporary Social Movement." *Health* 7 (3): 267–82. https://doi.org/10.1177/1363459303007003002.

Richards, E. 1988. "The Politics of Therapeutic Evaluation: The Vitamin C and Cancer Controversy." *Social Studies of Science* 18 (4): 653–701. https://doi.org/10.1177/030631288018004004.

Riskin, D., M. Longaker, M. Gertner, and T. Krummel. 2006. "Innovation in Surgery: A Historical Perspective." *Annals of Surgery* 244: 686–93. https://doi.org/10.1097/01.sla.0000242706.91771.ce.

Rogers, E. 2003. *Diffusion of Innovations*. 5th ed. New York: Free Press.

Rogers, W., M. Lotz, K. Hutchison, A. Pourmoslemi, and A. Eyers. 2014. "Identifying Surgical Innovation: A Qualitative Study of Surgeons' Views." *Annals of Surgery* 259: 273–8. https://doi.org/10.1097/SLA.0b013e31829ccc5f.

Ross, S., M. Robert, and A. Ducey. 2015. "The Short Lifecycle of a Surgical Device: Literature Analysis Using McKinlay's 7-Stage Model." *Health Policy and Technology* 4: 168–88. https://doi.org/10.1016/j.hlpt.2015.02.008.

Ross, S., M. Robert, M.-A. Harvey, S. Farrell, J. Schulz, D. Wilkie, D. Lovatsis, et al. 2008. "Ethical Issues Associated with the Introduction of New Surgical Devices, or Just Because We Can, Doesn't Mean We Should." *Journal of Obstetrics and Gynaecology Canada* 30 (6): 508–13. https://doi.org/10.1016/S1701-2163(16)32867-5.

Rothman, D. 1991. *Strangers at the Bedside: A History of How Law and Bioethics Transformed Medical Decision Making*. New York: Aldine de Gruyter.

Schlich, T. 2007. "The Art and Science of Surgery: Innovation and Concepts of Medical Practice in Operative Fracture Care: 1960s–1970s." *Science, Technology and Human Values* 32 (1): 65–87. https://doi.org/10.1177/0162243906293886.

Schubert, C. 2007. "Risk and Safety in the Operating Theater: An Ethnographic Study of Sociotechnical Practices." In *Biomedicine as Culture: Instrumental Practices, Technoscientific Knowledge and New Modes of Life*, edited by V. Burri and J. Dumit, 123–38. New York: Routledge.

Scott, J.C. 1998. *Seeing Like a State*. New Haven: Yale University Press.

Shojania, K., and M. Dixon-Woods. 2013. "'Bad Apples': Time to Redefine as a Type of Systems Problem?" *British Medical Journal Quality and Safety* 22 (7): 528–31. https://doi.org/10.1136%2Fbmjqs-2013-002138.

Silverman, D. 1981. "The Child as a Social Object: Down's Syndrome Children in a Paediatric Cardiology Clinic." *Sociology of Health and Illness* 3 (3): 254–74. https://doi.org/10.1111/1467-9566.ep10486744.

Tanenbaum, S. 1994. "Knowing and Acting in Medical Practice: The Epistemological Politics of Outcomes Research." *Journal of Health Politics, Policy and Law* 19 (1): 27–44. https://doi.org/10.1215/03616878-19-1-27.

Ulmsten, U., L. Henriksson, P. Johnson, and G. Varhos. 1996. "An Ambulatory Surgical Procedure under Local Anesthesia for Treatment of Female Urinary Incontinence." *International Urogynecology Journal* 7 (2): 81–6. https://doi.org/10.1007/BF01902378.

Waitzkin, H. 1993. *The Politics of Medical Encounters: How Patients and Doctors Deal with Social Problems.* New Haven: Yale University Press.

Whelan, E. 2009. "Negotiating Science and Experience in Medical Knowledge: Gynaecologists on Endometriosis." *Social Science and Medicine* 68 (8): 1489–97. https://doi.org/10.1016/j.socscimed.2009.01.032.

Whitbeck, C. 1996. "Ethics as Design: Doing Justice to Moral Problems." *Hastings Center Report* 26 (3): 9–16. https://doi.org/10.2307/3527925.

Wilde, S. 2004. "See One, Do One, Modify One: Prostate Surgery in the 1930s." *Medical History* 48 (3): 351–66. https://doi.org/10.1017/S0025727300007675.

Zetka, J.R. 2001. "Occupational Divisions of Labor and Their Technology Politics: The Case of Surgical Scopes and Gastrointestinal Medicine." *Social Forces* 79 (4): 1495–520. https://doi.org/10.1353/sof.2001.0056.

Zuiderent-Jerak, T. 2007. "Preventing Implementation: Exploring Interventions with Standardization in Health Care." *Science as Culture* 16 (3): 311–29. https://doi.org/10.1080/09505430701568719.

Zuiderent-Jerak, T., M. Strating, A. Nieboer, and R. Bal. 2009. "Sociological Refigurations of Patient Safety: Ontologies of Improvement and 'Acting with' Quality Collaboratives in Health Care." *Social Science and Medicine* 69: 1713–21. https://doi.org/10.1016/j.socscimed.2009.09.049.

Zussman, R. 1992. *Intensive Care: Medical Ethics and the Medical Profession.* Chicago: University of Chicago Press.

11 Seeking Disability Politics in Disability and Health-Related Non-profit Organizations

CHRISTINE KELLY

In October 2012, the national chairperson of the Council of Canadians with Disabilities, Tony Dolan, spoke to the federal Finance Committee. He described Canada's progress in relation to disability but was careful to specify, "To be blunt, these improvements came about because people with disabilities, their families and their organizations spoke out" (Council of Canadians with Disabilities 2012). At the time of Dolan's presentation, the Social Development Partnership Program-Disability (SDPP-D) was being reduced dramatically and transformed from a program that provided dedicated operating funds to national disability organizations to a managed competition open to an array of groups (Human Resources and Skills Development Canada 2009). Managed competition enacts neoliberal modes of governance by ensuring established organizations with strong measurement infrastructure gain time-limited access to funding, on which they must continually report. The resulting accountability relations allow government agencies to influence the activities of the non-profit sector. In 2013, the revised SDPP-D competition received 383 proposals and funded only 17. This is certainly a challenging landscape for disability organizations in Canada. If the national, rights-based groups are struggling to survive, where and how do disability politics surface in the non-profit sector?

This chapter considers how diverse disability organizations are adapting to and resisting this challenging landscape. Engaged in advocacy, political work, service provision, and other activities, these groups mobilize very different conceptions of disability. Drawing on a qualitative study of disability and health-related organizations in Ottawa, the chapter unravels how definitions of disability influenced by social movement histories are used by a spectrum of non-profit organizations. The findings from a website analysis of eighty-four organizations and three case examples demonstrate that there is a broad influence of disability politics evident among disability and health organizations. These politics are, however, sporadically enacted and are constrained by the sociopolitical landscape in Canada.

Further, this chapter finds that social and medical definitions of disability do not adequately capture the competing and sometimes muddled definitions at play in non-profit settings. A more complex "relational" model proposed by Kafer (2013) that leaves room for a politicized approach to health (rather than an outright rejection of medical models) may be more useful in considering the actions and ideas of disability and health non-profit organizations.

Context: Seeking Advocacy in the Non-profit Sector

Scholarship on the non-profit sector in Canada is challenged to define this complex and vast field (Hall and Banting 2000; Laforest 2011). The non-profit sector includes a wide range of organizations from religious groups, social movement organizations, hospitals, and long-standing charitable groups, among many others. This murkiness makes it particularly difficult to locate and understand the advocacy role of the non-profit sector. A number of scholars comment on the challenges organizations face in engaging in advocacy work, particularly under neoliberal governance (Laforest 2011; Young and Everitt 2004). Yet Bridge and Gilbert (2005) argue that non-profit organizations can and should play a vital role in informing the development of public policy.

Scott (2003) describes an "advocacy chill" experienced by the non-profit and voluntary sector where organizations are discouraged from participating in activist or advocacy activities. This is formally enshrined in the registration process for charitable status that limits "political activities" to 10 to 20 per cent of an organization's work (Canada Revenue Agency 2011). DeSantis (2010, 24) writes, "there is still a lack of clarity for NPOs that are registered charities regarding what does and does not constitute political activity. This lack of clarity leads to confusion in interpretation of laws for some NPOs, in turn stifling advocacy action for fear of government reprisals." Advocacy chill was further promoted through the Harper government's audit of the activities of charitable organizations towards the end of its final term, an audit that seemed to target organizations with social justice aims (CBC News 2014). In 2017, the Trudeau government announced its intention to end the practice of aggressively auditing these charitable organizations.

One unifying feature to the non-profit sector identified by Baines (2015) is an alternative "non-profit ethos" that includes altruism, advocacy, a commitment to inclusion, and a social justice orientation, among other features. She argues that this ethos is more prevalent among social service agencies and less common in health service organizations. The ethos is undermined by new public management discourses that emphasize measurement and accountability schematics. Disability and health-related non-profit organizations sit on the murky line between health and social services, making this sector an interesting example to consider.

Existing literature on disability organizations finds user-led organizations play a critical advocacy role that differs from professional-led and historical charitable disability groups and, further, that there is a need for new leadership in these groups (Hutchison et al. 2007). Neufeldt (2003a, b) documents the long history of disability organizations in developing services and advocating for change. This argument is confirmed by a qualitative study by McColl and Boyce (2003) that outlines the role of organizations that participated in policy advocacy (see also Stienstra 2003). Finally, Levesque's (2012, 17) interprovincial comparison of charitable tax returns of disability organizations found their innovative capacity is "undermined by the lack of stable core operating funds, which have long been called for." There is an urgent demand for disability organizations to participate in informing traditional policy formation as well as to disrupt normative cultural messages about disability. With this challenging landscape in mind, coupled with Baines's observations about the weaker non-profit ethos in health service organizations, this chapter now turns to some of the conceptual tensions around the social/medical divide related to disability.

Conceptual Debates: Models and Medicine

Attempts to distinguish between medical and social approaches to embodiment had long been the basis for disability activism and critical disability studies scholarship (Oliver 1983), and represents a valuable critique of biomedical modes of knowledge production that dominate the health sector. Most commonly, these discussions delineate a "social" model of disability from a "medical" one. The social model separates "disability" (physical and social barriers that cause disabling experiences) from "impairments" (mental or physical differences). Disability perspectives emphasize the dehumanizing presumptions of the medical model or, as contemporary disability justice activists suggest, a more complicated "medical industrial complex" (Mingus 2011). Treating disability as individual, medical problems to be solved by evidence overshadows the cultural, social, and physical exclusion of disabled people. Medical dominance in the realm of disability is linked to alarming responses to disabled people, including institutionalization, forced sterilization, cultural discourses of personal tragedy, and emphasis on "curing" rather than inclusion.

Proposing alternative models of disability is an essential disruption of medical dominance and scientific evidence: rather than viewing disability only through the lens of medical diagnostics, such models suggest that lived experiences situated in social, political, and economic contexts can and should inform our definitions of disability. Most commonly referenced, the "social model" suggests disability is caused by social and physical barriers in society, and not by individual medical issues (Oliver 1983). Yet Shakespeare and Watson (2002) and others (Dewsbury et al. 2004; French 1993; Gabel and Peters 2004; Thomas 1999) question whether these distinctions remain relevant in discussing disability in progressive and social settings. Feminist scholars highlight the ways in which the social model does not encapsulate all lived experiences of disability, especially for those with mental health issues, intellectual disabilities, and chronic pain (Garland-Thomson 2011; see also "impairment effects" in Thomas 1999).

It has become somewhat predictable to describe the field of disability studies with reference to the social model, as the establishment of this concept is often seen as the origin of the field. Even as the field evolves, newer understandings of disability continue to either build on or deconstruct the medical/social distinction. Swain and French (2000), for example, propose an affirmation model or pride model of disability that counters notions of tragedy. When developing this approach, Swain and French argue, "the social model has not, in itself, underpinned a non-tragedy view" (571). The affirmation model grows out of a critique of the social model, which begins to appear as a universal starting point for critical conversations about disability. Arguably, this concern with models restricts the field from more thorough explorations of geopolitics, racialization, and indigeneity, explorations that are sorely needed (Bell 2006; Erevelles 2011; Grech 2009).

On the one hand, a large proportion of the field seems prepared to move beyond the social model framework, as critiques of the model are cited as frequently as the definition. Perspectives drawing on specific strands of cultural theory, and developing independently from discussions of the social model, are gaining prominence (e.g., Fritsch 2015; Goodley, Lawthom, and Runswick-Cole 2014; Soldatic and Fiske 2009). On the other hand, the social model remains a minority understanding of disability, particularly in medical and non-academic settings, and can be seen as an important educational tool (Oliver 2004) that also represents a challenge to the applied turn in health and social services sectors.

Thus, we are faced with a conundrum of needing the social model as an educational and disruptive knowledge production tool but one that is theoretically limiting in more complex applications. Usefully, Kafer (2013, 7) develops a political/relational model that is a "friendly departure from the more common social model of disability." Kafer's model holds space for medicine in our approaches to disability, but calls for "a direct refusal of the widespread depoliticization of disability" (8). She explains the role of medical intervention in her framework:

> The political/relational model neither opposes nor valorizes medical intervention; rather than simply take such intervention for granted, it recognizes instead that medical representations, diagnoses, and treatments of bodily variation are imbued with ideological biases about what constitutes normalcy and deviance. In doing so, it recognizes the possibility of simultaneously desiring to be cured of chronic pain and to be identified and allied with disabled people. (6)

Some disabled people may desire cure and intervention, but these desires can be situated in broader, politicized frameworks for disability. Instead of generating a model that directly opposes medical understandings, Kafer's relational approach allows for an engagement and potentially critical reorientation to medicine and health care. Inspired by both Kafer's call to consider politicized relationships to medicine and Baines's observation regarding the milder non-profit ethos in health services, this chapter seeks definitions of disability in disability and health-related non-profit organizations. In doing so, it explores the relevance of medical and social definitions of disability in practical settings in order to echo Kafer's relational model, where health and politics interact with generative potential.

Methods

The findings for this chapter are embedded within a qualitative study that investigated how disability and health-related organizations were faring in light of shifting sociopolitical conditions, and how the organizations involved diverse youth with disabilities. The use of qualitative and participatory methods is informed by feminist and disability scholarship, and an intentional disruption of quantitative measurement and reporting that characterizes the non-profit sector, health services, and research. Through this disruption, alternative modes of knowledge production are privileged in order to generate a counter-evidence base that nuances and challenges quantitative metrics. The study was composed of four aspects in total; this chapter focuses on findings from the first and second components. The first was a mapping exercise and website analysis focusing on small and medium non-profit organizations in Ottawa. Organizations were eligible if they (1) used the word "disability" in their mission statement and/or (2) identified people with disabilities as a core audience or service users, and (3) had a mailing address in the city of Ottawa. The eligibility criteria intentionally aimed to include organizations beyond the rights-based or consumer-run groups that have been studied previously (Hutchison et al. 2007; Stienstra and Wight-Felske 2003). The inclusion criteria intended to reflect the expansive, inclusive definitions of disability promoted in the field of disability studies. The study did not include hospitals, foundations, or charitable organizations that did not have non-profit status.

As there is no public listing of non-profit organizations in Canada, the list of organizations was created through searching the Charity Village website, a list of non-profits released to Blumberg Segal LLP (Blumberg 2014), snowball referral, and a contact list from a disability service office at a local university. Eighty-four organizations were identified, although it is possible some organizations were accidentally missed. The eighty-four organizations were categorized into seven core audience groups: community living/intellectual disability (n = 18), health/chronic illness (n = 15), cross-disability (n = 14), mental health (n = 13), single impairment (n = 13), sport–cross-disability (n = 8), and sport–single impairment (n = 3). Websites from these organizations were then analysed with the help of NVivo qualitative data analysis software. When possible, information was collected on the year of founding, geographical scope, mission, vision, mandate, slogan, key activities, and other elements.

The second research component included semi-structured key informant interviews that were used to gather more in-depth perspectives of the challenges, strengths, and perceptions of representatives of non-profit organizations. Participants included executive directors or staff members from twenty-five organizations, selected to approximately reflect the audience categories identified in the website analysis. Twenty-five is close to one-third of the total organizations, and thematic repetition occurred in this set. The interviews took place between October 2014 and July 2015 and were conducted mostly by the author, with some by a graduate research assistant. Students in a graduate-level research methods class sat in on a few of the interviews with advance permission from participants. The participants were offered gift cards to recognize their time and contributions. Efforts were made to disguise their identities in dissemination activities, although it is possible some may be identifiable due to the public nature of their positions.

The third component of the study was focus group discussions with youth with disabilities (*n* = 46, ages seventeen to twenty-five, mean and median age of twenty-two). The fourth component was a participatory action project in which a volunteer subset of the focus group participants worked together to plan a community event at which preliminary findings were discussed. The results of the youth portion of this study are reported elsewhere (Kelly 2018; Kelly forthcoming).

All interviews and focus group recordings were professionally transcribed and analysed using NVivo software. A preliminary code book was developed by the researcher, a research associate, and graduate students based on themes in the literature and concepts from feminist disability studies.

Findings

The findings of the study reported below emphasize the definitions of disability utilized on official organizational websites as well as three cases from the key informant interviews.

DEFINITIONS OF DISABILITY: WEBSITE ANALYSIS

In order to consider the relevance of "models" of disability in practical settings and to situate disability politics in the non-profit sector, this chapter categorizes the organizational websites as employing four main definitions of disability (see Table 11.1). The most dominant definition is a social/activist one (*n* = 52). This includes key terms associated with activist histories such as "deinstitutionalization," "barriers," or "social model," and so on. What is perhaps disconcerting about this category is the frequency with which organizations use social/activist terms in their mandates and mission statements even as the activities and services they provide do not align with the values inherent in those movements. The key informant interviews, examples of which will be discussed in more depth below, reveal that some organizations are aware of these gaps, while others seem to be mis- or under-informed about the social histories of the frameworks they evoke. For example, there was one organization clearly influenced by deinstitutionalization but during one period of its history it ended up offering segregated day programs. The leadership re-evaluated this practice over the years and dramatically changed their programming to better align with the movements they referenced. On the other end of the spectrum, a more recent organization focused on developing an accessible recreational sporting venue. The organization drew on empowerment discourses and some phrases that can be associated with a social model understanding of disability, and yet their practices were rooted in charitable fundraising and pity narratives.

The second-most-common definition deployed by the organizations was medical (n = 14). This was less common than might be expected given the emphasis in critical disability scholarship on opposing medical understandings, although the social values of the non-profit ethos may also explain why this perspective is not as heavily emphasized (Baines 2015). Following this, there were nine organizations that used a mix of medical and social understandings. The mix did not necessarily represent Kafer's relational model, where disability is politicized and health perspectives are engaged with, but more an attempt to assimilate multiple perspectives. Finally, nine organizations did not offer a definition for understanding disability, mental health, or other health issues, but rather focused on the provision of services.

DEFINITIONS AND ACTIVITIES: KEY INFORMANT INTERVIEWS

The chapter now considers three case studies and related key informant interviews that use social/activist language on their websites. The three cases were selected to represent the diversity of the organizations and to investigate Kafer's relational model.

CASE 1: MAD MOVEMENTS IN PRACTICE

The study included an organization founded in the early 1990s made up of people with lived experience in the mental health system. It has a medium-sized operating budget that comes primarily from provincial government funding.

The organization carefully uses politicized language, with clear resonances to a broader mad, consumer, and/or survivor movement. Historically, the group started with a focus on advocacy and peer-help groups. The executive director (ED) said of this period, "I mean sometimes in movements, if we see the consumer/survivor situation as a movement, there is a place where you are angry and you are kind of railing against the system." The ED expressed frustration with this period in terms of not being able to get enough attention or accomplish the change she wished to see in policy related to mental health. She described a paradigm shift for herself and the organization, when she realized that "doing stuff, just doing it, goes a lot further than advocating for them." With this perspective, the organization transitioned into developing mental health programs offered within hospitals and other medical settings, and training people with lived experience to run them. The operating budget grew dramatically as a result of this shift. The organization is now recognized as a leader by more medically oriented perspectives, with the ED commenting, "nowadays we have psychiatrists referring to us all the time."

Table 11.1. Definitions of disability and health non-profit organizations

Definition	Description	Key terms	#	Examples
Social/activist	Working definitions of disability influenced by activist histories, including independent living, social model, community living, deinstitutionalization, or Paralympic sport * The term "community" was heavily emphasized	• barriers, obstacles, accessible/ity • citizen(ship) • community* • consumer • empower(ment) • equity, equitable, equal(ity) • inclusion/ive, integration/ed, acceptance • independent/ce • movement • (full) participation • peer • right/s	52	"Community Living Ontario envisions a society where everyone belongs, has equality, respect and acceptance. This gives people a sense of self-worth and opportunities for growth. The gifts, uniqueness and innate value of each individual are celebrated, supported and acknowledged as essential to the completeness of the whole community." "Our primary activity is public education and awareness about the social and physical barriers that prevent the full inclusion of persons with disabilities in Ontario."
Medical	Disability as an individual health issue rooted in the body, often in need of a cure or treatment	• care • cure • health • prevent(ion) • quality of life • treatment, treatable	14	"To enhance the lives of those affected with neuromuscular disorders by continually working to provide ongoing support and resources while relentlessly searching for a cure through well-funded research."

(Continued)

Definition	Description	Key terms	#	Examples
Multiple	Combination of social and medical definitions as outlined above		9	"To work toward the necessary changes that will improve the quality of life of Canadians with Autism Spectrum Disorders across their lifespan. We promote current understanding of ASD issues and respect for differences." Goals: • "Increase awareness and understanding of ASD and participation of individuals with ASD • Promote federal policies, programs, and legislation that respond to the needs of the Autism community • Promote evidence-based services/ treatment, best practices and standards • Promote targeted ASD research"
Service recipients	People with disabilities as only service recipients Organizations in other categories may mention services *in combination with* other indicators of social/ medical understandings. In contrast, these organizations emphasize only service provision and fundraising to support services they offer	• activities • program • serve/ing • services	9	"ICSS will be an excellent provider of quality services to people with developmental disabilities and their personal networks." "The Distress Centre of Ottawa and Region is a 24/7 volunteer-based organization offering confidential, emotional mental health support, crisis intervention, information referral and education services."

In terms of definitions of disability, this organization easily falls into the "social/activist" category utilized in Table 11.1. Histories of disability and mad activism are clearly present in the language, operating structures, and activities of the organization, and these understandings have evolved and shifted over time. The social movement language is not merely rhetoric, and the ED presents a complex, nuanced understanding of what it means to have lived experience of the mental health system. She comments:

> I don't want to make it sound like it is all some kind of movie where being crazy is charming. Because it is not, people suffer and they have really hard times and sometimes they lose everything. But there is also the potential to have amazing things to share with other people coming out of that. And I think that is probably true of everyone who would be considered to have a disability. So I guess we would identify with them in that sense. That we have these dubious gifts. Really sometimes exceedingly dubious.

The organization continues to evolve and push forward understandings of mental illness that differ greatly from that of the medical research world.

CASE 2: SINGLE IMPAIRMENT AND THE BLURRING OF MODELS

The second example organization is a single-impairment group that operates in one of four regions. It employs eleven full-time and four part-time staff and has a large operating budget, about ten times the amount of the first case's. Uniquely, this organization does not rely on government sources for their funding, but on charitable fundraising campaigns, including a large campaign run by a partner association. It provides information, education, systemic advocacy, and an equipment program. The national board is composed of researchers, clinicians, clients, family members, representatives of the fundraising organization, and corporate sponsors.

While categorized in the website analysis under the "social/activist" category, this single-impairment organization had a complex and at times conflicting set of practices that reflected other definitions of disability. For example, when speaking about the expanded membership criteria they had adopted in recent years, the regional executive director used a medically informed framework:

> [Our growing scope] is really directed by the medical scientific advisory committee, who is made up of researchers and also people who are affected ... Even though [the conditions] are very different in terms of the bio-

> medical piece. But there are definitely a lot of connections around the diagnosis and the symptoms ... You know, with the better diagnosing that it definitely has enhanced our disorder list, that's for sure.

Including medical practitioners on the volunteer board is another indicator of this type of framework. The organization was a vocal advocate for a number of policy issues, drawing on independent living approaches to disability. For example, the regional executive director explained the advocacy work they do related to home care:

> If you have a disability you are sick. And that is how you are treated, right. You have [home care] and somebody comes in and does a care model. So doing a lot of advocacy around the right to risk and independence. And you know people who have a disability aren't sick. So a lot of work around that.

The group also engaged in advocacy related to access to specific medical treatments and health care. The organization's ability to engage in advocacy so extensively was linked to having non-governmental sources of funding. In yet another paradox, while they used independent living discourses in their advocacy work, their charitable campaigns, especially the one run by an outside association, drew heavily on pity narratives.

CASE 3: SERVICE PROVIDER ADVOCACY

The third example comes from the intellectual disability audience category, a large service provider that runs group homes, employment services, and day programs. It had the largest staff and operating budget of the organizations in this study, and its funds came almost entirely from the provincial government. The organization has a very long wait list for their services, with the executive director commenting, "we are talking years, if not decades, for services."

The organization has a prominent role in provincial advocacy and is often called to comment in the media on issues related to intellectual disabilities. It draws on social and community living terminology on its website. However, the executive director explicitly distances the organization from other parts of this sector that he characterizes as "radical":

> I don't see us as being radical though. And there are many people in [the] community living movement, if I can put it that way, that would be very philosophical about certain aspects. We are much more of a holistic approach, if something makes sense and works for this individual we are going to consider it and implement it. We are not going to be wedded to a certain style or a certain approach or a certain way of interacting.

The executive director was alluding to the highly criticized, sheltered workshops they offer, where workers, rather than being paid minimum wage, are given an honorarium so they remain eligible for disability income support.

The executive director also described consulting and participating in a national campaign related to disability income that has faced some criticism from rights-based organizations, and perhaps represents a shift in disability activism towards increasing levels of service-provider advocacy that does not necessarily align with the goals of user-run organizations.

Discussion and Concluding Thoughts

The website analysis above demonstrates the reach and lasting influence of disability movements, including deinstitutionalization, mad movements, independent living, and others. This is evidence that these movements have been successful in what Fraser (1995) terms the "recognition" aspect of collective action, activities that have changed terminology and representation of certain groups. Organizations that fall far out of what would be defined as "user-led" (Hutchison et al. 2007) or social movement organizations (Carroll and Ratner 2001) are incorporating politicized language into their work. In the United Kingdom, Shakespeare (2006, 165) observes a similar phenomenon among historically charitable organizations, leading him to argue controversially that "disability rights is not incompatible with charity." It is also possible that the frequency of phrases that resonate with disability movement histories could be a coincidental shift in language patterns. Regardless, the high proportion of organizations using concepts that are possibly linked with social movement histories raises important questions about the co-optation of Canadian disability movements by groups with drastically different histories and goals.

With the relational model, Kafer (2013) asks us to see "disability as a site of questions rather than firm definitions" (11). The case studies above pose three questions related to disability in practical settings: (1) Are service provider organizations taking up more space (perhaps in co-opted ways) on the advocacy landscape? (2) Can we interpret disability service development and provision as a form of social action rather than as opposed to advocacy/activist work? and (3) What does the blurring of medical/social distinctions among these groups mean for disability movements?

In terms of co-optation, there are certainly questions raised by the activities of the second and third case study examples that are not user led. The single-impairment group draws on independent living language and engages people with lived experiences when it is convenient, but as a larger organization, is involved in activities that deploy narratives of pity and situate disability as a predominately medical issue. As Kafer (2013) points out in her work around medical intervention, this advocacy can be useful *as long as* the approach to medicine remains in a broader politicized framework, which is lacking in this example. The broad inclusion in the organization's board does not privilege social or activist messaging, but tends to privilege parents and medical clinicians. This is similar to trends around interdisciplinarity in research contexts that merely end up reproducing the values of evidence-based health research rather than social justice or social science epistemologies (Albert, Paradis, and Kuper 2015; Mykhalovskiy et al. 2008). The service provider group for people with developmental disabilities has a lot of resources relative to other organizations, and takes up a lot of space in the advocacy realm. This group does not endorse social movement perspectives and engages in certain programming that actually counters messaging from deinstitutionalization and community living movements. This could be linked to the diminishing capacity of rights-based or social justice disability organizations that are struggling to survive, and have a decreased presence.

Second, the case studies raise the issue of seeing service development and delivery as a form of activism. As indicated by the developmental disability service organization's sheltered workshops, there are values embedded in the way services are designed and delivered. Conversely, the expansion of peer-support counselling promoted by the mad organization suggests that crafting services around specific values can disrupt representations and experiences of madness – although Voronka's (2016) work found that sometimes inclusion in mainstream organizations can discourage critique. The idea of designing disruptive services is present in other elements of the disability movement, for example independent living attendant services (Kelly 2016). DeSantis' (2010, 40) qualitative research on non-profit organizations and advocacy found across thirty-nine organizations that "daily service delivery work informs advocacy strategies." Beyond informing advocacy, at times organizations can see their services as a less traditional form of activism, in that the programming is a message in itself. This is clearly supported by the shift in the mental health group from advocacy to service provision. It is thus possible that shifting to service provision is not only and always a survival mechanism used by struggling organizations, but can represent an intentional and strategic politicization of health services called for by Kafer's relational model.

Finally, both the website analysis and all three case studies demonstrate a blurring of medical and social models of disability, or social and health services in a more practical sense. At times this blurring implies Kafer's relational model of disability, while at other times it represents confused messaging. The mad organization provides services within medical settings, including hospitals, and works in close collaboration with medical professionals. This most closely resonates with Kafer's model, which calls for a social view of both disability and the health sector, without relying on an outright rejection of the medical industry or interventions. The single-impairment group oscillates between social discourses and clinical medical work in a way that is not well incorporated, as the clinical medical work is disconnected from the social efforts. The large service provider organization for people with developmental disabilities does not draw on many medical definitions in their work, nor does it provide health services, but it does at times deploy conflicting understandings of disability. In this context, distinctions between medical and social approaches to health remain paradoxically useful as well as difficult to identify as the organizations seek to maintain unique roles within the sector.

Michael Prince (2016, 22) observes, "Disability activism as a social movement is an ontological multiplicity. Working in, through and around disability organizations are competing power/knowledge configurations." As the website analysis and case studies included in this chapter demonstrate, this observation can be extended to even within organizations themselves. While social movement frameworks can influence the vision and mandate of different groups, as with all social justice initiatives it is difficult to enact these frameworks consistently, especially in light of a constrained and shifting sociopolitical landscape for the non-profit sector. What becomes clear through reflecting on the insights of this study is that there is a cultural and practical pull towards medical understandings of disability and, in fact, these approaches are concretely rewarded in terms of funding, stability, and credibility with a broad audience. Politicizing approaches to health and health services may in fact be a strategic way to continue disability politics under the limitations of neoliberal governance models.

ACKNOWLEDGMENTS

This research was supported by the Social Sciences and Humanities Research Council of Canada, grant number 430-2014-00237. I am grateful to the key informants who shared their time and insights while participating in this study. I also wish to acknowledge the work of Abbie Sizer, Kate Grisim, and Banke Oketola – brilliant graduate students who supported many aspects of this study – and to thank Dr. Yuns Oh for ongoing research support.

REFERENCES

Albert, M., E. Paradis, and A. Kuper. 2015. "Interdisciplinary Promises versus Practices in Medicine: The Decoupled Experiences of Social Sciences and Humanities Scholars." *Social Science & Medicine* 126 (0): 17–25. https://doi.org/10.1016/j.socscimed.2014.12.004.

Baines, D. 2015. "Neoliberalism and the Convergence of Nonprofit Care Work in Canada." *Competition & Change* 19 (3): 194–209. https://doi.org/10.1177/1024529415580258.

Bell, C. 2006. "Introducing White Disability Studies: A Modest Proposal." In *The Disability Studies Reader*, edited by L.J. Davis, 275–82. New York: Routledge.

Blumberg, M. 2014. "List of Ontario Non-Profit Corporations Finally Released by Ontario Government to Blumberg Segal LLP." http://www.globalphilanthropy.ca/images/uploads/List_of_Ontario_Non-Profit_Corporations_finally_released_by_Mark_Blumberg.pdf.

Bridge, R., and N. Gilbert. 2005. "Helping Charities Speak Out: What Funders Can Do." *The Philanthropist* 20 (2): 153–7. https://thephilanthropist.ca/2005/07/helping-charities-speak-out-what-funders-can-do/.

Canada Revenue Agency. 2011. "Factors That Will Prevent an Organization from Being Registered as a Charity." http://www.cra-arc.gc.ca.

Carroll, W.K, and R.S. Ratner. 2001. "Sustaining Oppositional Cultures in 'Post-Socialist' Times: A Comparative Study of Three Social Movement Organizations." *Sociology* 35 (3): 605–29. https://doi.org/10.1177/S0038038501000311.

CBC News. 2014. "'Preventing Poverty' Not a Valid Goal for Tax Purposes, CRA Tells Oxfam Canada." http://www.cbc.ca/news/politics/preventing-poverty-not-a-valid-goal-for-tax-purposes-cra-tells-oxfam-canada-1.2717774.

Council of Canadians with Disabilities. 2012. "Tony Dolan's Speaking Notes for an October 2012 Presentation to Finance Committee." http://www.ccdonline.ca/en/socialpolicy/poverty/tony-dolan-finance-committee-october-2012.

DeSantis, G. 2010. "Voices from the Margins: Policy Advocacy and Marginalized Communities." *Canadian Journal of Nonprofit and Social Economy Research* 1 (1): 23–45. https://doi.org/10.22230/cjnser.2010v1n1a24.

Dewsbury, G., K. Clarke, D. Randall, M. Rouncefield, and I. Sommerville. 2004. "The Anti-Social Model of Disability." *Disability & Society* 19 (2): 145–58. https://doi.org/10.1080/0968759042000181776.

Erevelles, N. 2011. *Disability and Difference in Global Contexts: Enabling a Transformative Body Politic.* New York: Palgrave Macmillan.

Fraser, N. 1995. "From Redistribution to Recognition? Dilemmas of Justice in a 'Post-Socialist' Age." *New Left Review* 1 (212): 68–93. https://newleftreview.org/issues/I212/articles/nancy-fraser-from-redistribution-to-recognition-dilemmas-of-justice-in-a-post-socialist-age.

French, S. 1993. "Disability, Impairment or Something in Between?" In *Disabling Barriers – Enabling Environments,* edited by J. Swain, V. Finkelstein, S. French, and M. Oliver, 17–25. London: Sage/Open University Press.

Fritsch, K. 2015. "Gradations of Debility and Capacity: Biocapitalism and the Neoliberalization of Disability Relations." *Canadian Journal of Disability Studies* 4 (2): 12–48. https://doi.org/10.15353/cjds.v4i2.208.

Gabel, S., and S. Peters. 2004. "Presage of a Paradigm Shift? Beyond the Social Model of Disability toward Resistance Theories of Disability." *Disability & Society* 19 (6): 585–600. https://doi.org/10.1080/0968759042000252515.

Garland-Thomson, R. 2011. "Misfits: A Feminist Materialist Disability Concept." *Hypatia* 26 (3): 591–609. https://doi.org/10.1111/j.1527-2001.2011.01206.x.

Goodley, D., R. Lawthom, and K. Runswick-Cole. 2014. "Dis/ability and Austerity: Beyond Work and Slow Death." *Disability & Society* 29 (6): 980–4. https://doi.org/10.1080/09687599.2014.920125.

Grech, S. 2009. "Disability, Poverty and Development: Critical Reflections on the Majority World Debate." *Disability & Society* 24 (6): 771–84. https://doi.org/10.1080/09687590903160266.

Hall, M., and K.G. Banting. 2000. "The Nonprofit Sector in Canada: An Introduction." In *The Nonprofit Sector in Canada: Roles and Relationships,* edited by K.G. Banting, 1–28. Kingston: School of Policy Studies, Queen's University.

Human Resources and Skills Development Canada. 2009. "Summative Evaluation of the Social Development Partnerships Program." Ottawa: HRSDC.

Hutchison, P., S. Arai, A. Pedlar, J. Lord, and F. Yuen. 2007. "Role of Canadian User-Led Disability Organizations in the Non-Profit Sector." *Disability & Society* 22 (7): 701–16. https://doi.org/10.1080/09687590701659550.

Kafer, A. 2013. *Feminist, Queer, Crip.* Bloomington: Indiana University Press.

Kelly, C. 2016. *Disability Politics and Care: The Challenge of Direct Funding.* Vancouver: UBC Press.

Kelly, C. 2018. "A Future for Disability: Perceptions of Disabled Youth and Nonprofit Organizations." *Social Theory & Health* 16 (1): 44–59. https://doi.org/10.1057/s41285-017-0042-5.

Kelly, C. forthcoming. "Evolving Disability Scholarship and Activism in Canadian Contexts: Making Room for Intersectionality." In *Women's Health in Canada: Critical Perspectives on Theory and Policy,* 2nd ed., edited by M. Morrow, O. Hankivsky, and C. Varcoe. Toronto: University of Toronto Press.

Laforest, R. 2011. *Voluntary Sector Organizations and the State: Building New Relations.* Vancouver: UBC Press.

Levesque, M. 2012. "Assessing the Ability of Disability Organizations: An Interprovincial Comparative Perspective." *Canadian Journal of Nonprofit and Social Economy Research* 3 (2): 82–103. https://doi.org/10.22230/cjnser.2012v3n2a119.

McColl, M.A., and W. Boyce. 2003. "Disability Advocacy Organizations: A Descriptive Framework." *Disability & Rehabilitation* 25 (8): 380. https://doi.org/10.1080/0963828021000058521.

Mingus, M. 2011. "Changing the Framework: Disability Justice." *Leaving Evidence* (blog). 12 February. https://leavingevidence.wordpress.com/2011/02/12/changing-the-framework-disability-justice/.

Mykhalovskiy, E., P. Armstrong, H. Armstrong, I. Bourgeault, J. Choiniere, J. Lexchin, S. Peters, and J. White. 2008. "Qualitative Research and the Politics of Knowledge in an Age of Evidence: Developing a Research-Based Practice of Immanent Critique." *Social Science & Medicine* 67 (1): 195–203. https://doi.org/10.1016/j.socscimed.2008.03.002.

Neufeldt, A.H. 2003a. "Disability in Canada: An Historical Perspective." In *In Pursuit of Equal Participation: Canada and Disability at Home and Abroad*, edited by H. Enns and A.H. Neufeldt, 22–79. Concord, ON: Captus.

Neufeldt, A.H. 2003b. "Growth and Evolution of Disability Advocacy in Canada." In *Making Equality: History of Advocacy and Persons with Disabilities in Canada*, edited by D. Stienstra and A. Wight-Felske, 11–32. Concord, ON: Captus.

Oliver, M. 1983. *Social Work with Disabled People*. Basingstoke: Macmillan.

Oliver, M. 2004. "The Social Model in Action: If I Had a Hammer." In *Implementing the Social Model of Disability: Theory and Research*, edited by C. Barnes and G. Mercer, 18–31. Leeds: Disability Press.

Prince, M.J. 2016. "Reconsidering Knowledge and Power: Reflections on Disability Communities and Disability Studies in Canada." *Canadian Journal of Disability Studies* 5 (2): 1–31. https://doi.org/10.15353/cjds.v5i2.271.

Scott, K. 2003. "Funding Matters: The Impact of Canada's New Funding Regime on Nonprofit and Voluntary Organizations." Kanata, ON: Canadian Council on Social Development.

Shakespeare, T. 2006. *Disability Rights and Wrongs*. New York: Routledge.

Shakespeare, T., and N. Watson. 2002. "The Social Model of Disability: An Outdated Ideology?" *Research in Social Science and Disability* 2: 9–28. https://doi.org/10.1016/S1479-3547(01)80018-X.

Soldatic, K., and L. Fiske. 2009. "Bodies 'Locked Up': Intersections of Disability and Race in Australian Immigration." *Disability & Society* 24 (3): 289–301. https://doi.org/10.1080/09687590902789453.

Stienstra, D. 2003. "'Listen, Really Listen, to Us': Consultation, Disabled People and Governments in Canada." In *Making Equality: History of Advocacy and Persons with Disabilities in Canada*, edited by D. Stienstra and A. Wight-Felske, 33–47. Concord, ON: Captus.

Stienstra, D., and A. Wight-Felske. 2003. *Making Equality: History of Advocacy of Persons with Disabilities in Canada*. Concord, ON: Captus.

Swain, J., and S. French. 2000. “Towards an Affirmation Model of Disability.” *Disability & Society* 15 (4): 569–82. https://doi.org/10.1080/09687590050058189.

Thomas, C. 1999. *Female Forms: Experiencing and Understanding Disability.* Philadephia: Open University Press.

Voronka, J. 2016. “Researching the Politics of Inclusion.” *Vision Passion Action* (blog). 14 March. https://radssite.wordpress.com/2016/03/14/researching-the-politics-of-inclusion/.

Young, L., and J. Everitt. 2004. *Advocacy Groups.* Vancouver: UBC Press.

12 Medical Laboratories: For-Profit Delivery and the Disintegration of Public Health Care

ROSS SUTHERLAND

In a 2015 *Calgary Herald* opinion article David MacLean, vice-president of the Alberta Enterprise Group, a "business advocacy organization," argued that

> Albertans have proven time and again that private business – due in no small part to the motivation and discipline inspired by private profit – can perform most services more cheaply and effectively than government ... the field of medical laboratory services, with its fast-paced technical advancements, is incredibly complex and competitive. It needs private sector innovation more than any other. (MacLean 2015)

MacLean's assertion that medical laboratory services are a "poster child" for the neoliberal view that social goods, like health care, are best provided by for-profit companies is challenged by the history of for-profit laboratories in Canada.

False Positive: Private Profit in Canada's Medical Laboratories (Sutherland 2011, 126) examines the effects of fifty years of public funding of private laboratory services and argues that "for-profit [laboratory] provision costs more, negatively affects the public delivery of health care, decreases quality, provides unequal access and limits democracy."

This chapter builds on the work presented in *False Positive.* Alberta, British Columbia, and Ontario government reports and public documents are analysed and show that the assumption that competition is a relevant force for greater efficiency in private provision of laboratory services is questionable. Instead of generating competition as claimed, recent policy initiatives have suppressed competition and supported corporate consolidation and the virtual monopolization of the private laboratory market.

The documentation from governments and policy analysts recognizes the high cost of using for-profit providers and outlines attempts to address this problem. Research presented in this chapter shows that for-profit provision does not decrease costs or create more "effective" service delivery, as assumptions about competition would suggest. Rather, analysis shows that costs are more controlled and integration is more advanced in the monopolized markets. Further, I will argue that due to arrangements that benefit for-profit providers, such as fee-for-service payments, a tolerance for overutilization, and the creation of separate structures to support the private market, the cost of using for-profit companies is greater than that of providing these services in the public sector.

Case studies of the 2013 Edmonton Request for Proposals and of the nationalization of Medicine Hat's laboratory services provide additional data on the increased cost of for-profit provision and the fallacy of competition: data that are limited due to commercial trade secrets and state protection of significant corporate information.

Why Study For-Profit Medical Laboratories?

The fact that most essential medical services in Canada are paid for by a popular universal government insurance program shapes the struggle between private profit and the provision of accessible, publicly controlled, quality, cost-efficient health services. Accessing public insurance payments becomes an important method of private capital accumulation. The expansion of primary care conglomerates, corporate addiction and mental health treatment programs, expensive medications, high-tech interventions, and contracting for a wide variety of hospital services, from surgery and diagnostic imaging to security and housekeeping, bear witness to this process.

The longevity and breadth of private-sector involvement in publicly funded medical laboratory services provides an opportunity to examine how the funding and ownership of the delivery of an essential service affect the provision of health care.

Laboratory services are also important both as a main driver of technological advancement and as a key component of technical diagnosis in our biomedical health care system. One common estimate is that laboratory tests are involved in 80 per cent of medical decisions (Office of the Auditor General of Ontario 2007, 385). Medical labs employ over twenty thousand laboratory technologists (Canadian Institute for Health Information 2010, 13). For-profit corporations receive over 1.1 billion dollars a year in revenue from public sources, primarily in three provinces, Ontario, BC, and Alberta (Alberta Health Services 2015; Sullivan, Gordon, and Minto 2015; Lawson 2012). The exact value of public transfers to private labs is difficult to obtain due to significant payments hidden in individual hospital budgets, and payments from a variety of government departments besides health, including Indigenous health services, workers compensation programs, and the armed forces.

Nomenclature

Private medical laboratories became significant actors after the passage of the 1966 Medical Care Insurance Act, one of the legislative precursors to the Canada Health Act. Medical laboratories, both non-profit and for-profit, are primarily governed by provincial legislation within the national context of the Canada Health Act, international trade agreements, and federal funding transfers.

A common way to describe laboratory services is by the source of the specimen. The public hospital system processes specimens from patients staying in acute care hospitals. Specimens from patients living in the community, and primarily ordered by family doctors and nurse practitioners, are processed in the community system. Most often, in Canada, all patients in all sectors have their work done in a unified non-profit system, primarily using hospital laboratories. In areas where there are for-profit laboratories, the hospital system usually provides for inpatients and for-profit laboratories for some portion of the community patients. For-profit laboratories are also called private laboratories and community laboratories. The "community laboratory" label is most common in Ontario and hides the ownership and control of these services.

Market Realities: Competition Is Dead

Despite the emergence of de facto monopolies in the for-profit laboratory sector policy, discussions promoting privatization continue to rely on the concept of competition. In the neoliberal context Davies (2014, 27) calls competition a "flexible rhetorical project" that uses "appeals to 'the market' ... to defend monopolistic corporations." Developments in Canada's medical laboratory services support the argument that the rhetorical appeal to competition falsely describes current conditions and covers for both more privatization of the sector and increased monopoly delivery.

In 1968 when medicare was launched most laboratory services were provided in non-profit facilities. For-profit labs in all provinces were small in size and scope. Medicare provided the income, structure, and demand to fund the expansion of private medical laboratories, primarily owned by physicians, to serve community patients.

The rapid expansion of many small laboratories quickly raised government concerns about quality, conflict of interest, and rapidly escalating costs. In response to government pressures to control costs, improve quality, and maintain access, companies started to amalgamate and corporatize (Sutherland 2011). MDS, Canada's historical private powerhouse and the precursor of LifeLabs, formed in 1969. By 1975 it was the largest laboratory corporation, controlling 18.7 per cent of Ontario's commercial market.[1]

Competition among for-profit laboratories in Ontario was greatest in the mid-1970s, with 126 companies (Table 12.1). Eight were left in 2015, of which one company, LifeLabs (a subsidiary of Borealis, an investment holding company owned by the Ontario Municipal Employees Pension Fund) controlled 63 per cent of the private market. A distant second, with a 31 per cent market share, was Dynacare, a wholly owned subsidiary of LabCorp, the second largest American laboratory corporation.

There is some evidence, following a 2015 policy recommendation to cut fifty million dollars from payments to Ontario's private laboratories (Sullivan, Gordon, and Minto 2015), that the companies are dividing Ontario up into regional monopolies. The announced 2017 closure of LifeLab's processing laboratory in Ottawa (LifeLabs 2016b) would leave Dynacare with the main laboratory in the only district where it has significantly more specimen collection centres than LifeLabs.[2] LifeLabs has a virtual monopoly in most areas outside of the Greater Toronto Area and, mirroring its dominance in provincial payments, has twice as many specimen collection centres in Toronto as Dynacare.

All other provinces that use private laboratories have seen a similar shift to near monopoly provision. LifeLab's purchase of BC Biomedical in 2013 makes it the dominant private medical laboratory in British Columbia. DynaLIFE has a monopoly on community services in Edmonton and northern Alberta.

Competitive Delusions: State Policies Support Large Private Providers

The contrast between the language of competition and the reality of monopoly control of privatized laboratory services is accentuated by state policies that support the large providers. Recent policy proposals for long-term contracts with the remaining providers (Alberta Health Services 2013; Sullivan, Gordon, and Minto 2015) continue a long tradition of governments favouring larger companies at the expense of competition.

Two of the more notable examples of governments promoting concentration occurred in the middle to late nineties. In 1998 Ontario's Mike Harris government froze the market share of all for-profit laboratory companies (Donovan 1998), effectively guaranteeing the large corporations

Table 12.1. Consolidation of Ontario's for-profit (FP) laboratory industry

Year	# FP laboratory companies	# of FP labs	% government payments to top two companies
1975	126	253	26
1993	62	159	n/a
2005	11	49	63
2015	8	n/a	94

Sources: **1975**: From a confidential Ministry of Health study, "Monopoly Potential in Private Laboratories in Ontario," 28 September 1977. Accessed through Archives Ontario, RG 10-39, file: Legislation. Monopoly Studies. **1993**: Ontario Ministry of Health, "Laboratory Services Review Discussion Paper #2: System." **2005**: Information released in freedom of information award, Beamish, Brian, 2009, Order PO-2780, Appeal PA07-263: Ministry of Health and Long-Term Care; Toronto, Information and Privacy Commission of Ontario, Tribunal Services Department, 27 April. **2015**: From records released by the Ontario Ministry of Health and Long-Term Care after a freedom of information request in 2016.

long-term dominance. To add insult to injury, the government forced the smaller companies to pay compensation to the large firms for any market share increases the former had won between 1996 and 1998. Simultaneously, the government effectively shut down Hospital-In-Common Laboratories, a non-profit community laboratory (Watts 1997).

In 1995 Alberta's Ralph Klein government cut for-profit laboratory payments by 40 per cent (Fagg et al. 1999). Concurrent with this initiative the government cajoled laboratory providers to form two consortiums, one to provide all of the laboratory services in Calgary, the other in Edmonton, effectively ending local competition. The result, after numerous twists and turns, was one non-profit provider, Calgary Laboratory Services, providing all of Calgary's medical laboratory needs, and DynaLIFE, a partnership between Dynacare and LifeLabs, serving the community market in Edmonton and northern Alberta.

Smaller labs in Ontario, through the Coalition for Laboratory Reform, have put up a noisy fight for their continued existence. Their efforts did not go unnoticed, as the 2015 Expert Panel tasked with improving and modernizing the laboratory sector recommended subsidies to help small labs meet quality and performance objectives. The panel also identified, but did not act on, barriers to new market entrants (Sullivan, Gordon, and Minto 2015).

Regardless, the Expert Panel's major policy recommendation was to negotiate a seven- to ten-year contract with the current providers that included a fifty-million-dollar reduction in payment from current levels. Failing a successful contract settlement within six months, the panel recommended a competitive Request for Proposals (RFP) to determine an alternative private provider (Sullivan, Gordon, and Minto 2015, 6). Competition has shifted from being a process to maximize innovations and efficiencies to being a stick the government can use to gain compliance for its financial agenda. The active consideration of long-term contracts with one or two major providers indicates that competition is no longer a serious factor in the provision of this public service.

The Edmonton Request for Proposals

It could be argued that the RFP process, open to all providers, even if they are primarily a few large multinational companies, satisfies the requirements of competition. This was the contention of Alberta's conservative government in 2013 when it issued an RFP for a fifteen- to twenty-five-year contract to provide expanded privatized laboratory services in Edmonton (Alberta Health Services 2013).

An enquiry into the Edmonton RFP found the process to be plagued by conflict of interest, lack of transparency, poor record keeping, undue influence from second-hand information, and corporate confidentiality leading to "doubts about the validity of the selection of the preferred proponent" (Stiver, Sciur, and Gazdic 2015, 57). The failed RFP process illustrates some of the difficulties of maintaining a transparent and fair competitive process. Community activists (Kushner, Baranek, and Dewar 2008), academics (Armstrong 2001; Aronson and Neysmith 2001), and government reviews (Caplan 2005) also identified problems with Ontario's RFP process for home care delivery as well as difficulties in transferring contracts to new companies. The problems for companies entering the market and the instability in service delivery during transition will be compounded by long-term contracts in the more capital-intensive and technologically sophisticated laboratory system, which is integrally connected to most core health care operations.

In a rapidly changing diagnostic services sector with regular announcements of new tests and procedures, and a quickly evolving health care legislative environment, the more likely outcome of long-term contracts is not competition and innovation, but complex and expensive renegotiations with a sole-source provider and significant barriers to entry for all but a very few companies at the end of the contract.

The 2015 election of the New Democratic Party, a social democratic government more sympathetic to public health care, plus significant public opposition to privatizing laboratory services, an effective public-sector alternative in the Calgary Laboratory Services, and a flawed RFP process contributed to the Edmonton RFP's cancellation. DynaLIFE's contract was extended until 2022, when its operations will be purchased by the government for fifty million dollars and returned to the public sector.[3]

The difficulties with the RFP process, the reliance on a small number of transnational corporations, and the preference for long-term contracts create a significant dissonance between the rhetoric of competition and the reality of using RFPs. Evidence indicates that the resulting monopoly would not benefit the system in terms of cost or overall system efficiency.

For-Profit Delivery Cost Concerns

Cost savings and efficiency continue to be central arguments in favour of private delivery at the same time that the main cause of financial concern is the for-profit providers. A 2015 review in Ontario, echoing concerns in BC, "focused mainly on findings and recommendations relating to funding, funding supports and other issues pertinent to the community [for-profit] laboratory sector" (Sullivan, Gordon, and Minto 2015, 6). A secondary focus in both provinces was greater hospital laboratory integration.

Fee-for-service payments and inappropriate utilization, two factors closely linked to increased costs, continue to be highlighted problems. Broader systemic costs associated with the for-profit laboratory sector, including overcapacity, increased monitoring and bureaucracy, decreased quality, for-profit laboratories' preference for the easier work, and duplication and lack of integration tied to maintaining a parallel system for private delivery (Sutherland 2011), receive scant if any attention.

Fee-For-Service

Fee-for-service (FFS), a payment method based on the number of units of work paid at a fixed cost for each unit, is the main component of private-sector lab payments in BC, Ontario, and Alberta. No province uses a strict FFS system. Most involve contracts or caps that are based on FFS measurement; nonetheless, they are all grounded in the assumption that the more units of work done, the higher the payment. Yet the cost of individual tests, central to FFS pricing, is at best very hard to calculate. "What is a correct fee?" has for decades been a concern in many studies and auditors' reports (Bayne 2003; British Columbia 1993; Jones 2014; Kilshaw et al. 1992; Office of the Auditor General of Ontario 2007; Ontario Council of Health 1982; Ontario Ministry of Health 1994).

In 1973, the Ontario government instituted the LMS (labour, materials, supervision) method to determine the cost of individual laboratory tests. By 1976, a study on the high cost of commercial laboratory services found that "no reliable cost data is available on which to determine a new fee schedule" (Ontario Ministry of Health 1976, 33) and recommended "consultants be commissioned immediately to conduct a cost accounting study to identify the complete unit cost of laboratory services" (6).

This recommendation was echoed thirty-six years later in BC's Laboratory Reform Committee's (2013, 9) report: "Recommendation 20: implement and maintain a regular review for the Laboratory Fee Schedule, to ensure fees reflect current best practice, technology and costs" (Laboratory 2013, 9).

Although no provinces have enacted new payment policies for community laboratories, Ontario's Expert Panel identified that the payment caps on top of FFS have not limited costs and recommended long-term performance-based contracts. BC's minster of health, Tom Lake, envisioned in 2014 "a potential future where we don't have fee for service for diagnostic testing."[4] BC's SECOR consultant's report opened the door to reconsider FFS with a recommendation that hospitals no longer have access to FFS funding so they can focus on "efficiencies and optimal resource deployment" (Lawson 2012, 8), the implication being that FFS promotes inefficiency and less than optimal resource deployment. SECOR also recommend for-profit pilot projects to experiment with "alternative, non-volume based, payment mechanisms" (9). Alberta's Health Minister is also "not convinced that privatization provides the best level of care at the best price" (Bennet 2016).

The 2015 Ontario recommendation to cut for-profit laboratory payments by fifty million dollars (Sullivan, Gordon, and Minto 2015) and a 2013 BC proposal to cut twenty-five million dollars (Laboratory Reform Committee 2013) continue a history of unilateral government cuts to for-profit labs ranging from 11 per cent in 1993 in Ontario to 40 per cent in 1995 in Alberta. While detail is lacking to justify any of these figures, two reasons given to justify the 2015 reductions were the comparatively lower costs of hospital services and the "significant profit margins" and "generous" FFS structure applicable to the for-profit laboratories (Sullivan, Gordon, and Minto 2015, 15).

There is also evidence that FFS discourages the introduction of the most up-to-date technology. Providers tend to stick with the old tests as their company's costs, but not payments, fall, and hesitate to introduce new tests or methods that may not be costed appropriately (Sutherland 2011, 27).

Despite the breadth and longevity of concern about FFS, it has proven remarkably resilient as the foundation of private-sector payment. The section on integration below examines the importance of maintaining this payment formula in providing a market for for-profit companies.

Inappropriate Utilization

One of the consensus concerns of BC stakeholders in consultations on reforming laboratory services was "improving ordering practices for laboratory tests" (Lawson 2012, 11). Similar to test costing, inappropriate utilization of laboratory services – ordering either the wrong test or unnecessary tests – has been a primary concern in the laboratory sector for fifty years.

In 1977, Ontario made the first attempt to limit unnecessary community tests by changing the form doctors use to order tests.[5] Both Ontario's 2015 Expert Panel and BC's 2013 Laboratory Review Committee recommended similar proposals to affect test ordering (Laboratory Reform Committee 2013; Sullivan, Gordon, and Minto 2015). The lack of appropriate testing in the community sector is compounded by the fact that laboratory specialists are usually in physically separated locations from the practitioners who order tests, and commonly, in provinces with for-profit laboratories, in different cities. Proximity of specialists to those doing the test ordering has been cited as a key factor in quality and appropriate test utilization (Plebani 1999).

What is surprising is that some "experts" still adhere to the faulty argument that if there is the right pricing for each test and better ordering procedures, the best value will be achieved. This paradox is best explained as a reflection of neoliberal ideology that sees the problem as one of individuals, in this case doctors' ordering behaviours, rather than as a systemic problem with FFS and the use of for-profit providers.

The Medicine Hat Diagnostic Laboratories Business Case

The finding that for-profit providers cost the health care system a minimum of 25 per cent more (Sutherland 2011) is bolstered by the Alberta government's "business case" for closing Medicine Hat Diagnostic Laboratories (MHDL) and shifting that work to the Medicine Hat public hospital (Ward, Sieben, and Hetchler 2013). A public business case justifying the decision to nationalize, or "repatriate" in the government's language, the work done by MHDL was probably necessary due to this counter-intuitive action by a conservative government. While the business case does not provide information on the company's internal operations or profit rate, it stands out in its level of detail, compared to the lack of information on other components of Alberta's laboratory system.

MHDL was a small, locally owned, for-profit laboratory that provided services to 60 per cent of Medicine Hat's community patients as well as some of the collection and courier services for the Medicine Hat hospital. MHDL's costs had increased by 77 per cent from 2004/5 to 2009/10, and were 20 to 40 per cent above the benchmark data set by "comparing test costs with Calgary Laboratory Services, DynaLIFE, and other A[lberta] H[ealth] S[ervices] services of a similar size" (Ward, Sieben, and Hetchler 2013, 4). The actual comparative data for these benchmarks were not provided. After two years of negotiating no agreement was reached on a new contract, and it was decided that repatriating MHDL's work could "allow for greater economies of scale resulting in reduced costs" (4). The benefits of repatriation included streamlining laboratory information systems, reducing duplication of testing and data entry, and streamlining quality assurance, safety, and training programs.

The approved repatriation plan authorized a 2.2-million-dollar renovation of Medicine Hat Regional Hospital so it could absorb MHDL's workload. The estimated savings are 6.5 million dollars over five years with payback in 1.35 years (Ward, Johnson, and Rawlake 2015).

While the small, but clear, example in Medicine Hat, coupled with continued focus on FFS and overutilization, are compelling explanations of the extra costs of using for-profit providers, they miss the larger systemic costs of maintaining two laboratory systems. This problem is recognized by the focus in all provinces on greater integration of health services.

For-Profit Delivery and Integration Conflicts

Monopoly consolidation of for-profit providers has achieved a partial integration of laboratory services. Each company uses one information system; has standard protocols, quality controls, labour management practices, and testing procedures; and works for efficiencies in delivery, as any large chain would.

The public sector has also been working at greater integration of inpatient services. In 1968, Ontario's Hospital-In-Common Laboratories was formed to share expertise and equipment between hospitals and evolved to use underutilized hospital laboratories to process community specimens at a cost 25 to 29 per cent cheaper than the private community laboratories (Sutherland 2011, 43).

Hospitals continue to develop ways of integrating their inpatient services, from the more informal Kingston General Hospital Outreach Program, which provides services on a contract basis to smaller area hospitals, to the more formal integration of all hospital laboratories in the Eastern Ontario Regional Laboratory Association. In 2008, BC undertook to integrate the Lower Mainland Health Authority's laboratories to control costs (Accenture 2010), and is starting to restructure the Interior Health Authority's labs (National Union of Public and General

Employees 2015). Alberta's province-wide health authority is aimed at greater integration.

Despite these efforts, the lack of integration between community and inpatient laboratory services creates the larger problem. For-profit laboratories exist in a separate market. Ontario has gone the furthest in establishing two distinct silos, drawing a firm line between the two systems in 2005 with a prohibition on hospitals processing community laboratory specimens. DynaLIFE also has a protected market in Edmonton. BC has historically had the most fluid boundaries, with both hospitals and the private sector able to process community work, but the core community work is paid on an FFS basis and has a different governance structure than the Health Authority–based hospital budgets.

A separate market for the private sector has inherent inefficiencies. Inpatient and community workflow patterns create overcapacity in both systems. For example, hospital laboratories need to be large enough to meet the high early morning testing volume and tend to sit largely idle at night. With two systems, many specimens are transported long distances rather than going to the closest lab, creating cost and quality concerns. For-profit laboratories prefer to service more densely populated areas, leaving the costlier work in rural and northern communities to the public sector.

Each system has different organizational boundaries. Corporations are usually organized provincially, if not internationally, and resist regional integration (Sutherland 2011). Non-profit laboratories are under some form of regional health authority. Laboratories under different ownership have different payment authorities and are usually governed under different pieces of legislation. Ontario has identified the myriad of governmental organizations involved in laboratory services as an impediment to sustainability, quality, and cost control (Sullivan, Gordon, and Minto 2015). The business case for the closure of MHDL gives some concrete examples of the potential savings from greater integration.

BC has taken a significant step that could promote integration between the public and private systems with the passage of the Laboratory Services Act (LSA) in 2015. The LSA brings all hospital and community laboratories, essentially LifeLabs, under one arm's-length non-profit administrative organization, the BC Clinical and Support Services Society, controlled by the minister of health. In 2016 the Society took over payments for all laboratory services but has made no significant changes to funding or organization since it is still in a "consultation" phase (British Columbia Ministry of Health 2015).

Despite Ontario's rhetoric supporting integration, if the recommendations of the 2015 Expert Panel are followed, the market will be reshaped to be more profitable for the private sector. Ontario's 2005 closing of all hospitals to community laboratory work meant the for-profits had to establish a costlier collection network through northern Ontario and into many small towns. One recommendation from the Expert Panel report was that in smaller communities the province relax the rule prohibiting hospitals from processing community work. This policy change, if enacted, will benefit smaller hospitals. It will increase their volumes, allowing them to maintain more complete laboratories, provide better access for rural patients, and ensure greater integration between hospital services and community physicians. It will also make it possible for the for-profits to withdraw from providing costly services in remote areas. To provide more profitable work for the private sector, the Expert Panel raised the possibility of shifting some routine work from public health labs to the for-profit laboratories (Sullivan, Gordon, and Minto 2015).

Will greater administrative integration, as in BC and Alberta, lead to more privatized laboratories, including hospitals, as was intended with the 2013 RFP in Edmonton? Terry Lake, the BC health minister, in response to questions from Judy Darcy, NDP health critic, said the LSA left open the possibility that it could be an "entire public system ... or ... an entire private system."[6] The LSA also allows the government to move services back and forth between public and for-profit providers without having to come back to the legislature.

Another possibility is that with greater provincial integration and less reliance on FFS there will be a gradual shift into the non-profit sector. This is what happened in Calgary in 2005, in Medicine Hat in 2017, and is intended for Edmonton in 2022.

The shift from for-profit to non-profit provision is not an example unique to Alberta. Saskatchewan transferred all the work provided by for-profit laboratories into the hospital system in 1995. The 2016 announcement of the nationalization of Edmonton's services and Saskatchewan's actions were both taken by social democratic governments under financial pressure and with strong public movements in support of non-profit health services. But both the Medicine Hat and Calgary initiatives were taken by conservative governments. Governments that believed in the benefits of private profit in public services were able to make these decisions on the basis of the existence of a single public payer for essential laboratory services, as well as the economic and organizational instability caused by private provision and the benefits of greater integration.

These examples of turning for-profit provision back to the public sector illustrate the feasibility of that option and may partially explain the trend to longer contracts with private companies.

Transfers of laboratory work from the private sector to non-profit hospital labs also took place separately from direct government action.

In the 1990s, two attempts at public-private partnerships in Ontario, one between the Toronto Hospital and MDS and the other between Sunnybrook Hospital and Dynacare, eventually had the non-profit component buy out the for-profit providers, or the private providers withdraw, a process similar to that in the evolution of Calgary's laboratory services (Sutherland 2011). Also, an RFP issued by the Ontario government in 1999 to have all laboratory work within defined geographic regions provided by consortiums that included for-profit providers failed when no proposals met the mandatory requirements (Page and Kornovski 2000, 29).

A reasonable conjecture is that the private sector is not interested, without significant profit assurances, in providing laboratory services. Without long-term contracts, FFS, and some form of shared future risk, the profit margins are just not sufficient for a viable private-sector operation. All of these benefits were present in the Edmonton RFP where the government included a variety of mechanisms to change the value of the contract as well as paying with a modified FFS (Alberta Health Services 2013).

A Public Blindness – Neoliberal Hegemony

Regardless of the extra costs and lack of competition, BC and Ontario, and Alberta before the election of Rachel Notley's NDP government, had not recommended an end to for-profit laboratory services. Government documents indicate that these decisions were bolstered by the authority of private consultants that recognized but dismissed viable non-profit alternatives, reflecting a neoliberal preference for "expert" and elite decision making over democratic and value-based discussions (Davies 2014, 188; Harvey 2005, 66). The reason given in the 2013 RFP for seeking a "collaborative business relationship" for Edmonton's laboratory services was that it "could offer capabilities that we [AHS] could not replicate internally" (Alberta Health Services 2013, 8). Yet three hundred kilometres down the road, Calgary Laboratory Services (CLS), a wholly owned subsidiary of the AHS, provides a full-service non-profit laboratory system that integrates all inpatient and community laboratory work within a region larger than that proposed in the Edmonton RFP.

Robert Michel (2011), editor of the *Dark Daily*, a leading laboratory industry news service, commended the CLS for its "focused effort to use a single consolidated testing organization as a way to sustain a high quality of laboratory testing at a competitive price." Reinforcing Michel's enthusiasm, a 2015 article found that CLS was a leader in the integration of teaching and clinical laboratory services "while providing efficient, economical and excellent clinical service" (Wright 2015, 10). It is likely that

CLS's recognized capability was ignored in the 2013 document because the CLS was a viable non-profit alternative, though no official reasons were given for this omission.

In BC, the SECOR consultants highlighted as options for stakeholder consultations only jurisdictions with either a mix of public and for-profit providers or solely private provision for all services, including inpatients (Lawson 2012). SECOR's sins of omission might be explained by the practicality that they were presenting only options acceptable to the BC government, which poses the question: Are they experts in recommending laboratory services that maximize the goals of accessibility, quality, and cost control, or experts in translating the government's desires into "expert" opinion? No reasons were given for discounting the non-profit alternatives that they had outlined in the background documents prior to their stakeholder consultations.

It is a reasonable assumption that to increase the likelihood that the outcome would be in line with supporting private profit accumulation, SECOR's stakeholder consultations did not include any community organizations, (such as the laboratory technologists and health care workers' unions or the BC Health Coalition) that might have had a significantly different perspective on the provision of health services.

Ontario's 2015 Expert Panel reaches the same end point as the SECOR report by stating that "the challenge ahead lies not in a complete redesign of the community laboratory system, but in a reorganization of the system to more effectively manage competition, to derive the efficiency benefits of a private sector delivery partnership" (Sullivan, Gordon, and Minto 2015, 6). Ignoring the reality that competition is, at best, minimal, the report's starting assumption is that the benefits from for-profit provision can be teased out by better government management rather than simply managing an integrated non-profit system, as is done in many parts of Canada.

For-Profit Corporate Privilege and Democracy

For-profit companies have actively used their power to influence laboratory policy in their favour and undermine public health care in Ontario (Sutherland 2011). This process is often as simple as their participation as privileged stakeholders. Ontario's Expert Panel vetted their final draft recommendations with a panel of private-sector CEOs before issuing their report (Sullivan, Gordon, and Minto 2015, 12). LifeLab's recent hiring of Chris Carson, once chief of staff to Ontario's minister of health and long-term care, as vice-president in charge of "establishing renewed relationship with government" continues a long tradition of exchanging personnel between health ministries and private companies (LifeLabs

2016a). For-profit laboratories have also been involved in drafting legislation, undermining government non-profit initiatives, and negotiating for the closure of non-profit competitors in pursuit of their own private interests (Sutherland 2011).

The lobbying efforts of for-profit labs are primarily funded by profits made from public payments and, in Ontario, the industry lobby group has been receiving an operating subsidy of $900,000 dollars a year from the government (Sullivan, Gordon, and Minto 2015, 16). Community groups advocating for expanded public services do not receive the same support.

Restrictions on informed public debate also increase with private-sector involvement. All provinces have legislation that provides some level of privacy protection for confidential business information, making it hard to comment on profit rates, investment decisions, staffing allocations, facility closings, and the full impact of private delivery. Many examples in this chapter, like the business case of MHDL, the Edmonton RFP, and the decision to nationalize DynaLIFE, are limited by the lack of public information.

The existence of private corporations in public health care privileges their influence on public policy to support their private profit while simultaneously limiting public debate and undermining public health care. If companies seeking private profit were not present, consideration of how to organize health care could focus on the public interest benefits and have the flexibility to adapt to changing medical technologies and meet local concerns without having to buy out complex contracts or structure markets to protect private profit.

Conclusion

The use of for-profit providers has created fifty years of instability in Canada's laboratory finances and policy. Neoliberal arguments promoting for-profit delivery rely upon the benefits of competition despite the evidence that strong privatized medical laboratory services tend towards monopolization. Fee-for-service funding, overutilization, and the overarching systemic costs inherent in providing a parallel for-profit market are consistent problems adding to the extra costs of private provision and public-sector disintegration.

The history of for-profit medical laboratory provision provides evidence that private companies are interested in providing services only if they are given conditions that grant them an assured profit, usually guaranteed in a defined market with FFS payment and some form of public sharing, or extraordinary compensation, for the riskier aspects of service delivery.

The competitive delusions and public blindness that accompany laboratory policy in Alberta, BC, and Ontario have harmed open democratic debate and illustrate the pervasive acceptance of neoliberalism: in this case accepting as common sense that profit-driven services will provide the best value for money in health care.

NOTES

1 From a confidential Ministry of Health study, "Monopoly Potential in Private Laboratories in Ontario," 28 September 1977. Accessed through Archives Ontario, RG 10-39, file: Legislation. Monopoly Studies.

2 Data on the distribution of SSCs in Ontario was taken from the Ontario Association of Medical Laboratories website, http://oaml.com/find-a-location/, accessed July 2016.

3 Email from Carolyn Ziegler, assistant director, Media Relations, Alberta Health, 14 November 2016.

4 Legislature of BC, *Hansard*, 31 March 2014, vol. 9, no. 5, 2592.

5 "Cost Containment Project." Memorandum to W.E. Graham, acting director, Inspection Branch, Ontario Ministry of Health, from Paul J. Plant, chief, Laboratory and Specimen Collection Centre Inspection Service, 24 July 1978.

6 Legislature of BC, *Hansard*, 31 March 2014, vol. 9 no. 5, 2598.

REFERENCES

Accenture. 2010. *Lower Mainland Consolidation Project: Due Diligence Assessment.* 26 July. Victoria: BC Ministry of Health.

Alberta Health Services. 2013. "Alberta Health Services Request for Proposals for Laboratory Services: Request for Proposals no. AHS2013-1962." 11 December. Edmonton: Alberta Health Services.

Alberta Health Services. 2015. "AHS, DynaLIFE Extend Laboratory Services Contract: One Year Extension Means Continuity of Patient Care for Albertans." Media release, 14 October, Edmonton.

Armstrong, H. 2001. "Social Cohesion and the Privatization of Health Care." *Canadian Journal of Law and Society* 16 (2): 65–81. https://doi.org/10.1017/S0829320100006797.

Aronson, J., and S.M. Neysmith. 2001. "Manufacturing Social Exclusion in the Home Care Market." *Canadian Public Policy* 27 (2): 150–65. https://doi.org/10.2307/3552194.

Bayne, L. 2003. *BC Laboratory Services Review.* Victoria: BC Ministry of Health.

Bennet, D. 2016. "Alberta to Revamp Medical Lab Testing; Sets Higher Bar for Private Labs." *Winnipeg Free Press.* 3 May. https://www.winnipegfreepress.com/arts-and-life/life/health/alberta-to-revamp-medical-lab-testing-raises-bar-for-private-labs-378015091.html.

British Columbia Ministry of Health. 1993. *Review of Diagnostic Services: A Report to the Minister of Health Province of British Columbia.* Victoria: BC Ministry of Health.

British Columbia Ministry of Health. 2015. "Laboratory Services Act Implementation Update." Program newsletter 1 (1), 1 October. https://www2.gov.bc.ca/assets/gov/health/practitioner-pro/laboratory-services/lsa_implementation_update_vol1_issue1_1oct2015.pdf.

Canadian Institute for Health Information. 2010. "Medical Laboratory Technologists in Canada, 2010." https://secure.cihi.ca/free_products/MLT_2010_Report_EN_web.pdf.

Caplan, E. 2005. *Realizing the Potential of Home Care: Competing for Excellence by Rewarding Results.* Toronto: CCAC Procurement Review. https://www.hhr-rhs.ca/index.php?option=com_mtree&task=viewlink&link_id=5077&Itemid=64&lang=en.

Davies, W. 2014. *The Limits of Neoliberalism: Authority, Sovereignty and the Logic of Competition.* London: Sage.

Donovan, K. 1998. "Medical Labs Argue against Payment Limits." *Toronto Star,* 26 November.

Fagg, K.L., P. Gordon, B. Reib, J.T. McGann, T.E. Higa, D.W. Kinniburgh, and G.S. Cembrowski. 1999. "Laboratory Restructuring in Metropolitan Edmonton: A Model for Laboratory Reorganization in Canada." *Clinica Chimica Acta* 290 (1): 73–91. https://doi.org/10.1016/S0009-8981(99)00178-3.

Harvey, D. 2005. *A Brief History of Neoliberalism.* Oxford: Oxford University Press.

Jones, R. 2014. *Oversight of Physician Services.* Victoria: Office of the Auditor General of BC.

Kilshaw, M.F., 1992. *Review of Diagnostic Laboratory Services: A Report to the Minister of Health, Province of Saskatchewan.* Regina: Ministry of Health.

Kushner, C., P. Baranek, and M. Dewar. 2008. *Home Care: Change We Need, Report on the Ontario Health Coalition's Home Care Hearing.* Toronto: Ontario Health Coalition.

Laboratory Reform Committee (BC). 2013. *Laboratory Services Plan.* Victoria: BC Ministry of Health.

Lawson, J. 2012. *Options for Laboratory Transformation.* Vancouver: SECOR Consulting. https://www.health.gov.bc.ca/library/publications/year/2012/options-for-laboratory-transformation.pdf.

LifeLabs. 2016a. "Chris Carson to Join LifeLabs as Vice-President, Partner Relations and Transformation." Media release, 7 January, Toronto.

LifeLabs. 2016b. "Operation Adjustments in Ontario: Questions and Answers." Media release, 23 February, Toronto.

MacLean, D. 2015. "Cancellation of Lab Contract a Warning to Business Community." *Calgary Herald,* 21 August. https://calgaryherald.com/opinion/columnists/maclean-cancellation-of-lab-contract-a warning-to-business-community.

Michel, R. 2011. "Calgary Laboratory Services Represents One Model of Regional Consolidation of Clinical Laboratories." *Dark Daily.* https://www.darkdaily.com/calgary-laboratory-services-represents-one-model-of-regional-consolidation-of-clinical-laboratories-91611/.

National Union of Public and General Employees. 2015. "BC Interior Health Authority Announces Plans to Restructure Lab Services." Media release, 24 July, Vancouver.

Office of the Auditor General of Ontario. 2007. *2007 Annual Report.* Toronto: Queen's Printer.

Ontario Council of Health. 1982. *Report of the Task Force on Laboratory Services.* Toronto: Ontario Ministry of Health.

Ontario Ministry of Health. 1976. *Report of the Laboratory Study Committee.* Archives of Ontario, RG 10–39.

Ontario Ministry of Health. 1994. *Laboratory Services Review.* Toronto: Ontario Ministry of Health.

Page, J.S., and B. Kornovski. 2000. "Provincial Group on Laboratory Reform." Toronto: Ontario Ministry of Health.

Plebani, M. 1999. "The Clinical Importance of Laboratory Reasoning." *Clinica Chimica Acta* 280 (1–2): 35–45. https://doi.org/10.1016/S0009-8981(98)00196-X.

Stiver, L.J., G.D. Sciur, and K. Gazdic. 2015. *Alberta Health Services Vendor Bid Appeal Panel: In the Matter of An Appeal by DynaLIFEdx, Dated November 6, 2014, Regarding Laboratory Services for Alberta Health Services.* Edmonton: Alberta Health Services.

Sullivan, T., P. Gordon, and S. Minto. 2015. *Laboratory Expert Panel: Final.* Toronto: Laboratory Expert Panel Review. http://www.health.gov.on.ca/en/common/ministry/publications/reports/lab_services/labservices.pdf.

Sutherland, R. 2011. *False Positive: Private Profit in Canada's Medical Laboratories.* Halifax: Fernwood.

Ward, D., L. Johnson, and S. Rawlake. 2015. *South Zone Laboratory Service Model: Business Case – Addendum.* Edmonton: Alberta Health Services.

Ward, D., B. Sieben, and C. Hetchler. 2013. *South Zone Laboratory Service Model: Business Case.* Edmonton: Alberta Health Services.

Watts, M. 1997. "Laboratory Restructuring in Ontario." *Hospital News,* February.

Wright, J.R. 2015. "Calgary Laboratory Services: A Unique Canadian Model for an Academic Department of Pathology and Laboratory Medicine Succeeding in the Face of Provincial Integration of Public, Private and Academic Laboratories." *Academic Pathology* 2 (4): 1–11. https://doi.org/10.1177/2374289515619944.

13 Nail Salons, Toxics, and Health: Organizing for a Better Work Environment

ANNE ROCHON FORD

Discount nail salons are a rapidly growing feature of most urban centres in Canada. Their popularity is expanding as women of all ages discover that "a little pampering" can cost them less than an evening for two at the cinema. "Mani-pedi parties" are now commonplace in salons with girls as young as five or six; girls and women of all ages frequent nail salons on a regular basis for manicures, pedicures, and application of acrylic nails, often with a brief foot massage thrown in.

But there's a nasty side to all of this beauty enhancement, and it is felt far more by the women who spend their days working in the salons than by the many who frequent them as customers. Some of the chemicals that make up the stock and trade of the work of nail salon employees are endocrine disruptors and others are carcinogenic. The nail technicians[1] who work in discount salons are often new immigrants vulnerable to exploitation by salon owners, both while training and once employed.

This chapter is based on the outcome of cumulative work of researchers at the National Network on Environments and Women's Health (NNEWH) at York University and the Parkdale Queen West Community Health Centre (PQWCHC), a primary care organization largely servicing vulnerable populations in downtown Toronto. NNEWH's ongoing work on the social and policy dimensions of chemical exposures and women's health dovetailed in 2014 with PQWCHC's front-line health promotion initiative with women working in discount nail salons in the immediate geographic vicinity.

This population of women had been presenting with growing frequency at the PQWCHC with a range of health problems that had been identified in the literature as possibly linked to chemical exposures. The centre responded by conducting focus groups with local nail technicians to determine what their needs were and whether they might benefit from in-salon prevention workshops. NNEWH brought its expertise in research to develop a review of the health literature on nail salon workers and to add their experience in developing a plan for longer-term policy-based solutions to the health problems faced by this population.

Based on the focus group feedback and a review of the literature, programs (workshops) were designed and are being carried out in nail salons by nail technicians (trained by project staff) to help workers protect themselves as best as possible, in the absence of better legislation and Occupational Health and Safety measures.

An additional partner in this work has been the Centre for Research Expertise in Occupational Disease (CREOD), based at the University of Toronto. A team there has been involved in research in skin health of nail salon workers and developed the curriculum for the nail salon peer training sessions. As we go to print, they are completing research involving the measurement of select chemicals in a sampling of nail salons in Toronto, the first known research of its type in Canada.

From the inception of this partnership the goal has been to study both the larger systemic issues that are exacerbating health problems in this precarious line of work and to provide immediate shorter-term solutions to health issues through prevention-focused workshops in salons, run by peers who know the business and speak the languages of the majority of workers. The project has had evaluation components since its inception to determine if the workshops are meeting a need; results thus far have been positive.

With these three key partners as the foundational agencies, the Healthy Nail Salon Network (Toronto) was established in 2014. The network brings together, on a regular basis, nail technicians and partners from a range of related front-line agencies and programs covering women's health, occupational health, settlement services, multicultural health and legal clinics, workers' advocacy, and related disease-specific organizations. More recently (2019) the Nail Technicians' Network was formed in Toronto to provide opportunities for nail technicians to unite around common issues.

Research on the health of nail salon workers is relatively thin, and Canadian research even more so. A growing body of international work looks at the impact of chemicals commonly found in nail salon products on animal health, with a smaller component looking at human health. A research area of particular concern is endocrine-disrupting (or hormone-disrupting) chemicals that mimic or block the animal or human endocrine system, which governs fertility, behaviour, development, intelligence, metabolism, longevity, and more. By "tricking" or mimicking the normal processes of different species, these substances can cause damage to glands within the endocrine system (reproductive, including ovaries and testes, pituitary, thyroid, adrenal, etc.), leading to higher risks of cancer, diabetes, birth defects, infertility, obesity, ADHD, early puberty, and a range of other health problems (Diamanti-Kandarakis et al. 2009). Some chemicals found in nail salon products are known endocrine disruptors.

As more becomes known about human health impacts, interest in research on the health of nail salon workers is increasing. However, studying this area of occupational health and safety in a more comprehensive way is complicated given the involvement of all three levels of government in regulating the sector: the chemicals found in most of the products come under the legislation of the federal government; the occupational health and safety and the employment standards in salons are overseen by the province; and the licensing of salons as well as public health oversight (to protect the public) occurs at the municipal level.

The study of this area would be easier if all salons were licensed and required to report information to a central data-gathering source. Many are not and many do not. We do not know, for example, how many businesses there are in any given municipality or province, whether they are nail operations within larger businesses such as hair salons or spas, how many employees they have, whether they are owner operated, or what is the demographic make-up of their workforce. All of this makes research in this area challenging.

Given these complex and constricting parameters, how can we begin to make sense of the best way to make these environments healthier places to work? Which level of legislation should be the focus for the best or most expedient results? What is the best way to navigate the layers of employment standards infractions without alienating salon owners or putting employees at (further) risk? How do we convince salon owners that better ventilation – perhaps initially costly to install – is in everyone's best interest? How do we advise nail technicians on health prevention measures when there is little scientific literature on product toxicity? Finally, how can we turn around an industry (cosmetics manufacturing) that has benefited for so long from loose regulation around chemicals management, and with considerable product manufacturing taking place outside of Canada?

There are no quick or easy answers to any of these challenges, but there are some good models from which we can borrow and adapt. Advocates in other jurisdictions like San Francisco, New York, and Boston have been working for several years at addressing the health issues posed by nail salons and have had successes that go beyond their geographic boundaries. In this chapter, I will elaborate on this area of growing public health concern through the lens of our joint initiative underway in Toronto.

Precarity and the Labour of Nail Work

The custom of polishing one's nails with a coloured coating dates back to Babylonia in 3200 BC (when it was just as common for men to polish their nails as women) and later in China in 3000 BC. At these times, the components of polish included such everyday (and relatively innocuous) ingredients as beeswax, egg whites, gelatin, gum Arabic, flower petals, and vegetable dyes. Colour was generally a signifier of class and social standing: royalty preferred gold and silver polishes. Growing one's nails out was also a signifier of class; those who did manual labour could not afford to have long nails, while those of a leisure class could.

Modern-day polishes have their recent origins in high gloss enamel paint used on automobiles, which was found to have a similarly glossy effect when used on nails. The rise in popularity of coloured glossy polishes as we know them today coincided with a rise in automobile use and the availability of related compounds and mixtures. By the 1940s in North America, colourful, painted nails were a marker of high fashion, their popularity aided by the use of brightly coloured glossy polishes on the nails of Hollywood actresses. Today, painted nails are commonplace and the nail salon industry is a rapidly growing one (IBISWorld 2016).

American sociologist Miliann Kang offers some interesting insights into the rapid development in popularity of women "having their nails done." From her feminist and ethnographic lens on nail salons and nail salon workers in New York, she has contributed significantly to the literature in this area. She writes, "No individual woman suddenly wakes up with the idea that manicured nails are central to her identity" (Kang 2010, 9). Rather, she argues that it takes years of socialization and messaging from the social world around her to come to the conclusion (conscious or otherwise) that nails "say something important about who she is and that it is worth paying someone to make the statement that she desires." A subject in the documentary film *Painted Nails* (Jordan and Griffin 2016) who drives a bus in San Francisco and gets her nails done regularly comments, "Some people are into shoes. Some people are into hair. I'm just into taking care of my nails ... [it] express[es] my feminine side."

Kang's social context provides an important backdrop for us to consider the broader social, economic, and health parameters of the world of nail salon workers. She adds, "While most customers insist on seeing their manicures as purely private rituals, their manicuring practices emerge at the nexus of historical and contemporary forces that have fostered a booming global niche in nail products and services" (Kang 2010, 10).

As noted, sound statistics on the nail salon industry and its employees in Canada are scant at best; what data gathering there is varies from municipality to municipality and from province to province. There are nonetheless some details we know anecdotally (and from some data sources) with a degree of certainty. Most nail salon workers in Canada and elsewhere earn low incomes and work in non-unionized environments. We have been told by nail technicians working in discount nail salons in Toronto that there is a high degree of financial exploitation, particularly in the training phase. Although higher-end spas and beauty salons that offer nail services usually require training from college or beauty school programs for cosmeticians, manicurists, and pedicurists, discount nail salons usually only require on-the-job training. Service Canada classifies this work under "Estheticians, Electrologists and Related Occupations," and notes that in addition to programs in schools, "on-the-job training" is sanctioned (Statistics Canada 2011).

> The conditions in the salons are the bitter fruit at the end of a long food chain that includes customers' desire for cheap, fast services, toxic cosmetic products, and a broken immigration system that depends on the mobile, contingent labor of young immigrant women ... but does not recognize or protect these workers. (Kang 2016, 32)

Because language proficiency in Canada's official languages is not a formal requirement, discount nail salons can be an attractive option for a woman who is new to Canada. We know from the program director that inspectors who visit the salons for the City of Toronto Department of Public Health's BodySafe program[2] (a public protection and infection control initiative) observe that the majority of staff they see in the city's discount salons are Asian (Chinese, Vietnamese, Korean), with fewer numbers of some other immigrant groups (Tibetan, Eastern European, Latin American). Language competency varies, but many have a fairly poor command of English.[3]

We also know from focus groups carried out with nail technicians in 2014 in Toronto (David 2014) that immigration concerns are an issue for some. Toronto journalist Denise Balkissoon, in her investigative research on nail salon workers in 2012, found that women working in this industry in Toronto did not want to be interviewed about their health for fear of repercussions stemming from their immigration status or from the owners of the salons where they worked (Balkissoon 2012).

In short, the community (or communities) of nail technicians working in discount salons in Toronto and elsewhere fit a classic profile of precarious workers. Ng et al. (2016, 9) describe precarious work as "working conditions that are characterized by increased economic insecurity, reduced entitlement to ongoing employment, limited control over work schedules, low pay, limited benefits and few opportunities for career advancement." Nail technicians' work is difficult (see the following section): as employees they are subject to exploitation, and the extent to which they are protected by existing legislation (occupational health and safety/toxic exposures, employment standards, etc.) is questionable.

We have benefited in Canada from a rich body of work in feminist political economy and in labour studies providing us with a context for understanding the place of nail salon workers (Armstrong 2010; Cohen and Pulkingham 2009; Fudge and Owens 2006; Vosko 2002). Vosko (2002, 3) speaks to the notion of "gendered precariousness" in her 2002 lecture in the Robarts Canada Research Chairholders Series, referring to "an insecure labour market situation, shaped, in the current context, by deregulation, the deterioration of full-time full-year employment, the erosion of the standard employment relationship as a norm and the spread of non-standard forms of employment." All of these conditions apply to the working lives and realities of many nail salon workers in discount salons.

Vosko contends that "social reproduction" – including the mostly invisible and unpaid work of women in the home and the family context – must be factored into any discussion of precarious work, and that women bear a disproportionate burden of social reproduction work, adding to what Ng et al. (2016) refer to as "the precarity capture." While good data on this are scant, Ng et al.'s preliminary study, including interviews with Toronto women, confirms that the added burden of social reproduction work adds a layer of mental and physical strain to an already stressful work life. This is further compounded by a flagging social safety network in Ontario with a weakening of employment insurance, welfare, and childcare.

From what we know about the nail salon industry in Toronto and elsewhere, it ticks off all or most of the boxes for defining precarity: small businesses with limited control for workers over their working conditions (hours, breaks, wage negotiations, etc.), few if any benefits, poor adherence to employment standards, highly sex-segregated, and largely immigrant and racialized. Compounding this portrait is the fact that on key factors in the work of nail technicians (occupational health and safety, labour standards, licensing) oversight is generally weak in most Canadian jurisdictions and discount salon owners, like many small business owners, are free to exploit that weakness. For example, with respect to protecting workers from exposure to hazardous chemicals, jurisdiction over small businesses with fewer than ten employees imposes minimal requirements of owners. Salon owners in Toronto are not obliged, therefore, to provide any training to new employees on the handling of hazardous products, as they would be in a larger work environment with more employees (such as plastics manufacturing in a plant). With licensing of salons (only a recent practice in Canada's largest urban centre) handled at the municipal level, and health and safety requirements dictated at the provincial level, there is a disconnect between what is expected of a new salon owner. Because of varying levels of responsibility for oversight, nail salons fall between the cracks, and their workers are its victims.

Kang offers an additional consideration, which adds to both the complexity and the nuance in the study of this profession. She refers to the work performed by nail technicians as "body labour ... catering to the needs of customers, but complicated by differences of language, culture, class and race. This form of body labour enforces the treatment of white women's bodies as both special and normative, thereby upholding these women's racial and class privilege. Simultaneously, it disciplines Asian women's bodies to display deference and attentiveness in line with the controlling image of the Asian 'model minority'" (Kang 2010, 9).

This "required behaviour" was also noted in Ng et al.'s (2016, 17) study: a nail salon worker interviewed for their research commented that "you are under constant pressure to work faster, to chat and make customers happy!" A peer educator who is part of our Healthy Nail Salon Network in Toronto shared a text message from her salon owner boss about the upcoming holiday season, underscoring the need to always be on time and to keep breaks short because, she wrote, "customers are generally more impatient at this time of year."

Those who own their own salons, while having more autonomy than hired technicians, can also be rigidly bound by the dictates of the nature of this work. The main subject of the documentary film *Painted Nails*, Van Hoang, a Vietnamese salon owner in San Francisco, notes, "We cook and eat here. The only thing we don't do is sleep here. We get here early in the morning and we leave here late at night ... I don't have many friends. I just work here all day" (Jordan and Griffin 2016).

The deference and attentiveness Kang (2010) refers to above are critical features of nail salon work, bringing their own set of unique stressors to the women who work in this business.

Health Challenges and the Added Burden of Toxic Exposures

Ng et al.'s (2016, 3) study of the health impacts of precarious work on racialized refugee and immigrant women in Toronto calls the situation "a looming but largely invisible public health crisis." The authors and community researchers shine light on both the physical and mental health effects of precarious work and speak of an emerging consensus that "precarious working conditions have become a determinant of poor health" (7): "the negative health effects of precarious work are a matter of when, not if" (22). Nail salon workers were part of this study.

Compounding the general conditions of precarity noted above – conditions that nail technicians in discount salons share with many other immigrant women workers in urban settings like Toronto (retail sales, housecleaning, personal service workers, childcare, etc.) – nail technicians also have the added burden of working in physically toxic environments. Nail technicians in a focus group in Toronto in 2014 were asked about their level of knowledge of toxic exposures, and some acknowledged fear about learning more because it "might make them feel they need to leave their job, on which they depend for their salary" (David 2014, 5).

As with labour force and demographic research on the nail salon industry in Canada, research on the chemicals used in nail salons is not as robust as one might hope. One of the most recent comprehensive studies of chemicals found in nail salons was conducted by the New York State Department of Health in July 2016, where it was noted that "there are about 30 chemicals or chemical categories that appear to be commonly used in nail products" (4). Because the data have not been gathered, we cannot say with complete certainty that this number is an accurate capture of typical salons in Toronto, or if there are fewer or more chemicals of concern. We can only assume, by the services that are offered and the products that are visible in the workplace, that there is probably a similar number in Toronto salons.

As noted earlier, our focus and concern have been with discount salons in Toronto that offer the cheapest services and tend to use the cheapest (and therefore most toxic) products. The standard products used in salons are dictated by the services those salons offer, but most salons have polishes, enamels, gels, solvents, cuticle softeners, and acrylics as part of their stock and trade, all containing chemicals that put human health at risk (Ford 2014; Quach et al. 2011; Women's Voices 2015). The chemicals of particular concern are formaldehyde, toluene, and dibutyl phthalate, commonly known as "the toxic trio."

Formaldehyde, a known human carcinogen (Agency for Toxic Substances and Disease Registry 2011a), is used as a preservative and is an irritant to the eyes, nose, and throat, causing both respiratory and dermatological conditions of concern. Exposure occurs through inhalation and skin exposure.

Toluene, a solvent and a known endocrine-disrupting chemical, is used to reinforce colour and smoothness in nail products. It is rapidly absorbed when inhaled and can also enter the bloodstream through the skin. Researched effects include kidney and liver toxicity at high exposures; central nervous system conditions such as confusion, weakness, dizziness, and memory loss (Agency for Toxic Substances and Disease Registry 2011b), and impacts on newborns following fetal exposure, including increased risk of spontaneous abortion (Figa-Telemanca 2006).

Dibutyl phthalate is part of a large family of plasticizers and softeners with known endocrine-disrupting properties (TEDX n.d.). It is used as a plasticizer in nail products; and in addition to findings that it provokes asthma through inhalation, animal research has established a connection with reproductive effects in male offspring (Foster 2005). Although phthalates are explicitly regulated only in soft vinyl articles for children in Canada, their use in the Canadian cosmetics industry is largely unregulated.

Other chemicals found routinely in nail salon products include acrylamide, acetone, parabens, triphenyl phosphate, ethyl, and methyl methacrylate (acrylics, false nails, and gels involve some of the most toxic chemicals). In Canada, manufacturers are not required to label cosmetic products unless they are distributed in industrial-size quantities. This oversight poses problems at a couple of levels: for researchers who are wanting to study the products and their ingredients, and for nail technicians using the products and not knowing exactly what chemicals they are being exposed to at any given time.

Other problems less directly linked to chemical exposure have also been identified, such as musculoskeletal issues that result from the ergonomic challenges the job entails. Constant bending over in restrictive and long-held positions can cause repeated aches and pains, and constant holds against hard contact surfaces can cause pressure on joints and blood flow disruption. Mental health issues stemming from the challenges faced by those in precarious work have also been identified.

As with other aspects of studying this population, the scientific literature on exposures faced by this group of workers is relatively small but growing. Most research done to date has been on animals, although some research has been done in salons and among salon workers. An additional challenge in researching health effects for this population is that in this and related environments, a worker is never exposed to just *one* chemical. Exposure to a mixture of chemicals has not been studied for the synergistic toxic effects that can result.

Focus: Reproductive Health Issues

At a recent meeting of the Toronto Healthy Nail Salon Network, one nail technician commented, "We come from China where the government says one baby only. We come to Canada and hope to have more babies, but we cannot get pregnant because of our work."

Issues relating to reproduction (fertility, pregnancy, fetal development) are not as easily discussed as other health issues such as skin or respiratory problems. Most of the nail technicians we come in contact with through our project work in Toronto are of reproductive age, and many are concerned about exposure during pregnancy (David 2014). Animal research has drawn many links from nail salon chemical exposures to problematic reproductive outcomes (Quach et al. 2014): parabens and phthalates, for example, are endocrine disrupters, and exposure to phthalates in pregnancy has been linked to problems in male reproductive development (Swan 2008) and pre-term birth (Ferguson, McElrath, and Meeker 2014). Table 13.1 below provides more detail.

To address nail technicians' concerns related to toxic exposures in pregnancy, we have developed a teaching module (to be taken into the salons by peer outreach workers) that provides basic, easily understood information on exposure prevention, pregnancy planning, and knowledge about chemicals of concern. This involves our taking the best of the scientific research on exposures in conception and pregnancy and synthesizing it into easily understood information to best protect this population. We recognize that limiting personal exposure in the workplace is only a first step in improving reproductive outcomes; broader, more systemic changes that are noted above are needed for optimum protection of nail salon workers.

A Hopeful Model for Change

For the community of people attempting to improve the health of women employed in nail salons, there are examples of work undertaken in certain North American municipalities that serve both as models for adaptation and as inspiration to continue the challenge. The work being done in Toronto is comparatively recent, and while feedback on our work to date has been positive,[4] we need to look to the model used in municipalities such as San Francisco for help in determining our next steps.

One key element that distinguishes the work being done in San Francisco from that in other municipalities (e.g., New York) is that they have made a concerted effort to work *with* salon owners to improve health in nail salon environments (e.g., rewarding for good behaviour),

Table 13.1. Reproductive health effects of chemicals used in nail salons

Chemical	Use	Concern for reproductive health
Formaldehyde	Used in nail polish and nail hardeners	Carcinogen; associated with low birth weight in several studies (Figa-Telemanca 2006); reduced fertility (Duong et al. 2011)
Toluene	Used as a solvent (aromatic hydrocarbon) in nail polish, polish remover, and fingernail glue	Endocrine disrupter; breathing high levels in pregnancy can cause birth defects, slow growth, and retard mental abilities of offspring (Donald et al. 1991); increased risk of reduced fertility and spontaneous abortion (Figa-Telemanca 2006)
Dibutyl phthalate	Used in nail polish to make it more flexible	Endocrine disrupter (Figa-Telemanca 2006); female reproductive toxicity in mice research (birth defects and reduced birth weight) (Marsman 1995); problems in male genital development (Kortenkamp et al. 2011); can have permanent effects on development of central nervous system (World Health Organization 2012)
Parabens	Used as a preservative in cosmetics	Endocrine disrupter (Figa-Telemanca 2006); diminished fertility in animal studies (Kortenkamp et al. 2011)
Acrylamides	Used as a nail strengthener, topcoat	Carcinogen; decreased sperm count in male rats (Sakamoto and Hashimoto 1986)
Methanol	Used in non-acetone polish removers	Reproductive toxin;[a] adverse effects on developing fetus (Center for Environmental Health 2016)
Triphenyl phosphate (TPP or TPHP)	Used as plasticizer in nail polish; considered a replacement for dibutyl phthalate	Endocrine disrupter; developmental toxicity in offspring

[a] Reproductive toxicity is defined as "adverse effects on sexual function and fertility in adult males and females, as well as developmental toxicity in the offspring" (Kortenkamp et al. 2011, 72).

as opposed to taking a more antagonistic or adversarial approach (e.g., reporting violations to municipal authorities). This is an approach we endeavour to replicate in Toronto.

Much of the work that has been done in San Francisco over the past ten-plus years can be attributed to the California Healthy Nail Salon Collaborative (HNSC), a collection of health, environmental, social service, and legal agencies that works closely with not just nail salon owners and technicians but product manufacturers and state officials. The

HNSC's mission is "to improve the health, safety, and rights of the nail and beauty care workforce to achieve a healthier, more sustainable, and just industry."[5]

Their persistent lobbying and advocacy efforts on behalf of nail technicians over many years has paid off: through their collective efforts, they have created a model for a voluntary recognition program to promote healthy practices – the state established a Healthy Nail Salon Recognition Program in 2013 – and developed a program that outlines ten requirements to protect the health of workers and clients. Salons that meet the ten requirements for a healthier salon are recognized by the respective county and can display a sign in their window indicating they have been accredited as a healthy nail salon. In 2016, the state governor expanded the program to cover salons in the entire state.

HNSC's work has gone beyond the establishment of the recognition program. In 2016, in collaboration with the US Environmental Protection Agency, banks, and local counties, they piloted a microloan project that makes available loans with zero per cent interest, enabling salon owners to purchase less toxic nail products and ventilation equipment. They have also been involved in implementing hazardous waste management programs to reduce chemical exposure in nail salons. In recognition of their ground-breaking work, the HNSC received the prestigious 2016 Roy Family Award for Environmental Partnership from the Kennedy School of Government at Harvard University.

There are some critical reasons for the success of the San Francisco model:[6]

1 The HNSC has always put the nail technicians at the centre of any and all of their work.
2 They forged strong ties with key players in the Vietnamese community at the beginning of their work and have since maintained those ties.
3 A non-antagonistic model was favoured wherein salon owners were not treated as "bad guys" but rather given incentives to make their salons healthier places to work.
4 They engaged a base of customers as critical allies in the fight for healthier nail salons.
5 They have demonstrated that the personal is political.[7]

While the San Francisco model offers other municipalities like Toronto great opportunities for study and implementation, it also poses challenges. We have noted that data collection is inconsistent and patchwork in all municipalities in Canada, making it difficult to present an accurate picture of the current situation. In addition, the San Francisco experience benefited from having an almost homogeneous community of salon workers with which to work – immigrant women from Vietnam (Quach et al. 2011). Toronto, for example, has a more varied nail salon population, necessitating the establishment and nurturing of relationships with a broader range of immigrant community organizations and opinion makers. Nonetheless, the San Francisco group had their own set of challenges to face, and they have shown that these were not insurmountable.

Conclusion

Women who work in the discount nail salon industry in Canadian urban settings represent canaries in the coal mine of health challenges. In addition to being precarious workers as a result of their often insecure immigration status, their vulnerability to exploitation in a small-industry environment, and their experiences of racism as new immigrants, they have the additional challenge of being exposed to hazardous chemicals that put their overall health at risk. This cluster of precariousness should make them, and people in related work situations, a high priority for health care in Canada. But we have observed that, as with the multitudes of people who have worked with asbestos, many of them ultimately dying from exposure, work-related chemical exposures have not been a priority of any Canadian federal or provincial governments, and change – when it happens – usually comes only after many years of persistent lobbying and advocacy efforts.

The direct involvement of nail technicians in the Healthy Nail Salon Network project, and the more recent Nail Technicians' Network, has been central to this work. Despite the lack of clear scientific evidence linking their health problems to their work environments, nail salon workers presented at a community health centre with a range of health problems known from the animal literature to be linked to the very chemicals with which they work. We maintain that there is enough known about the harms caused by the chemicals to which nail technicians are exposed that we should be practising the precautionary principle. The New York State Department of Public Health (2016, 11) report concurs, concluding that "in the absence of a complete understanding of the exposure potential and toxicity properties of the variety of chemicals found in nail salon products, actions to minimize chemical exposures should be emphasized." More specifically, our governments, in their regulation of these chemicals, in the establishment of occupational health and safety standards, and in the licensing of these work venues, should be practising the precautionary principle.

NOTES

1 I use the terms "nail salon employees," "nail salon workers," and "nail technicians" interchangeably in this chapter.
2 Conversation with Cecilia Alterman, director of BodySafe program, City of Toronto, Department of Public Health, 10 October 2016.
3 Our in-salon health promotion and prevention workshops in Toronto are conducted in Vietnamese and Mandarin.
4 See "Healthy Nail Technician Program Evaluation: Survey Results," 2015, Centre for Research Expertise in Occupational Disease, Dalla Lana School of Public Health, University of Toronto. (Document available from author upon request.)
5 California Healthy Nail Salon Collaborative, https://cahealthynailsalons.org/.
6 The following list is based on a presentation in Toronto in 2014 by leaders from the California Healthy Nail Salon Collaborative and on conversations with these leaders. An audio file of the public presentation is available at http://www.cwhn.ca/sites/default/files/Beyond%20the%20Mani-Pedi%20Audio.mp3.
7 In the film *Painted Nails* (Jordan and Griffin 2016) we follow the development of a San Francisco salon owner, who starts by acknowledging health issues caused by her day-to-day salon exposures and later is assisted by the HNSC in testifying in Washington at national public hearings on a bill related to toxic chemicals in the workplace.

REFERENCES

Agency for Toxic Substances and Disease Registry. 2011a. "Toxic Substances Portal: Formaldehyde." http://www.atsdr.cdc.gov/substances/toxsubstance.asp?toxid=39.

Agency for Toxic Substances and Disease Registry. 2011b. "Toxic Substances Portal: Toluene." https://www.atsdr.cdc.gov/substances/toxsubstance.asp?toxid=29.

Armstrong, P. 2010. *The Double Ghetto: Canadian Women and Their Segregated Work.* Toronto: Oxford University Press.

Balkissoon, D. 2012. "Your Manicure Looks Beautiful. But the Health Effects Are Ugly." *Globe and Mail,* 13 July. https://www.theglobeandmail.com/life/health-and-fitness/health/your-manicure-looks-beautiful-but-the-health-effects-are-ugly/article4416784/.

Center for Environmental Health. 2016. "Review of Chemicals Used in Nail Salons." http://www.health.ny.gov/press/reports/docs/nail_salon_chemical_report.pdf.

Cohen, M., and J. Pulkingham. 2009. *Public Policy for Women: The State, Income Security, and Labour Market Issues.* Toronto: University of Toronto Press.

David, L. 2014. "Focus Group Results: How Training and Employment Conditions Impact on Toronto Nail Technicians' Ability to Protect Themselves at Work." https://pqwchc.org/wp-content/uploads/Focus-Group-Summary.pdf.

Diamanti-Kandarakis, E., J.-P. Bourguignon, L.C. Guidice, R. Hauser, G.S. Prins, A.M. Soto, R.T. Zoeller, and A.C. Gore. 2009. "Endocrine Disrupting Chemicals: An Endocrine Society Scientific Statement." *Endocrine Reviews* 30 (4): 293–342. https://doi.org/10.1210/er.2009-0002.

Donald, J.M., K. Hooper, and C. Hopenhayn-Rich. 1991. "Reproductive and Developmental Toxicity of Toluene: A Review." *Environmental Health Perspectives* 94: 237–44. https://doi.org/doi:10.2307/3431317.

Duong, A., C. Steinmaus, C.L. McHale, C.P. Vaughan, and L. Zhang. 2011. "Reproductive and Developmental Toxicity of Formaldehyde: A Systematic Review." *Mutation Research* 728 (3): 118–38. https://doi.org/10.1016/j.mrrev.2011.07.003.

TEDX. n.d. "Endocrine Disruption Exchange: Phthalates." https://endocrinedisruption.org/interactive-tools/critical-windows-of-development/about-the-timeline/phthalates. Accessed 30 December 2019.

Ferguson, K.K., T.F. McElrath, and J.D. Meeker. 2014. "Environmental Phthalate Exposure and Preterm Birth." *Journal of the American Medical Association Pediatrics* 168 (1): 61–8. https://doi.org/10.1001/jamapediatrics.2013.3699.

Figa-Telemanca, I. 2006. "Occupational Risk Factors and Reproductive Health of Women." *Occupational Medicine* 56 (8): 521–31. https://doi.org/10.1093/occmed/kql114.

Ford, A.R. 2014. "Overexposed, Underinformed: Nail Salon Workers and Hazards to Their Health: A Review of the Literature." National Network on Environments and Women's Health. https://nnewh.files.wordpress.com/2016/01/literature-review-nail-salon-project-january-2014.pdf.

Foster, P.M.D. 2005. "Disruption of Reproductive Development in Male Rat Offspring Following In Utero Exposure to Phthalate Esters." *International Journal of Andrology* 29: 140–7. https://doi.org/10.1111/j.1365-2605.2005.00563.x.

Fudge, J., and R. Owens. 2006. *Precarious Work, Women and the New Economy: The Challenge to Legal Norms.* Oxford: Hart.

IBISWorld. 2016. "Hair and Nail Salons in Canada: Market Research Report." http://www.ibisworld.ca/industry/hair-nail-salons.html.

Jordan, E., and D. Griffin, dirs. 2016. *Painted Nails* (documentary). DigiAll Films. http://www.paintednailsmovie.com/.

Kang, M. 2010. *The Managed Hand: Race, Gender, and the Body in Beauty Service Work.* Berkeley: University of California Press.

Kang, M. 2016. "Is It Possible to Get a Safe, Fair Manicure?" *Women and Environments International* 96–97 (Summer/Fall): 30–3.

Kortenkamp, A., O. Martin, M. Faust, R. Evans, R. McKinlay, F. Orton, and E. Rosivatz. 2011. "State of the Art Assessment of Endocrine Disrupters: Final Report." December. European Commission, DG Environment. https://

ec.europa.eu/environment/chemicals/endocrine/pdf/sota_edc_final_report.pdf.

Marsman, D.S. 1995. "NTP Technical Report on Toxicity Studies of Dibutyl Phthalate." NIH Publication 95-3353. March. https://www.ncbi.nlm.nih.gov/pubmed/12209194.

New York State Department of Health. 2016. "Review of Chemicals Used in Nail Salons." July. NYS Department of Health. http://www.health.ny.gov/press/reports/docs/nail_salon_chemical_report.pdf.

Ng, W., A. Sundar, J. Poole, B. Karpoche, I. Abdillahi, S. Arat-Koc, A. Benjamin, and G.E. Galabuzi. 2016. "A Public Health Crisis in the Making: The Health Impacts of Precarious Work on Racialized Refugee and Immigrant Women." October. Ryerson University, Toronto.

Quach, T., R. Gunier, A. Tran, J. Von Behren, P.-A. Doan-Billings, K.-D. Nguyen, L. Okahara, et al. 2011. "Characterizing Workplace Exposures in Vietnamese Women Working in California Nail Salons." *American Journal of Public Health*, supp. 1, 101 (S1): S271–S276. https://doi.org/10.2105/AJPH.2010.300099.

Quach, T., J. Von Behren, D. Goldberg, M. Layefsky, and P. Reynolds. 2014. "Adverse Birth Outcomes and Maternal Complications in Licensed Cosmetologists and Manicurists in California." *International Archives of Occupational and Environmental Health* 88 (7): 823–33. https://doi.org/10.1007/s00420-014-1011-0.

Sakamoto, J., and K. Hashimoto. 1986. "Reproductive Toxicity of Acrylamide and Related Compounds in Mice – Effects on Fertility and Sperm Morphology." *Archives of Toxicology* 59 (4): 201–5. https://doi.org/10.1007/BF00290538.

Statistics Canada. 2011. "Estheticians, Electrologists and Related Occupations." National Occupational Classification. Government of Canada. https://www23.statcan.gc.ca/imdb/p3VD.pl? Function=getVD&TVD=122372&CVD=122376&CPV=6562&CST=01012011&CLV=4&MLV=4.

Swan, S.H. 2008. "Environmental Phthalate Exposure in Relation to Reproductive Outcomes and Other Health Endpoints in Humans." *Environmental Research* 108 (2): 177–84. https://doi.org/10.1016/j.envres.2008.08.007.

Vosko, L. 2002. "Rethinking Feminization: Gendered Precariousness in the Canadian Labour Market and the Crisis in Social Reproduction." Robarts Canada Research Chairholders Series. 11 April. York University, Toronto.

Women's Voices for the Earth. 2015. "Nail Products and Polishes That Contain Chemicals of Concern." http://www.womensvoices.org/2015/05/18/nail-products-polishes-thatcontain-chemicals-of-concern/.

World Health Organization. 2012. "Endocrine Disrupters and Child Health: Possible Developmental Early Effects of Endocrine Disrupters on Child Health." Geneva: World Health Organization.

14 Conclusion – Health Matters: Research in Practice

PAT ARMSTRONG, HUGH ARMSTRONG, JACQUELINE CHOINIERE, AND ERIC MYKHALOVSKIY

Drawing on a broad literature, the introductory chapter of this volume explains the editors' perspective on evidence, critical social science, and health care in Canada. We approached authors to write chapters because we knew they take a critical perspective, although they address significantly different areas and are not united by a single theoretical approach. After their chapters were completed, we interviewed the authors about their topics, their approaches, their evidence, their challenges, and their ways of sharing research. Perhaps surprising, given the range of issues they address and methods they use, our analysis of the interviews reveals many common themes. This final chapter draws out those themes, relying on the words of the individual chapter authors taken from our interviews with them.

Context Matters

The emphasis on generalizability and the search for "best practices" are elements that most often seek to transcend the specific locations of individuals and/or communities in order to identify universals. The contributors to this volume take a different approach that is in keeping with emerging scholarship on the importance of context for conceptualizing, designing, delivering, and evaluating health practices and interventions (Hawe 2015; Shoveller et al. 2015). They stress that context and relations of power matter in ways that lead to the recognition of specificity. The context is layered and interacting, stretching from the international and the national to the local, the group, and the individual.

As Christianne Stephens explains, her research on Indigenous peoples' experiences of health care "explores how historically rooted processes of colonization, assimilation, and industrialization have impacted and transformed Indigenous health and well-being. There are many challenges to doing this type of work, ranging from theoretical and methodological considerations to ethical concerns. One of the shortcomings of biomedicine is its tendency to view diseases as distinct phenomena that exist apart from social groups and contexts."

Understanding the context shapes both the research and the identification of practices worth sharing. In their exploration of code work in long-term residential care, Tamara Daly, Jacqueline Choiniere, and Hugh Armstrong began their ethnographic studies of long-term care by developing "clear notions of local and national contexts to conduct the ethnographies." This background research "focused on understanding the broad financing and ownership, accountability, approaches to care, and work organization models in each of the jurisdictions where we studied"; "by reminding ourselves of the importance of context, and [that] what works in one place may not work in another, we could focus on practices that are promising without advancing one clear way."

The importance of context for particular populations is further illustrated by Alisa Grigorovich in her chapter on home care:

> Lesbian and bisexual women have unique experiences of quality that are tied to being not only older, female-identified, and needing care, but also being a sexual minority within a heteronormative health care system. Their experiences illustrate the fallacy of constructing a "universalist" quality-of-care standard, as this ignores the ways in which social location or context matters for enabling the quality of care. My suggestion for how to construct quality in ways that are more sensitive to social location is to start with listening to the perspectives of diverse care recipients about what enables good care, for whom, and under what conditions.

As Christine Kelly explains, this is also the case with age and disability: "There seems to be a different perspective when you are aging into disability [rather] than aging with a disability."

Taking context into account is important for not only those who need care but also those who provide care. Although Craig Dale was "initially heartened that health managers were interested in supporting preventative nursing hygiene," it quickly became clear that "patient-identified needs and nursing knowledge development in preventative oral care" were peripheral to fiscal imperatives. Nurses were "characterized as wilfully neglectful of their patients' oral and bodily hygiene, a discourse that ascribes blame for costly patient and system problems to a less powerful group in the health care hierarchy." Dale's research on nurses' mouth care in ICU settings exposes a discourse of neglect that focuses on individual nurses rather than on the conditions that prevent them from doing preventative work. "On the one hand, this discourse circulates nursing accountability through a purported dereliction of duty. On the other hand, such language [deflects] attention [from] the contextual barriers impeding this work. A discourse of neglect is not informing the practical delivery of oral care."

Power relations play out in all these contexts, and evidence – even of the sort traditionally in high regard – may be ignored in the process. Vicki Van Wagner and Elizabeth Darling talk about these struggles in relation to midwifery:

> It can be more difficult to discuss evidence that illustrates the benefits of a model of care associated with one profession than to discuss the benefits of a new drug or procedure. All of the provider groups involved in offering care for childbirth are deeply committed to the role of their profession, and this can evoke conflict as well as collaboration. Suggestions for change, no matter how evidence based, can be challenging, particularly when current systems are stressed. As the newest profession involved in maternity care, it is always a challenge to be a midwifery researcher in a Canadian context. We may be perceived as having a bias towards our profession or towards a low-intervention approach to birth, while a physician or nurse researcher is seen as more neutral.

Tensions Matter

There is a tendency in social science research to simplify in ways that reduce complexity and to avoid the ongoing tensions both in doing the research and in the processes or subject of the research. In contrast, the contributors to this collection draw out the tensions and contradictions that are not only part of health and care but also part of the research process.

Some authors highlighted the tensions among researchers. Daly, Choiniere, and Armstrong, for example, explained that in their international, interdisciplinary project "differences, in terms of analysis, can result in productive tensions. Harnessing rather than suppressing these tensions has helped us to productively identify the boundaries around issues to produce nuanced and textured analysis."

More than one author highlighted the tensions for researchers themselves, especially when they are practitioners in the fields they are studying. Mary Ellen Macdonald and David Kenneth Wright, for example, spoke about the "tensions in both what is studied and in the position as insider/outsider." For Wright, the

> ethnographic imagination caused me to think about the ways that certain palliative care practices and discourses – the same ones that I found so inspiring –

> might paradoxically cause harm. My conversations with family members who were disturbed by the tranquil hospice environment, or who felt that pain management practices had hurt rather than helped their loved one, were key moments in uncovering this tension. In essence, a main "challenge" was navigating insider-outsider positionings over the course of data collection, analysis, and dissemination. During fieldwork, my identity as a member of the palliative care community enabled a certain level of access and insight that I might not have otherwise enjoyed. At the same time, it took conscious effort to maintain a necessary distance to question and challenge experiences and practices that might otherwise seem familiar and unproblematic.

Similarly, Van Wagner and Darling are midwives who "practice, teach, and do health systems research. Balancing these roles brings insight but can also be challenging to juggle."

Then there is the tension involved in balancing competing pressures. For Stephens,

> one of the most challenging questions that I've had to ask myself during my research is: How do I reveal the devastating health impacts of social inequalities and lifelong traumas without pathologizing those whose story I am telling? One solution has been to strike a balance between reporting on the factors that cause disease, hurt, and trauma and those elements that promote good health, healing, and a sense of well-being. For example, my full ethnographic account of the Wilson family's health genealogy also illuminates the positive aspects of the family's life experiences and includes Rachel and her son Paul's advocacy work on behalf of residential school survivors and the active involvement of Rachel's daughters in environmental stewardship initiatives that have had a positive impact on their community.

There can also be tensions related to pressures for researchers to take a particular position on their research. Kirsten Bell talks about the challenges others bring to the values held by a researcher. She has, for instance, been "accused of 'parroting' or supporting the tobacco industry." She notes:

> I get very tired of defending myself against these kinds of accusations, which have probably been my biggest challenge. I mean, there's a history there that I understand – lots of folks in the field of tobacco control have been "fighting the good fight" since the 1970s and have witnessed some extremely underhand tactics on the part of the tobacco industry – but this context has resulted in a rather unfortunate "if you're not with us, you're against us" mentality. This environment makes it difficult to approach the topic of smoking in a way that tries to grapple with it beyond the very

limited cessationist frame – as we are currently witnessing in the heated debates about e-cigarettes.

While such tensions faced by researchers often go unacknowledged, it is even more likely that the tensions and contradictions in the findings are left out of or minimized in standard reporting. In contrast, these researchers seek to make such tensions and contradictions visible. Bell, for example, asks, "What's left when we strip away these models of human being that treat 'the smoker' as a simultaneously rational and irrational being?" For Macdonald and Wright, it is important to capture the tensions between approaches to care of the dying:

> Palliative care providers are not wrong to derive meaning and satisfaction, even pride, from the work that they do. But they should never lose sight of the *value-laden* nature of their field, and they should recognize that some people hold different values about life, death, and care. We both believe that palliative care providers should continuously reflect on how to better meet their responsibilities toward *all* people who face end-of-life situations, particularly people whose preferences, priorities, expectations, or hopes do not align with the palliative care vision of what it means to die well. Surely these people deserve a "good death" too? We hope that our research contributes to deliberate reflection about and examination of the moral experiences of this latter group of people.

Methods Matter

The individual authors in this volume share the conviction that we need to hear from those who live the health care system on a daily basis. For most, this means an ethnographic approach that allows researchers to take context, complexity, and contradiction into account.

Dale describes how he chose a "critical ethnographic" approach:

> I wanted to move underneath health reform discourses in the investigation of oral care. The "critical" part was an invitation to question the status quo, while the "ethnographic" part offered the opportunity to immerse myself in the intensive care unit context amongst real people and everyday problems. Ultimately, ethnographic description offered a counterpoint to undignified characterizations of nursing and the ability to articulate a contrasting account ... We need novel ways of engaging seriously ill patients and their caregivers in the identification of problems and opportunities. I envision direct observation and first-hand experience as essential sources of evidence. It should not be a radical idea to directly observe patients and inquire whether they've been washed, offered fluids, or had their pain addressed.

> The frequent inability of Canadian nurses to provide such care is hidden in the numbers. Accountability in my mind means keeping people, and not just statistics, in view.

Like a number of other authors in this volume, Dale uses ethnographic data to challenge the numbers that are given such authority. Drawing on their ethnographic research in long-term residential care, Daly, Choiniere, and Armstrong ask what's missing from the numbers and what shapes the numerical data that are collected:

> We link the administrative record keeping in the sector to broader gendered, and neoliberal or market-based, forces. We also critique how accountability for the care received by the increasingly vulnerable residents in this sector has become mostly about measuring clinical indicators to better – as in more efficiently – manage care. While recognizing the importance of clinical factors, we suggest that "quality of life," identified as a priority by residents and their families, suffers with this preoccupation. Residents want and need human engagement as much as a precise measurement of their fluid intake. In arguing for a broader notion of quality, one recognizing the relational aspects of care and its prerequisites, we are strengthening the argument that the conditions of work are the conditions of care.

Similarly, based on her ethnographic work Grigorovich offers a critique of the way numbers are used in home care:

> There are at least two problems with how quality of care in home care is currently assessed. The first is that it is assessed very narrowly, using a limited set of population-based numerical indicators that artificially flatten out variability among diverse care receivers across Ontario. Even if we accept that (some) numerical indicators can be useful for providing direction for how to enhance the quality of care, it is clear that the current metrics reflect neoliberal priorities and offer very little in terms of evidence of whether home care services are equitably distributed and/or meet individuals' needs and care situations. At a minimum, recognition of this problem suggests the need for developing other indicators that can enable us to better understand variation in how services are distributed across population groups and geographic settings, as well as whether these reflect structural and social inequalities ...
>
> However, the use of numerical metrics and the "evidence" created from them also needs to be more transparent in terms of public reporting; their use should include a discussion of what such indicators can and cannot measure, and they should be more critically applied in terms of using this

> evidence to inform health policy decisions. This brings us to the second problem, which is that in privileging counting, current systems of accountability ignore aspects of quality that cannot be reduced to numbers, such as the care relationship, emotional labour, and women's experiences of being cared for and being cared about. Recognition of the limitations of numerical accountability systems that prioritize standardization demands that we also make room for qualitative ways of assessment that are more sensitive to local complexity and can better capture these relational aspects of care. Thus, one practical implication of my research is that we need to create a more participatory approach to quality improvement and knowledge production regarding quality of care. This would require facilitating intersectoral collaborations between academics, health care users, health care professionals, and policymakers, with the aim of co-creating a quality assessment and improvement system that is more responsive to local care priorities and needs.

Doing ethnography does not exclude employing other methods. Indeed, most authors in this volume took other kinds of evidence into account or combined methods in their own primary research. Kelly Holloway and Matthew Herder are a case in point:

> We approached the research in several ways – through a survey, qualitative interviews, and ethnographic work at conferences and events. Our survey data allowed us to identify increased exposure of commercialization over time across Canadian universities. These early findings influenced our approach to qualitative interviews with emerging and established researchers, where we decided to not only identify exposure, or even views on commercialization, but also what kinds of tensions exist for academic health researchers who lived through a shift in structures that increasingly valued commercialization compared with those that have entered into their scientific training with these structural forms and exposures in place already. With our qualitative interviews at Dalhousie University, we were able to gain insight into the tensions that academic health scientists describe at different stages of their careers. Researching across these generations also allowed us to understand what is communicated from established to emerging researchers about the commercialization of research.

Relying on existing data sources can be challenging, as Ross Sutherland explains about his search for information on for-profit medical laboratories:

> It was often difficult to come up with firm conclusions. You had to make reasonable conjectures, for instance about why the private firms don't like

> to operate in integrated systems. There's a lot of data to indicate that they sabotage integration and that they back out of it. But you can't get direct access to their motivation. You deal only with outcomes, examining the hard data on the winners and losers of government policy. The effect of the research on me had to do with the small-l liberal faith in regulation. My research showed me how ineffective regulations have been over the years. Privatization has an inherently destabilizing effect.

At the same time, pioneering research by others can provide the basis for new research, as Anne Rochon Ford makes clear in talking about her collaborative research on nail salons and the workers in them:

> There is so much work to do here, but we are encouraged by others who have been at this much longer than we have, such as a group in California. The women we work with who are salon technicians or who are well connected in the Chinese and Vietnamese communities have been the backbone of this project. Were it not for the opportunity to work with them, and to see that the workshops they are doing in salons can have an impact on nail technicians' health, I would have lost interest by now! ... Inasmuch as this work has had a research focus, we have worked as a group to respond to the articulated needs of this community set out at the beginning through focus groups. From that, we merged those findings with a review of the literature to create a plan for on-site health education workshops for nail salon workers. We have additionally involved a professional evaluator in this current educational stage of the work to assess whether our workshops are having an impact.

Dissemination Matters

Science, especially in the health field, is most often understood as value free and based on research undertaken by those distant from the issues at stake so that they can take an objective view. In contrast, the contributors to this volume are engaged scholars. As public intellectuals, they seek to involve throughout the process those who will benefit most from the research. For the most part, they make their values and their advocacy work explicit, setting up yet another contrast with more traditional research in the field.

Stephens makes her position clear:

> Unlike "top-down" approaches that maintain a distanced and apolitical stance, I utilize my research findings strategically to bring attention to pressing issues and to actively advocate on behalf of community residents. I share my expertise and analyses with community partners and assist in

> developing community-based deliverables such as technical reports and needs assessments. I have been invited by community leaders to present my research at symposia and other notable gatherings. I was honoured to present keynote speeches on the topic of intergenerational trauma and community health at the 2016 Shingwauk Gathering and Conference at Algoma University and the 2017 Lambton-Kent District School Board's professional development day. A less recognized yet equally important form of advocacy is public service that involves assisting others to produce and document their own knowledge and experience. I "ghost write" a lot – meaning I help people put their thoughts [in] to words. Sometimes this work takes the form of straight transcription of people's personal stories. Other times, it involves drawing on my own anthropologically informed situated knowledge and ethnographic evidence to provide contextual information that will support their viewpoints. From writing speeches that allow the community's political leadership to convey key messages to high-level government officials, to assisting elders in documenting their testimonies of residential school suffering and abuse, I provide the prose and epistemological framework that help people advocate for themselves. This is one of the most powerful and gratifying aspects of my work.

Dale too is quite explicit about research providing a basis to "advocate for a new material accountability in health services management and evaluation." But these researchers also recognize that this must be done with care. As Macdonald and Wright put it, "During dissemination, an ongoing challenge is in portraying the findings of this study in a way that is honest and critical, but without eclipsing the deep respect I continue to feel for the participants of this research who taught me so much."

Holloway and Herder understand that their scholarly work

> has contributed to knowledge, discussion, and debates about the commercialization of health research in Canada, and the tensions and contradictions facing scientific researchers. Our research has also had an impact at multiple levels beyond the scholarly literature in this area. During our investigation we presented early findings from our work to an international group of emerging scientists at the Gordon Research Seminar in the United States; we published a blog in *University Affairs* entitled "The Trouble with the Entrepreneurial Mindset" problematizing how some public discourse in Canada undermines science in the public interest; and we held a public meeting at Dalhousie University on the topic of commercialization with guest speaker Dr. David Healy, a well-regarded scholar on the topic of commercialization and pharmaceuticalization in medicine. Finally, we were contracted to write a report for the Canadian Association of Graduate

Studies entitled "Emerging Researchers and Intellectual Property: Law, Policy and Practice" in which we compared intellectual property [IP] policies for emerging academic health researchers at seventeen Canadian research universities, and offered an extensive set of recommendations to address gaps and shortcomings of IP policies for Canadian universities. In these multiple ways we have engaged Canadian academic health researchers in a discussion about the commercialization of biomedical research and its implications for the types of questions health researchers are encouraged to and choose to pursue.

Ariel Ducey's research on vaginal mesh seeks to have an impact on a tough audience, creating research that faces particular kinds of barriers:

I think local practices that encourage practitioners to be more reflexive about their own choices and preferences and create opportunities for practitioners to share their successes and failures are crucial. Exposing health care providers to a sociological perspective could help with this. There are surgeons who work in environments where this kind of collegial process is more common and accepted – where patient cases are discussed by interdisciplinary teams, where cases are routinely reviewed, and where practitioners can regularly "scrub in" with one another. I believe surgeons who say that some of the attempts at rationalizing, standardizing, and surveilling medical practice have made it more difficult to learn from one another. But I also recognize surgery as a profession that has not been sufficiently good, in many instances, at weeding out the "bad apples" or controlling who performs which procedures and when for the benefit and safety of patients. This problem is sometimes downplayed or disguised when surgery is depicted as an "art." It's good to remember, however, that such problems occur with most self-regulating professions, including university professors. But we, of course, do not have scalpels in our hands. Surgery is also a profession in which "failures" can be judged particularly harshly, or problems with specific procedures and devices are readily and conveniently imputed to the inadequacy of the surgeon using them, which creates a strong cultural disincentive to openness and exchange.

Our team did organize a workshop on ethics and surgical decision making for a major international conference of pelvic floor specialists, but it was cancelled because no one signed up for it. We plan to repackage the workshop and try again and may have more participants for such an event when we are better known (through publications) for this work. But there are few incentives for surgeons to spend time and money studying ethical and social issues around their practice. The surgeons we have talked to informally about this research do seem to find it interesting and important. I also suspect that when many surgeons hear the words "ethics" or "morals" they

> equate them with the sort of profound dilemmas that make up textbooks in clinical ethics, and as therefore largely irrelevant to the everyday decisions about which devices and techniques to use in which patients – decisions that also consume almost all their time. One of the key contributions of this work, therefore, could be to convince surgeons that decisions and actions they might tend to view as technical or mundane or routine are in fact moral and social, to make visible to them a register of everyday differences and distinctions that do in fact matter for individual patients and that when ignored can result in a great deal of harm.

Like Stephens, Kelly set out to include various communities in her work. "I hosted a community forum with the organizations that participated in my research. I wanted to broaden the understanding and approach to disability, moving beyond notions of physical impairment. I hoped to move away from single-impairment issues to see connections between, for example, HIV and Downs Syndrome. The research helped change the way we think about disability, leadership, and activism. It changed the way I think about disability and what Canadian disability movements are, allowing me to see that the movement is not dying; it is just changing." At the same time, the process has had an impact on her conceptual approach and her methods:

> I am also changing the way I think about research on care and aging, my other research focus. I have become more open to quantitative methods, in part because I am in a faculty of medicine. I see the potential for a participatory component in research, but I also see how participatory research uses up the resources of individuals and organizations with little compensation. I try to be thoughtful and to give back in other ways, for example sitting on boards. Participatory research is an important challenge to expertise. On the other hand, this can require researchers to defend theory and the need for conceptual frameworks. There can be pushback about the theoretical choices made by the researcher, and it can be challenging to balance the multiple perspectives out there.

A long-time community activist, Sutherland talks about how his research supports resistance against for-profit care:

> My research is being used in a series of ways to fight privatization and to encourage governments to bring lab work back into the public sector. In Alberta, the hospital unions and public-sector interest groups used *False Positive* and then got my articles into local papers, including the *Edmonton Journal*. That played into the provincial government being able to nationalize

> the Edmonton labs. In Ontario, the research informed recommendations to allow small hospitals to start doing community lab work. Managers, workers, and communities all used it, because to have a small hospital leave your community is pretty devastating. You need a good lab, with reasonable volume and sufficient staffing, to keep emergency and other services that rely on prompt lab work going. Without them, you lose the hospital. I did a lot of work to prepare an academic article for the *CMAJ*, but in the end they rejected it, unofficially because it was "too political." *Open Medicine* did publish it, but the research's impact has primarily come from the newspaper articles that sprang from it.

Like Sutherland, Rochon Ford is embedded in an activist community. Unlike most others in this volume, she does not have an academic job but rather conducts research with advocacy groups:

> The "activism" or "advocacy" component of our work has always been foremost in the minds of our project organizers, but we have been circumspect in how we discuss this, for funding/political reasons. It has been very clear, though, that our educational work has limitations without advocacy action happening in tandem. While it is easier to get funding to do educational workshops, we acknowledge that this is not primary prevention. Primary prevention changes – eliminating toxic chemicals from the products, having mandatory ventilation regulations tied to licensing, for example – will only happen with continued pressuring of those who hold those strings of control (industry, government regulators). A challenge for our project has been building capacity in those who are most directly affected, i.e., the nail technicians, many of whom do not have the level of confidence or language facility to speak with those in power (i.e., to be their own advocates, rather than having project organizers advocating on their behalf). Working with the nail technicians to help build some of that capacity is our next area of focus.

Critical Conclusions

Increasingly, those who fund health care research are looking for documented impact. However, the forms of evidence created by a critical social science perspective are often resisted, in part because such evidence challenges established practices not only of creating evidence but also of "relations of ruling," to use Dorothy Smith's (1987) phrase.

Asked how she gets her work taken up by policymakers, Bell responded:

> The short answer is that it *doesn't* get taken up as evidence in any meaningful way. The primary problem with evidence-based policymaking, which

> sounds great in theory, is that it's based on a very particular view of what constitutes evidence that draws a conceptual separation between "real" and "anecdotal" evidence, with anthropological fieldwork and qualitative research effectively falling into the latter category. Although efforts have been made to try and broaden its evidence hierarchies, I don't think they've dislodged these assumptions. In fact, I'd say that such efforts have been partly responsible for *impoverishing* qualitative research, especially in the field of health, which has become increasingly prescriptive and standardized in terms of how it's carried out, framed, and evaluated. For instance, I've seen countless papers where the authors draw attention to the inadequacy of their findings (e.g., their lack of generalizability), which I think social scientists need to stop doing – I suspect that translation is potentially part of the problem here. In a recent co-authored paper on cigarette packaging, we basically argued that ethnographic research *is* generalizable if the parameters of this concept are expanded along the lines that various anthropologists suggest – e.g., Kirsten Hastrup on "horizontal" verus "vertical" generalization and Didier Fassin's distinction between "extensive" and "comprehensive" generalization.

Bell, along with the other authors in this collection, clearly illustrates why resistance to critical scholarship on health care must itself be resisted. Critical social science, with its attendant critical approach to the forms of medico-administrative knowledge that are increasingly produced within the health care system and used in health care decision making, is a unique and important voice within the field of health research. It is a much-needed counter-discourse to the applied instrumental turn in Canadian health research and the forms of research that it promotes and values. The research studies presented here do not cover the full range of issues that present challenges to the Canadian health care system, nor do they represent all of the traditions of social science critique of health care produced by Canadian health scholars. Taken as a whole, what they do offer are ways of thinking about the problems of health care and how to address them that stand as an alternative to health research in neoliberalism and that challenge established policy perspectives. This volume is not "anti-evidence," but it does call into question what counts as "evidence." *Health Matters* casts a critical eye on managerial ways of knowing and the forms of commodification of health care and relations of accountability with which it is associated. The contributors to this volume produce knowledge about health care in context. They explore tensions and contradictions in relations of power in health care and take seriously the experiences of providers and health care users. They make their values explicit while creating health research that matters.

REFERENCES

Hawe, P. 2015. "Lessons from Complex Interventions to Improve Health." *Annual Review of Public Health* 36: 307–23. https://doi.org/10.1146/annurev-publhealth-031912-114421.

Shoveller, J., S. Viehbeck, E. Di Ruggiero, D. Greyson, K. Thomson, and R. Knight. 2015. "A Critical Examination of Representations of Context within Research on Population Health Intervention." *Critical Public Health* 26 (5): 1–14. https://doi.org/10.1080/09581596.2015.1117577.

Smith, D.E. 1987. *The Everyday World as Problematic: A Feminist Sociology*. Toronto: University of Toronto Press.

Contributors

Hugh Armstrong is distinguished research professor and professor emeritus in social work, political economy, and sociology at Carleton University. He has served as a board member for the Ottawa-Carleton Community Care Access Centre and the Council on Aging of Ottawa, and as a member of the Community Advisory Committee for The Ottawa Hospital. His research outputs include articles on state workers, the privatization of long-term care, and neoliberalism and official health statistics. With Pat Armstrong he has published several books, including *The Double Ghetto: Canadian Women and Their Segregated Work*; *Universal Health Care: What the United States Can Learn from the Canadian Experience*; *Wasting Away: The Undermining of Canadian Health Care*; *Critical to Care: The Invisible Women in Health Services*; and *About Canada: Health Care.* His current research includes participation in the "Re-imagining Long-Term Residential Care: An International Study of Promising Practices" project and in several spin-off projects.

Pat Armstrong is distinguished research professor in sociology at York University and a fellow of the Royal Society of Canada. She has co-authored and co-edited many books in the fields of social policy, women, work, and health and social services, including *Creative Team Work: Developing Rapid, Site-Switching Ethnography*; *Wash, Wear, and Care: Clothing and Laundry in Long-Term Residential Care*; *Troubling Care: Critical Perspectives on Research and Practices*; *Thinking Women and Health Care Reform in Canada*; and *Wasting Away: The Undermining of Canadian Health Care.* She has served as Chair of Women and Health Care Reform and as acting director of the National Network for Environments and Women's Health, and is currently a member of the board of the Canadian Health Coalition and the Canadian Centre for Policy Alternatives. Pat is principal investigator of "Re-imagining Long-Term Residential Care: An

International Study of Promising Practices" (SSHRC) and "Changing Places: Unpaid Work in Public Places" (SSHRC).

Kirsten Bell is professor of social anthropology at the Centre for Research in Evolutionary, Social and Inter-Disciplinary Anthropology in the Department of Life Sciences at the University of Roehampton (UK). Her research has focused primarily on bringing an anthropological lens to bear on smoking, on both tobacco use itself and efforts to eradicate it (especially tobacco "denormalization" strategies). She has a similar interest in cancer – both how it is experienced and how it is intervened into – especially in the "survivorship" phase. She is also interested in procedural research ethics and scholarly publishing and the processes that shape academic knowledge production more broadly, and has been involved in efforts to intervene into both – most recently via her participation in Libraria, a collective of anthropology, archaeology, and related journals exploring cooperative alternatives to the current ecology of academic publishing. Her most recent book is *Health and Other Unassailable Values: Reconfigurations of Health, Evidence and Ethics* (Routledge, 2017).

Jacqueline Choiniere is associate professor and graduate program director, School of Nursing, York University. She has a long history of involvement in health, health care, and health care policy. Since she arrived at York in 2008, Jacqueline's research has focused on the influence of political, economic, and social forces on the quality of care and quality of work and life for nurses and other health care providers. Her work critically examines the influence of current reforms on the conditions and relations of care, most recently in settings where older adults receive care. Jacqueline has been co-investigator and co-theme leader on "Re-imagining Long-Term Residential Care: An International Study of Promising Practices," headed by Pat Armstrong. More recently, she is a participant in "Changing Places: Unpaid Work in Public Spaces," also led by Pat Armstrong, and a co-applicant on "Imagining Age-Friendly 'Communities within Communities': International Promising Practices," led by Tamara Daly.

Craig Dale is assistant professor at the Lawrence S. Bloomberg Faculty of Nursing, University of Toronto. He is also an advanced practice nurse in Adult Intensive Care (ICU) at Sunnybrook Health Sciences Centre in Toronto. The inability to recognize his own nursing experiences in health reform narratives attracted Craig to theoretical perspectives that acknowledge the influence of political, social, and economic interests in the patient-nurse encounter. His research explores fundamental aspects of nursing care for ventilator-assisted patients, including oral hygiene, symptom management, and communication. He has employed qualitative and ethnographic methods in both single and multicentre studies to advance issues of importance to patients, families, and clinicians. Craig has published in *Qualitative Health Research, Critical Care Medicine, American Journal of Critical Care,* and *Intensive & Critical Care Nursing,* among other journals.

Tamara Daly is professor at York University, director of the York University Centre of Aging Research and Education, and director of the SSHRC Partnership for Age-Friendly Communities within Communities. She held a CIHR Research Chair in Gender, Work and Health (2013–18). Her focus is on gender and health equity, social care policy quality work, and aged care in international cities. She employs multiple methods to conduct comparative, historically situated, and critically oriented policy research in the areas of seniors' care, access to care by immigrants and women, and care work organization. Her theoretical contributions are in health services research, feminist political economy, and labour process theory. She has authored numerous academic and plain-language publications, is the recipient of teaching and research awards, and actively supervises graduate students in research and publication.

Elizabeth Darling is associate professor in the Department of Obstetrics and Gynecology at McMaster University. Her research focuses on maternal-newborn health services. Areas of interest include midwifery services, health disparities, access to care, health policy, and perinatal health surveillance. She has particular expertise in the midwifery data collected in Ontario's perinatal registry (BORN Ontario). Elizabeth holds a PhD in population health from the University of Ottawa. She has been an active representative of the midwifery profession at the provincial and national level, including serving as a member of the Expert Advisory Committee for the Canadian Perinatal Surveillance System. From 2008 to 2015 she chaired the Clinical Practice Guidelines Committee at the Association of Ontario Midwives. She is currently a member of the Research Standing Committee of the International Confederation of Midwives.

Ariel Ducey is associate professor in the Department of Sociology, University of Calgary. Her research centres on issues of responsibility, ethicality, knowledge, and emotions in the institutions and practices of health care and medicine. Her book *Never Good Enough: Health Care Workers and the False Promise of Job Training* (Cornell 2009) examined the creation and justification of a billion-dollar industry for training, upgrading, and multiskilling unionized, front-line health care workers in New York City. In addition to her research on pelvic floor surgery, Ariel has been collaborating on related research on the adoption and regulation of medical devices, the gendered dimensions of medical knowledge and practice, and the nature of technologically mediated senses in contemporary health care.

Anne Rochon Ford is a researcher, writer, and activist in women's health. She is the former executive director of the Canadian Women's Health Network and past co-director of the National Network on Environments and Women's Health, York University. She is co-editor of *The Push to Prescribe: Women and Canadian Drug Policy* (Women's Press, 2009). On the occasion of the one-hundredth anniversary of the admission of women into the University of Toronto, she authored *A Path Not Strewn with Roses: 100 Years of Women at University of Toronto, 1884–1984* (University of Toronto Press, 1984). In 2014 she received the Constance E. Hamilton Award, which recognizes recipients' significant social, economic, or cultural contribution to securing equitable treatment for women in Toronto. Anne's recent work involves studying the environment that nail salon staff work in and the impact that it has on their health.

Alisa Grigorovich is an interdisciplinary health services and policy researcher and a CIHR Health System Impact postdoctoral fellow at the Kite Research Institute – UHN. Her postdoctoral research explores the social, ethical, and policy implications of implementing intelligent monitoring technologies in institutional care spaces. Broadly, her research interests include the politics of care, structural violence and stigma, health equity and ethics, and cultural imaginaries of sexuality and gender.

Matthew Herder is currently the director of the Health Law Institute at Dalhousie University in Halifax, Nova Scotia, and is also associate professor at Dalhousie University's faculties of medicine and law. Matthew's research focuses on biomedical innovation policy, with a particular emphasis on intellectual property rights and the regulation of biopharmaceutical interventions. He was appointed by federal cabinet as a member of the Patented Medicine Prices Review Board, Canada's national drug price regulator, and became a member of the Royal Society of Canada's College of New Scholars, Artists and Scientists in 2019.

Barry Hoffmaster is professor emeritus of philosophy at the University of Western Ontario. Most recently, he and Cliff Hooker co-wrote *Re-Reasoning Ethics* (MIT Press, 2018).

Kelly Holloway is a postdoctoral fellow at the Institute for Health Policy, Management and Evaluation at the University of Toronto. She is currently studying the political economy of molecular diagnostics. Her doctoral work in sociology at York University explored pharmaceutical industry influence in medical education in the United States and Canada. She has also completed a postdoctoral fellowship at Dalhousie University, studying emerging health researchers and the commercialization of academic science.

Christine Kelly is assistant professor in community health sciences at the University of Manitoba. Informed by feminist and critical disability scholarship, she uses qualitative methods to explore the politics of care, aging, and Canadian disability movements. She is co-editor of *Mobilizing Metaphor: Art, Culture and Disability Activism in Canada* (UBC Press, 2016) and author of *Disability Politics and Care: The Challenge of Direct Funding* (UBC Press, 2016). Christine presently co-edits a book series for UBC Press, is leading a national CIHR study on directly funded home care, and is involved in initiatives related to disability, aging and care. For more information, see www.christinekelly.ca.

Mary Ellen Macdonald is a medical anthropologist with doctoral training in Indigenous health and postdoctoral training in palliative care. She is associate professor in the Faculty of Dentistry at McGill University, associate member of the McGill Institute for Health Sciences Education, chair of the McGill Qualitative Health Research Group (mcgill.ca/mqhrg), and program head of Pediatric Palliative Care Research at the McGill University Health Centre. Her current research program focuses on the health of vulnerable populations in Canada, looking across three main domains: palliative care, Indigenous peoples' health, and oral health. She works mainly with qualitative (especially ethnographic) and participatory methodologies. A central focus of her research program is on the various ways the social, the cultural, and the political intersect to both produce and respond to particular forms of vulnerability within Canadian society.

Eric Mykhalovskiy is a sociologist of health and illness and professor of sociology, York University. His research explores the role that formal discourses of knowledge play in contemporary forms of health governance. Much of his work explores public health issues, especially related to HIV, from a critical social science perspective. His current projects include research on the public health implications of HIV criminalization and a new study of the governance of residential "nuisance noise" in downtown Toronto. He is co-author, with Lorna Weir, of *Global Public Health Vigilance: Creating a World on Alert* (Routledge, 2012) and co-editor, with Viviane Namaste, of *Thinking Differently about HIV/AIDS: Contributions from Critical Social Science* (UBC Press, 2019). In 2017, Eric received the Canadian Association for HIV Research/Canadian Foundation for AIDS Research Excellence in Research Award for the Social Sciences. He is a senior editor of the *Canadian Journal of Public Health.*

Magali Robert is professor in the Department of Obstetrics and Gynaecology and the Department of Anesthesiology, Perioperative and Pain Medicine, Cumming School of Medicine, University of Calgary. She began her career in urogynecology researching surgical outcomes with Dr. Sue Ross. This led to collaborations that extended from exploring pessary use in rural Nepal to identifying outcome measures for chronic pain. She is presently medical director of the Calgary Chronic Pain Centre.

Sue Ross, a health services researcher, is currently the Carvazan Chair in Mature Women's Health Research at the University of Alberta. Her research focus is on improving the patient experience and ensuring the safety and efficacy of treatments available to mature women for pelvic floor disorders and menopause. She has undertaken research using a wide variety of research methods from randomized clinical trials (principally in pelvic floor disorders) to qualitative research involving surgeons and surgical practice. She has also undertaken database work to determine the prevalence and impact of pelvic floor disorders using data obtained by family physicians from across Canada. Sue also works with local menopause clinics to expand upon the factors that contribute to mature women's wellness, including measuring quality of life and the impact of menopause on their lives.

Christianne Stephens is a medical anthropologist and faculty member at York University. She specializes in the anthropology of health and Indigenous health and is also trained as a health geographer. Christianne has been conducting ethnographic fieldwork and collaborative, community-based research in Indigenous contexts for the past seventeen years. Her current project (body mapping) utilizes a visual medium for documenting structural violence, syndemic suffering, and intergeneration trauma in an Ontario First Nation community. Christianne's scholarship combines theoretical innovation with critical analysis, long-term ethnographic fieldwork, collaborative research, and the use of mixed methods in order to explore various dimensions of health, including mental health issues, historical trauma, and cultural epidemiology. She supports the use of *citizen science* (the collection and analysis of data relating to the natural world by members of the general public) in health knowledge production and recognizes its potential for empowering marginalized populations.

Ross Sutherland has a master's degree in political economy from Carleton University and is a registered nurse with a long history as a health care and union activist. He is a co-chair of the Administration Committee of the Ontario Health Coalition. He has been a grievance coordinator in the Ontario Nurses Association, chair of CUPE Ontario's Community Health Committee, and an executive assistant at the Labour Council of Metropolitan Toronto. Before his work on for-profit medical laboratory corporations he wrote on the effects of using private companies to deliver home-care services and diagnostic imaging services. As a nurse Ross worked in emergency, home care, and community health and addictions settings; he has retired from nursing and become a township councillor in South Frontenac.

Vicki Van Wagner is a midwife and educator in Toronto and at the Inuulitsivik Health Centre in Nunavik, Quebec. She is associate professor in the Ryerson University Midwifery Education Program and a member of the Provincial Council on Maternal and Child Health. Vicki earned her master's and doctoral degrees at York University in Toronto. Her PhD explored unexpected effects of evidence-based practice in maternity care. Her research publications have focused on midwifery outcomes; on midwifery in remote, northern, and aboriginal communities; and on clinical education. In 2014 Vicki was one of two recipients of the first Lifetime Achievement Awards from the Association of Ontario Midwives.

David Kenneth Wright is a registered nurse with doctoral training in palliative care and ethnography, and postdoctoral training in ethics. He is associate professor of nursing at the University of Ottawa and academic lead for palliative care and nursing ethics at the Centre for Research on Health and Nursing. His current research program questions the relational ethics of palliative care, with a specific focus on notions of moral identity and moral agency in end-of-life-care nursing. David is the inaugural director-at-large for research with the Canadian Hospice Palliative Care Nurses Group (2016–20). He also holds specialty certification in hospice palliative nursing from the Canadian Nurses Association and maintains an active clinical practice as a palliative care nurse in Montreal.